FIFTH EDITION

PATIENT EDUCATION

in Health and Illness

FIFTH EDITION

PATIENT EDUCATION
in Health and Illness

Sally H. Rankin, RN, PhD, FAAN
Professor and Chair
Department of Family Health Care Nursing
University of California, San Francisco
San Francisco, California

Karen Duffy Stallings, RN, MEd
Associate Director
North Carolina AHEC Program
The University of North Carolina at Chapel Hill
Chapel Hill, North Carolina

Fran London, MS, RN
Health Education Specialist
The Emily Center, Phoenix Children's Hospital
Phoenix, Arizona

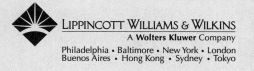

LIPPINCOTT WILLIAMS & WILKINS
A **Wolters Kluwer** Company
Philadelphia • Baltimore • New York • London
Buenos Aires • Hong Kong • Sydney • Tokyo

Senior Acquisitions Editor: Quincy McDonald
Managing Editor: Joseph Morita
Editorial Assistant: Marie Rim
Production Editor: Danielle Michaely
Director of Nursing Production: Helen Ewan

Art Director: Carolyn O'Brien
Senior Manufacturing Manager: William Alberti
Indexer: Coughlin Indexing Services
Compositor: Lippincott Williams & Wilkins
Printer: R.R. Donnelley-Crawfordsville

9 8 7 6 5 4 3 2 1

Library of Congress Cataloging-in-Publication Data

Rankin, Sally H.
   Patient education in health and illness / Sally H. Rankin, Karen Duffy Stallings, Fran
London.— 5th ed.
      p. ; cm.
   Rev. ed. of: Patient education : principles & practice / Sally H. Rankin, Karen Duffy
Stallings. 4th ed. 2001.
   Includes bibliographical references and index.
   ISBN 0-7817-4849-6 (alk. paper)
   1. Patient education. 2. Nurse and patient. I. Stallings, Karen Duffy. II. London, Fran. III.
Rankin, Sally H. Patient education. IV. Title.
   [DNLM: 1. Nursing Process. 2. Patient Education—Nurses' Instruction. WY 100 R211p 2005]
RT90.R35 2005
61.5'071—dc22
                                                                          2004013289

Care has been taken to confirm the accuracy of the information presented and to
describe generally accepted practices. However, the authors, editors, and publisher are not responsible for errors or omissions or for any consequences from
application of the information in this book and make no warranty, express or
implied, with respect to the content of the publication.

   The authors, editors, and publisher have exerted every effort to ensure that
drug selection and dosage set forth in this text are in accordance with the current recommendations and practice at the time of publication. However, in view
of ongoing research, changes in government regulations, and the constant flow of
information relating to drug therapy and drug reactions, the reader is urged to
check the package insert for each drug for any change in indications and dosage
and for added warnings and precautions. This is particularly important when the
recommended agent is a new or infrequently employed drug.

   Some drugs and medical devices presented in this publication have Food and
Drug Administration (FDA) clearance for limited use in restricted research settings. It is the responsibility of the health care provider to ascertain the FDA status of each drug or device planned for use in his or her clinical practice.

   LWW.com

Contributors to Previous Editions

Barbara E. Hollinger, RN-C, MS, FNP
Associate Clinical Professor
Family Health Care Nursing
University of California, San Francisco
San Francisco, CA
Chapter 3: Integration of Cultural Systems and Beliefs

Ronna E. Krozy, EdD, RN
Associate Professor, Community Health
William F. Connell School of Nursing
Boston College
Chestnut Hill, MA
Chapter 6: Community Health Promotion: Assessment and Intervention

Karen S. Zeliff, MLS
Director
Education Technology Services
Greensboro Area Health Education Center
Greensboro, NC
Chapter 10: Patient Education Resources on the Internet

Marilyn P. Verhey, PhD, RN, CS
Professor
San Francisco State University
School of Nursing
San Francisco, CA
Chapter 13: Community-Based Patient Education Programs

Reviewers

Katharine C. Cook, RN, PhD-C
Associate Professor of Nursing
College of Notre Dame of Maryland
Baltimore, Maryland

Elaine L. Gross, RN, MSN
Assistant Professor
Temple University
Philadelphia, Pennsylvania

Dolores M. Huffman, RN, BSN, MALS, MS, PhD
Associate Professor of Nursing
Purdue University Calumet
Hammond, Indiana

Brenda M. (Arnett) McLean, MEd, BScN, RN
Faculty Lecturer
University of Alberta
Edmonton, AB, Canada

Linda J. Patrick, RN, PhD(c)
Assistant Professor
University of Windsor
Windsor, ON, Canada

Beth Perry, RN, BScN, PhD
Associate Professor
Athabasca University
Athabasca, AB, Canada

Donna M. Romyn, RN, BScN, MN, PhD
Director and Associate Professor
Athabasca University
Athabasca, AB, Canada

Pamela Starcher, RN, MSN, PhD
Director of Nursing
Pennsylvania College of Technology
Williamsport, Pennsylvania

Lisa AJ Sykes, OTR, MEd
Adjunct Faculty
Ithaca College
Ithaca, New York

Jill E. Winland-Brown, EdD, ARNP
Professor and Undergraduate Program Coordinator
College of Nursing, Florida Atlantic University
Boca Raton, Florida

Preface

In 1983 the first edition of *Patient Education: Issues, Principles, and Guidelines* reflected our youthful enthusiasm for an area of health care and nursing practice that was in its infancy. We were certain that patient education was the panacea for frustrated patients and dissatisfied nurses, and we naively believed that we could improve health care through the publication of the text. We continue to believe patient education provides patients with the self-care skills to optimize health and independence, while enhancing health care provider satisfaction. We have revised earlier editions to reflect the increasing complexity of interdisciplinary health care, and the integration of electronic technology.

The text is designed to be helpful to students in all health care disciplines, in both generic and advanced practice programs. We believe that professionals in all health care disciplines will find the book valuable, but since the authors are nurses practicing in nursing arenas, the work draws heavily on nursing examples and the science and research of our discipline. Since all health care providers share a central interest in the welfare of patients, this patient-centered approach can be applied universally.

This fifth edition has been titled *Patient Education in Health and Illness* to reflect the applications of patient education throughout the continuum of care, in all health care settings. Current research findings in patient education have been integrated throughout the text. In response to nursing educators' requests, the fifth edition includes more in-depth coverage of theory, and more references to Canadian resources. In addition, research from a range of health care disciplines, beyond nursing, has been included.

The text has been updated to reflect current trends in patient education. Discussions of health literacy and readability have been strengthened. More information has been provided to help the student better tailor teaching to the learner's needs, considering aspects such as development, culture, and physical factors that make learning difficult. Information about how to use consumers to help design group and community educational programs has also been enhanced.

The fifth edition also includes more resources accessible through the Internet. Since electronic resources update more quickly and more often than print resources, some of the web addresses current at the time of printing may not be accurate when the reader tries to access the content. Consequently, key searching terms have also been provided to help the reader find the same content at new locations, or more recent information.

To succeed in today's health care environment, it is essential that interdisciplinary health care providers communicate and collaborate across the continuum of care. We need to share information about assessments, interventions, and evaluations to provide efficient and effective health care. We need to collaborate with our learners to develop the plan of care, so it can and will be implemented. Patients and families need clear, consistent, unambiguous instructions. Economic constraints mean they are increasingly responsible for more of their own care, and we need to be sure they understand what to do, are willing and able to do it, and know when and who to ask for help. In our evolving health care environment, the delivery of quality patient education is more crucial than when this book was first written.

Sally H. Rankin, RN, PhD, FAAN
Karen Duffy Stallings, RN, MEd
Fran London, MS, RN

Acknowledgments

Our years in nursing education and practice have provided us with a deep appreciation of our profession. The jewel in the crown of nursing practice is without doubt patient education; we are proud to be able to elucidate this jewel for continuing generations of students and practicing nurses. As we speak to audiences on the topic of patient education, we are encouraged by the comments of staff nurses who are working across all health care settings. In particular, we recognize the expertise of nurses who assume leadership roles in managed care, making patient education its centerpiece. We are awed by the dedication of nurses working in acute and primary care settings who struggle to clarify the intricacies of complex medical regimens, and we appreciate the educators who speak to the utility of our textbook.

We would also like to express our appreciation to the Medical Librarian at Phoenix Children's Hospital, Kathy Zeblisky, for her help in identifying and gathering the updated research in this edition. Despite the ease of Internet searching, professional librarians are still essential to ensure a thorough search and full access to resources.

We appreciate the guidance offered by nursing editors at Lippincott Williams & Wilkins during the revisions of this book: Joe Morita, Margaret Zuccarini, Susan Rainey, and Quincy McDonald. Lastly, we gratefully acknowledge the love and support of our families, which is visible to us between the lines of the text. A special note of gratitude goes to Amy Rankin Williams; Bill and Rob Rankin; Frank, Sarah, and Emily Stallings; and Jay London.

Contents

Section I: **Principles of Contemporary Patient Education 1**

1. Patient Education in Clinical Practice 3
Introduction 4
Overview of Nursing Practice and Patient Education 6
Changing Environment of Health Care Delivery 7
Challenges in Patient Education 20
Summary 24

2. Health Promotion: Models and Applications to Patient Education 27
Introduction 28
Health Promotion, Disease Prevention, and Health Maintenance 28
The Health Belief Model 30
The Health Promotion Model 31
Other Health Promotion Frameworks 33
Summary of Models and Implications for Patient Education 36
Healthy People 2010 39
Guide to Clinical Preventive Services and Clinician's Handbook of Preventive Services 39
Clinical Relevance of Health Promotion to Patient Education 40
Summary 43

3. Integration of Cultural Systems and Beliefs 47
Introduction 48
The Cultural Assessment Framework 49
The Kleinman Model 59
Cultural Relevance 60
Summary 69

4. Educational Theories for Teaching and Motivating Patients 72
Introduction 73
Patient Education: A Process of Influencing Behavior 73
The Agenda of Education 75
Patient Decision-Making 76
Models and Theories as the Research and Practice Foundation of Patient Education 76
Developmental Frameworks: The Bases for Patient Education 81
The Process of Teaching and Learning 87
Clinical Relevance: Patient Advocacy and Promotion of Change 90

Theories of Learning   92
Summary   98

5. **Staff Development in Patient Education 100**
Introduction   101
Beyond Meeting JCAHO Standards: Principles and Strategies for Staff
   Development   103
Clinical Applications   122
Summary   129

6. **Community Health Promotion: Assessment and Intervention 132**
Planning, Assessment, Outcomes, & Evaluation Resources   133
Introduction   133
Community Health Promotion and Education 133
Improving the Success of Community Health Programs 134
Political and Legal Influences on Health Promotion 136
Community Empowerment   136
The Influence of Marketing   138
Global Health Promotion   139
Summary   153

Section II: **Application of the Principles in Nursing Practice   155**

7. **Assessment for Patient Education   157**
Introduction   158
The Assessment Process 161
Case Studies   175
Summary   186

8. **Planning: Shared Goals for Patient Education   189**
Introduction   190
Patient-Centered Goals for Teaching and Learning 192
The Learning Contract   207
Clinical Relevance of Planning   209
Summary   213

9. **Educational Interventions for Patients and Families   216**
Introduction   217
Setting the Stage for Teaching and Learning   218
Strategic Use of Instructional Methods   224
Strategic Use of Learning Activities   228
Strategic Use of Educational Media   231
Designing Patient Education Programs   252
Summary   265

10. Patient Education Resources on the Internet   268
Introduction   269
Applying the Information Retrieval Process to the Internet   270
Using the Information Retrieval Process to Meet Patient Needs   283
Summary   287

11. Evaluating Patient Education Outcomes   290
Introduction: Assessing Outcomes   291
Scope of Evaluation   291
The Four Levels of Patient Learning Outcomes   293
Evaluating Patient Education Interventions   296
Documentation of Patient Education   302
Clinical Application of Evaluating Patient Education Outcomes:
    Case Studies   305
Summary   310

12. Case Management and Patient Education Programs   313
Introduction   314
Products of Case Management   315
Process Issues in Case Management   319
Evaluating Patient Education Programs   329
Health Outcomes Research and Patient Education   330
Developing Research Proposals to Study the Efficacy of
    Patient Education   333
Summary   336

13. Community-Based Patient Education Programs   339
Introduction   340
Community-Based Health Education Programs   340
Clinical Relevance: Two Community-Based Health Education Projects   346
Summary   351

Index   355

Principles of Contemporary Patient Education

Patient Education in Clinical Practice

LEARNING OBJECTIVES

After reading this chapter, the student should be able to:

1. Describe patient education as a dimension of caring.

2. Define patient education.

3. Discuss the role of patient education in a reformed health care system.

4. Describe the relationship between patient education and discharge planning.

5. Describe the process of integrating patient education into clinical practice.

The goal of patient education is to assist patients in the improvement of their own health.

(FREDA, 2002)

INTRODUCTION

Patient Education as a Dimension of Caring

Patient education is the process of influencing patient behavior and producing the changes in knowledge, attitudes, and skills necessary to maintain or improve health (American Academy of Family Physicians, 2000). Nurses clearly see themselves as advocates, as persons who stand alongside of, and empower, patients and their families to have a voice when they are weak and vulnerable (Benner, 2001).

Caring is an integral part of nursing practice. However, studies show that this hidden work may go unrecognized by patients and their families, except when the behaviors and attitudes associated with caring are missed. Caring—which helps to heal, cure, and improve a patient's health—is the essence of nursing. In several studies that describe the process of caring, shared vulnerability between the nurse and the patient and activities directed toward the welfare of the patient are identified. Nurse caring includes behaviors such as active listening, comforting, getting to know the patient as a person, respecting the patient, touching the patient, providing information to the patient to help decision-making, recognizing that patients know themselves best, perceiving patient needs, and providing good physical care (Wolf, Giardino, Osborne, & Ambrose, 1994).

Caring includes being a patient advocate, enabling the patient to make informed decisions, and promoting autonomy. Simultane-ously, caring includes making the patient feel safe, comforted, and valued (Tanner, Benner, Chesla, & Gordon, 1993). The accuracy and fidelity of clinical and caring knowledge are clarified through scientific knowledge, clinical outcomes, and personal and social understandings as they become available. Thus, clinical reasoning and caring practices are socially embedded (Benner, Tanner, & Chesla, 1996).

Patient education is a dimension of caring when it considers the best interests of the patient and recognizes that the best case manager for a patient is ultimately the patient himself or herself. Caring is a delicate balance of comfort and challenge and a creative ability to maximize resources for the patient's benefit (Sanford, 2000). Research shows that as novice nurses move through the developmental stages of advanced beginner, competent, proficient, and expert practice, patient education becomes an integral part of nurse caring (Benner, 2001).

We hope that the issues, principles, and practices addressed in this text will help students and novice nurses develop survival skills for teaching. For nurses working toward expert practice, we hope the text will promote a creative integration of patient education with various practice and patient populations. Furthermore, we hope expert nurses will discover validation for their teaching efforts and a call to provide leadership in research, education, and practice arenas. The stereotypical images of a caring nurse, developed early in childhood, can influence the willingness and effectiveness of nurses to become patient teachers.

We are aware, as educators, that much literature is available on patient education. When we first planned this book, we thought strongly that another how-to approach to patient education was not needed. Instead, we examined issues that arise in our own practice environments and issues suggested by our colleagues. The first six chapters present principles of contemporary patient education and address pressing concerns around leadership issues and administrative support for patient education, influencing and understanding patient decisions, effective work with high-risk populations, legal and ethical concerns related to patient education, and motivational theories.

As we designed the remaining chapters, we responded to students' questions about applying the principles of patient education. Faculty members also identified specific needs of their students in the implementation of patient education. In summarizing these evaluations, we developed Chapters 7 to 13 to guide students from all types of practice settings as they integrate patient education into their clinical practice. We found that students wanted realistic approaches that consider the pressures of time, extensive patient care responsibilities, and paperwork overloads. Health care providers find they must possess teaching skills, astutely define patient learning needs, and know how to involve patients' families. In addition, they want reassurance that patient education can be an integral part of patient care. We have attempted, throughout the text, to offer practical, realistic approaches.

How Does Patient Education Begin?

It was a rainy Saturday. In an upstairs bedroom, four sisters opened a doll hospital. Dolls of various sizes were placed carefully in shoe boxes, and each box was labeled with the patient's name. The patients were all sick, but the specific illness did not matter. The four little nurses scurried busily among the patients, giving baths, administering shots with pins from their mother's sewing basket, and applying scarf bandages and Band-Aids. They reassured their patients they would take care of everything and make them better soon. Eventually, the sisters' mother called the girls to lunch. This completed the recoveries of all the patients. The sisters dressed the dolls, put them back in their usual places, and cleaned up the messy bandages to prevent discovery of their magic treatments.

Years later, the four sisters went off to college. One sister chose to study nursing, and her first day of clinical was, in many ways, as full of adventure as that rainy Saturday. The nursing student walked onto the floors of hospitals with excitement, fear, and a certain reverence. She watched the nurses rush about, answering calls and caring for sick patients. Each nurse was assigned a patient, and the young student reached anxiously for the chart. She hoped for a patient who needed dressing changes, injections, or treatments she had never performed. She hoped she would be able to decipher the doctor's handwriting and understand the medical jargon. Would she have to make an occupied bed? Would there be an intravenous or central venous pressure line?

Many nurses are first attracted to the profession during childhood, perhaps prompted by the desire to help people become healthier and happier and to end their pain. They may view the fields of medicine and nursing as cloaked in mystery and may hope to evoke cures. During nursing school, or early in one's nursing career, a nurse may discover that he or she cannot fix everything or relieve all the pain. Most nurses come to terms with their own strengths and limitations and realize that the effectiveness of one's work is determined more by the ability to influence, rather than by the ability to control people. Also, most nurses learn that the control exercised in the hospital does not necessarily help patients or their families adjust after discharge. Despite well-meaning and knowledgeable advice, patients do not always follow a nurse's directions.

Patients often have many health problems, are sicker than imagined, and may be discharged from the hospital earlier than a nurse wishes. Nurses must provide care in various settings, including ambulatory care, acute care, home care, and long-term care.

Educating patients is part of the care nurses provide in all these settings. Rarely is there enough time to teach patients and families all they need to know, and often patients are too sick to participate. Nurses must be skilled in assessing each patient's needs and in setting priorities to meet the most critical of these needs before the patient's discharge from care (see Chapters 7 and 8). Moreover, patients are influenced by beliefs and values often different from the nurse's. Many patients have limited reading or writing skills; others do not speak English fluently. Nurses must be open, flexible, and creative (see Chapters 3 and 8).

Nurses as Part of a Team

The health care delivery system is driven by economic reality (ie, limited financial resources in the era of managed care) and nursing care must be defined, qualified, and quantified. Nurses must communicate with administrators and patients and must learn to provide effective interventions and quality, cost-effective care through nursing care management systems (see Chapter 12). Thus, nurses do not interact with patients in a vacuum. Rather, nurses are members of a larger team, which includes various health care professionals. Each team member has a special expertise or contribution, and learning to work in harmony with other team members can be more challenging than learning technical skills.

Changing one's view of patients is another challenge. Patients are not just recipients of care; instead, they and their families are at the head of the health care team. By recognizing their right to choose their own futures and by willingly sharing our knowledge with them, a nurse can shift his or her focus to true patient education—a practice based on influence, not control. The nurse also learns to appreciate the roles of the other team members and to find ways to articulate the contributions of each team member in helping patients and their families.

OVERVIEW OF NURSING PRACTICE AND PATIENT EDUCATION

Increasingly, the general public is becoming more health conscious. As the threat of most communicable diseases decreased, the health message that began to take root and grow in the collective psyche of the American public was that no longer would an immunization, a pill, or a legislative act result in major impacts on morbidity and mortality. Individuals had to reduce risk factors such as diets high in fat, sedentary lifestyles, stress, smoking, alcohol use, and unsafe sexual practices before diseases such as cardiovascular disease, diabetes, many cancers, and AIDS could be conquered. Self-responsibility for health and wellness offered the best option for optimizing wellness and preventing disease.

(BOYD, GRAHAM, GLEIT, & WHITMAN, 1998)

During the past three decades, patient education has become widely recognized as a professional role of health care providers. The growth of consumerism and the self-help movement has motivated people to take responsibility for their own health. Simultaneously, this growth and self-help movement has motivated nurses and other health care professionals to implement patient education and to recognize its importance in patient care.

Providing patient education is central to the role of every clinician who provides patient care, regardless of job title or clinical setting. Current models of education should address basic skills needed for contemporary clinical practice: critical thinking, relationship skills, care management skills, primary care skills, and community-focused skills (Balik, 1998).

CHANGING ENVIRONMENT OF HEALTH CARE DELIVERY

Today, more than ever, individuals are responsible for their own health maintenance, for modifying their behavior to reduce the risks of various chronic diseases, and for managing multiple chronic illnesses with complex therapeutic regimens, some of which require technologically sophisticated equipment. Providers have less time to teach and counsel patients on a one-to-one basis. At the same time the consumer movement and microcomputers have helped many patients, particularly of the baby boom generation and younger, to become increasingly more sophisticated about health care and seek information about health problems.

(KRAMER, ET AL., 1999)

Because of the changing environments of health care delivery, clinicians practice in various settings, and patient education is integrated in the care delivered in these settings. The expertise health care providers develop as patient teachers is carried to new roles and practice settings. Although each setting has unique challenges, the core competencies needed to teach patients are relevant to providing quality care in hospitals, subacute settings, rehabilitation and long-term care facilities, retirement communities, health maintenance organizations, preferred provider organizations, specialized inpatient and outpatient settings (including ambulatory care, urgent care, birthing centers, and day care centers), schools, mental health centers, rural health centers, and home health and hospice agencies. Emerging integrated delivery systems welcome nurses with the following skills:

- Competency to practice in settings with little direct supervision

- Ability to integrate care with other providers across multiple care settings
- Qualitative and quantitative research skills
- Telephone case management
- Use, development, and evaluation of care protocols
- Strong skills in physical assessment and patient teaching for complex and chronically ill populations (Balik, 1998)

Patient care increasingly takes place in the home, where home health care nurses provide skilled, efficient care to patients with complex and chronic illnesses. Under the constraints of managed care (eg, limited number of approved visits, limited time for visits because of heavy caseload), this care must be administered within a short time. Nurses must adapt to the logistical and clinical components of caring for a patient at home and to the patient's resources and needs, as well as the patient's and family's learning capacity. Nurses gain autonomy as they adapt the equipment, procedures, themselves, and their own resources to the situation. Nurses must be creative, innovative, and flexible (Neal, 1999).

The knowledge and skills to provide patient education and the ability to work as a member of an interdisciplinary team are critical factors to a nurse's effectiveness in various practice settings. Nurses describe patient education as a key to enhancing job satisfaction because it creates greater patient and nurse autonomy. In addition, nurses in advanced practice attribute success in obtaining new employment positions to possessing skills and experience in patient education.

Patient Education in Advanced Practice

Advanced education provides expanded career options for nurses, who can become nurse practitioners, clinical nurse specialists, and nurse midwives. The roles of advanced practice nurses (APNs) change rapidly with increased authority in primary care settings and more patient management in the inpatient setting. Managed care, which promotes use of the least costly provider to deliver care, explains the growth in career options for APNs. Implementing preventive and health promotion interventions, counseling and patient education expertise, and providing family support to people with chronic illness and disability are some of the factors that make APNs valued providers (Gilliss & Mundinger, 1998).

The public has been highly satisfied with nurse practitioner care. Double-blind comparisons of physician and nurse practitioner practice indicate that management of uncomplicated, primary care problems has the same, if not better, outcomes for nurse practitioners (Mundinger, 1994). One of the reasons cited for public approbation of the nurse practitioner role is the amount of patient teaching performed by nurse practitioners. One physician explained that he preferred to hire nurse practitioners instead of physician assistants because of the patient education preparation that nurses have in their educational programs. Health education, preventive care, and counseling have become valued by health care consumers and purchasers of health care. Nurses must be part of health care teams for patients to have access to these visible services (Mundinger, 1996).

One nurse practitioner describes her collaborative practice with a physician at a large, university medical center: "We work well together and we comanage all of the prenatal patients. The physician sends the client for her first prenatal visit to me, because I will do the physical examination and prenatal workup and all of the necessary teaching related to diet, physical and environmental factors associated with pregnancy, guidelines for management of common problems, and instructions related to subsequent visits. The physician I work with is more interested in the problems and pathology, whereas I'm more interested in the day-to-day management of the prenatal patient."

Certified nurse midwives also bring a nursing background and preparation to advanced clinical practice. Patients frequently state that they chose midwifery services because of excellent patient education and the encouragement they offer patients to participate in preventive care, prenatal care, and the delivery experience.

Nursing centers, nurse-managed centers, and community nursing centers have become recognized providers of ambulatory health care. Often affiliated with schools of nursing, they employ a combination of registered nurses (RNs), APNs, and other health professionals. Centers that employ APNs can provide an array of high-quality and cost-effective services. Health education and risk reduction are key components of the care that is provided (Bellack, 1998).

As the objectives of *Healthy People 2010* (U.S. Department of Health and Human Services, 2000) are incorporated into preventive care and health promotion, research in the area of patient education should receive additional attention. Nursing has embraced Healthy People 2010 and has incorporated it into curricula, especially for advanced practice nurses.

An example of the use of Healthy People 2010 objectives in research and practice is evident in a pediatric and family clinic owned, managed, and run as a faculty practice by the Department of Family Health Care Nursing at the University of San Francisco, California. In an effort to gauge the effectiveness of patient care at the faculty practice, Healthy People 2010 objectives were examined in light of the achievement of such objectives within the San Francisco Bay area. When it was determined that San Francisco has lagged nationally in the achievement of focus areas related to mental health, sexually transmitted diseases, and immunizations, the clinic staff instituted a database that will, in the future, provide concrete measures of the desired outcomes. These outcomes are predicated on effective patient education; therefore, the faculty who practice in this clinic will be measuring the effectiveness of their patient education interventions.

A Tradition of Teaching

Clearly patient education holds historical significance within the profession, is important to nurse theorists, and is incorporated into professional standards for practice.

(SANFORD, 2000)

Teaching was recognized as a function of nursing when Florence Nightingale wrote her significant treatises on nursing in 1859 (Nightingale, 1992). Throughout the history of nursing, nurses have helped patients take responsibility for their own health. Some of this power has been returned to nursing, thereby increasing the profession's credibility and viability.

In the words of Virginia Henderson, "The unique function of the nurse is to assist the individual, sick or well, in the performance of those activities contributing to health or its recovery (or to peaceful death) that he would perform unaided if he had the necessary strength, will or knowledge. And to do this in such a way as to help him gain independence as rapidly as possible" (Henderson, 1966). Patient education ensures such individualized care.

Although teaching has always been an integral part of nursing practice, nursing education has not always prepared nurses for the teaching role. In the early part of this century, the National League for Nursing (NLN) voiced concern that nursing education dealt only with disease and not with preparation for teaching (National League for Nursing Education, 1918). The NLN continues to advocate the importance of educating nurses to teach.

The American Nurses Association (ANA) also supports the professional nurse's responsibility to teach the patient and family relevant facts about specific health care needs and supporting appropriate modification of behavior. The ANA (1999) identified 10 nursing-sensitive quality indicators for acute care settings that capture care or its outcomes most affected by nursing care. One of these identi-fied indicators is patient satisfaction with educational information. The quality of nursing care can be measured, in part, by the quality of patient and family education provided.

References to patient education are found in health care agency policies, nursing job descriptions, and the ethics codes of nursing organizations. Furthermore, the courts have consistently upheld the rights of patients to know about their health problems and treatments. Patient education has become a professional expectation and a legal duty of nurses.

Patient Partnership Versus Patient Compliance

Patients have a right to receive appropriate education and to use the knowledge they gain to participate in decision-making. However, patients also have a responsibility to participate in their own care decisions and care processes.

(JCAHO, 2001)

A recent nursing graduate shared the following: "I think patient education is an important part of the care patients receive. We should be willing to teach patients what we know and help them to understand what choices they have. Sometimes I feel that it really makes a difference and I can tell that the patient understands. But my experiences are not all positive ones and I end up feeling frustrated and angry. After all, patient education takes time from an already busy schedule of patient care. It requires patience and extra effort to explain procedures and answer questions. I usually have to repeat the information several times or try to explain it in a different way so the patient can understand. After all my effort, some patients still don't take medications or treatments as they should. I end up wondering if they just don't want to be well or if they would have taken the information more seriously if it came from a doctor. Then I ask myself: What did I do wrong?"

Physicians express similar feelings of frustration when patient education fails. Although we all recognize that patients have the right and free will to make choices, we also question our own skills in teaching our patients. We wonder, "Should I have done things differently?"

Many health care professionals describe patient education as giving patients information about their problems and treatments. The quality of patient education is perceived to have a direct correlation with the availability of audiovisual programs and patient education materials and resources, and the informative posters in the physician's office. Patient education programs and materials stress the importance of multiple behavior changes, such as taking medications on an appropriate schedule and with correct dose, changing diet, starting exercise programs, and stopping smoking. Nurses and other health care providers tend to prescribe these changes freely to patients by simply instructing patients what they need to do. The clinician may think his or her job is completed once the instruction is given, and that it becomes the patient's responsibility to make these behavior changes. When patients fail to perform the desired behaviors, the clinician may assume the patient was not given enough information or that the patient failed to assimilate it. The health care provider may respond by repeating the information or by providing it in a different form. When the behaviors of patients fail to change, should the health care provider assume that patients have not learned the facts impressed on them?

Therapeutic movement is one stage at a time. Assessing the patient's readiness to change is the first task of the provider. Once we have determined where our patients are along the continuum, our task is to facilitate movement from their current position to the next stage.

(SHINITZKY & KUB, 2001)

The behaviors health care providers prescribe for patients involve not a single decision, but many difficult daily decisions that often involve pain, expense, social isolation, a perceived loss of independence, and the difficulty of breaking old habits. Changing a single behavior pattern, such as what one eats, is difficult. Clinicians frequently ask patients to change two or more behaviors (eg, diet, exercise regimen, and smoking cessation) simultaneously. The term compliance not only oversimplifies the way patients are educated but also overlooks the needed negotiation, coaching, and integration of health practices in the patient's and family's daily life. Chapter 8 provides strategies for goal setting and for supporting patients in behavior change.

When health care providers discuss obstacles in providing patient education, they often identify problems motivating patients to change current behaviors to improve the patient's health status. When asked to elaborate, it becomes evident that they see motivation and compliance as closely related. The implication is that a sufficiently motivated patient will comply with the doctor's or nurse's instructions.

Many health professionals have justified their involvement in patient education by asserting that it would increase patient compliance; in other words, it would convince patients to follow instructions. Despite teaching, patients frequently do not make the choices recommended to them by nurses, physicians, and other health care professionals (termed as noncompliance).

The term compliance implies that clinicians may dictate to the patient what is to be done or changed and that the patient must obey. A clinician may be uncomfortable with the patient's right to choose not to follow advice or to change his or her behaviors. Clinicians should strive to enlist the patient's partnership—rather than compliance—and view patient education as a process of influencing behavior in ways that are acceptable to the patient. An orientation toward cooperation helps the health care provider think about his or her own effectiveness in patient education in a different light. Patient education successes have more to do with the patient's preparation to make informed choices than they do with acts of compliance. In fact, if patient education acknowledges the patient's free will to make choices, it must afford understanding of the importance of his or her values and wishes and the ability to participate in decision-making. Chapter 8 provides an in-depth discussion of the issues surrounding patient decision-making.

Compliance with a medical regimen is an important goal of patient education, but it is not the only goal. A significant process occurs between education and compliance, one in which the patient internalizes the teaching and then makes informed choices about applying the teaching to his or her life. Compliance is a product not only of learning about the medical regimen, but also of the patient's lifestyle, a complex group of behaviors including social and family patterns, activities of daily living, and dietary, exercise, and sleep patterns.

The term compliance is so ingrained in discussions of patient education that it is difficult to replace it with another term that reflects mutuality. However, we suggest the terms alliance, concurrence, and cooperation as alternatives. These terms suggest choice, mutuality of goals, and a patient–provider relationship based on respect and trust.

Adherence refers to making the behavior change identified in the mutually defined goals. Behavior change is an elusive variable because researchers cannot always assume that patient teaching is responsible for the behavior change. Additionally, because evaluation of behavior change usually hinges on the patient's self-report, the data may be unreliable. Adherence is measured more easily in some disease processes, such as diabetes, because nearly all patients with type 1 and most patients with type 2 diabetes use home blood glucose monitoring devices. Many of these devices store the blood glucose levels with the date and time the reading is obtained. When the devices are downloaded into a computer, the researcher can obtain a 30-day history of blood glucose readings. The blood glucose monitor, therefore, not only allows the health care provider to obtain an indication of adherence to the medical regimen but also reveals whether the patient has monitored the blood glucose level as recommended. These devices are both useful data collection tools and an intervention that may induce desired behavior change.

Reforming Health Care: A Central Role for Patient Education

General Considerations

An intense debate about health care delivery in the United States will continue on both state and national levels. Questions about how to provide universal access to basic health services and how to finance rising health care costs are central to the debate. Millions of Americans have no health care insurance, and therefore appropriate and early medical treatment is often avoided or deferred. Uninsured patients often present for treatment only in the event of acute episodes or exacerbation of chronic illness, thereby increasing costs, complications, disability, and mortality.

The hopes for a reformed health care system hold promise of the availability and access to early detection and improved management of chronic health conditions, with lower cost and better outcomes. Nursing views itself as a valuable and visible contributor to managed health care systems of the present and future. The ANA is a voice for nursing in the United States, promoting a changed delivery system and featuring consumer responsibility for self-care, informed decision-making, and choices in the selection of health care providers and services (American Nurses Association, 1991). The ANA believes that improving the health of Americans provides a solid foundation for building a strong nation for the 21st century.

The image of a reformed system calls for increasing patient involvement in the health care team and for increasing emphasis on the patient's role in improving health status. Patient education provides patients with the knowledge and skills to assume these responsibilities.

Reforms in Education

Although it is difficult to achieve a national consensus on basic health care benefits and on how to finance a comprehensive system, health care reforms are sweeping across traditional settings in which nurses are employed and are influencing nursing education. The downsizing, or right sizing, of hospitals moves nurses into community-based practice. The delivery of patient care continues to move closer to home. In nursing schools, increasing emphasis is placed on preparing students for public, community, and home health settings and for delivering preventive health services in the context of managed care. Nursing school curricula emphasize patient education as an integral part of nursing practice. RNs who pursue bachelor of science in nursing (BSN) degrees gain new knowledge of patient education based in many practice settings.

In addition, nurses enrolled in nurse practitioner and advanced degree programs should refine patient education skills needed for practice. To meet the public's needs for primary care, the expanded training of medical students for generalist roles is accompanied by an increased amount of training in rural, underserved, and community-based sites. Nursing programs are expanding student exposure to include similar clinical training sites. A growing demand for nurse practitioners, nurse midwives, and physician's assistants is also related to improving the access and cost of primary care services to meet the public's needs. Patient education must be a critical component of graduate nursing education programs that prepare nurses to assume advanced practice roles.

Beyond Informed Consent

Nurses who were prepared to practice in the 1970s witnessed the importance of providing for the informed consent of the patient. The patient's right to know includes the right to know what illness he or she has, the right to know what diagnostic and therapeutic processes will be used, and the right to know the prognosis for physical recovery. The patient has a right to refuse treatment and to be informed of the consequences of those actions. The nature of this contractual agreement guarantees a patient's right to know what he or she can do to effect physical recovery and includes necessary patient education (Edwards, 1998, 1999, and Office for Protection from Research Risks, 1993).

Discharge Planning and Patient Education

By the end of the 1970s, patient teaching witnessed a shifting and an expanding list of priorities. No longer were new nurses educated solely for hospital-based practice. Practice in ambulatory care, long-term care, and home care settings helped nurses gain greater appreciation for the vital link between patient education, discharge planning, and continuity of care. Patients were discharged from hospitals to other settings sicker and quicker.

Discharge planning begins on the day of admission; this is a golden rule taught to all nursing students. Until the past decade, however, the number of days a patient stayed in the hospital was flexible and often could be extended to prepare patients and families to assume self-care. As health care costs continued to increase, hospitals were blamed for inefficiency and the amount of money spent to care for patients. American industry and government agencies pressed for changes in health care reimbursement that would build incentives for efficiency and containment of costs to third-party payers.

Medicare began using a prospective payment system called diagnosis-related groups

(DRGs). This major trend in reimbursement became law in 1983. With DRGs, payments were no longer made to hospitals based on the costs of services or on the number of days of care provided to a patient. Instead, a predetermined payment was assigned to each of the DRGs. Each DRG has an assigned mean length of stay (ie, the number of days Medicare would pay for services). An *outlier* cutoff (ie, the maximum number of days for which a hospital can bill Medicare) was set. To negotiate payment, the hospital had to prove that the patient's condition was complicated. Since then, the health insurance industry has introduced sweeping changes, and new alliances for managed health care evolve daily. Cost and quality are the key components of managed health care.

With the advent of DRGs, discharge planning assumed a new meaning. Financial incentives were tied to the discharge date because hospitals were reimbursed fixed amounts based on these DRGs. The strategies developed for fiscally managing patient care range from new approaches to preadmission screening to inpatient case management, and from outpatient specialty clinics to high-technology home care. Health care systems emerged, linking providers across a continuum of health care settings. Case management involved ensuring continuity of patient care services, maximizing the quality of care, and minimizing the costs. With the advent of each new approach, patient education has taken center stage.

The primary focus of patient education in the 1980s shifted from provider outcomes to patient and family outcomes. Successful patient education could not be guaranteed based solely on the ability and willingness of health care providers to deliver understandable information about diagnosis, treatment, and prognosis. Discharge planning, in most cases, implies patient education and is viewed as part of routine patient care—an interdisciplinary process to help patients and their families develop and implement a feasible posthospital plan of care. The goals

for education of all patients must include learning survival skills, recognizing problems after discharge, and making decisions that contribute to self-care management. Special discharge-planning services are warranted when posthospital needs are expected to be complex. Guidelines and methods for integrating discharge planning and patient education planning are covered in Chapter 8.

Growing Needs of Older Patients and People with Chronic Health Conditions

The fastest growing segment of our society is our older population. Health care advances and medical technology have helped these patients to live longer; nevertheless, they continue to have chronic health conditions, physical disabilities, and functional limitations. Therefore, they depend heavily on health care services, particularly nursing care. With increases in the number of older patients and the arrival of prospective payment has come a boom in the home health care industry and rehabilitative programs of long-term care institutions. Many treatments and technologies are now used in the home. More acute care is being provided in the home, and the discharge of patients from the hospital, sicker and quicker, demands the provision of patient and family teaching and continuity with caretakers in the home.

Recognizing the growing threats of acquired immunodeficiency syndrome (AIDS) and tuberculosis, nurses employed in public health departments have assumed an active role in new prevention and detection programs for high-risk populations. Patient education for prevention is targeted to the homeless, migrant farm workers, and prison populations. Nurses have augmented their skills in patient education with a new understanding of how culture and poverty can influence patient behavior.

A Gallup poll funded by the Robert Wood Johnson Foundation revealed that although one of seven Americans faces major limitations because of chronic illness, one-third of these patients do not seek routine or preventive health care; they receive care only for acute problems. The exacerbation of chronic illness is the only time they may access the health care system. Without patient education and patient involvement in care to prevent acute episodes, health care is costlier and quality of life suffers. Chronic disorders account for much of U.S. expenditures on health care in a health care system geared to cure acute diseases. The number of Americans living with chronic health conditions (eg, diabetes, cancer, emphysema, heart disease, muscular dystrophy, spina bifida, AIDS, chronic mental illness, dementia, disabling injuries, alcoholism, blindness, and disabling arthritis) continues to increase.

Heart disease is a major cause of mortality and morbidity among adults who are older than 65 years of age. Structured educational programs that include exercise and modification of risk factors have been shown to reduce the risk of subsequent coronary events. A comprehensive approach can result in optimal care, and can help ensure patients in rehabilitation return to the highest functional level possible (Resnick, 2002).

The following problems, from which older people and persons with chronic health conditions are especially at risk, are priorities in discharge planning and patient teaching:

- **Medications.** Does the patient know what to take, how much, when, and why?
- **Nutrition and hydration.** Healing of wounds and infection require good nutrition. The patient may not be motivated to prepare meals or drink fluids as needed.
- **Unintentional injury.** The patient may fall, which is often related to weakness or side effects of medication.
- **Mobility and transportation.** Can the patient get transportation to return for appointments, to pick up medications, to get groceries?
- **Support services needed at home.** Is assistance needed with meals, treatments, social services?

- **When and how to seek appropriate treatment.** Do the patient and family recognize danger signs that need treatment (eg, pain, medication side effects)? Do they know how to get help? Do they know when to see the physician and when to go to the emergency room?

Health care providers also recognize that the caregivers of older patients need support and possible assistance from community agencies to help them succeed in their caregiving roles. They should be alert and attuned to the language and behaviors related to maintaining control, and should teach caregivers about taking a break, provide information about respite services, and encourage caregivers to talk openly about their caregiving experiences so nurses can help them to find the best solutions to caregiving problems. This is especially important in the home care of patients with Alzheimer's disease and other dementias (Szabo & Strang, 1999).

Disease Management: Pediatric Asthma

Patient education is a large piece of the disease management for pediatric asthma. Unless patients and families accept their responsibility to change behaviors, the goals of disease management cannot be met. In these cases, patient education requires much more from providers than simply providing patients and families information. The education must be tailored to individual needs and circumstances.

The National Cooperative Inner-City Asthma Study (NCICAS) used an innovative approach, with four key components:

1. Clinical care, including primary care services (improve access to care, get asthma care plans, improve communications with their primary care providers).
2. Patient education, to help families and children understand the asthma care plan and to identify asthma triggers.

3. Psychosocial services, including counseling, and help with resolving problems with housing and health insurance.
4. Providing referrals to appropriate community resources, including smoking cessation and strategies to minimize exposure to cockroach and pet allergens.

This multifaceted asthma intervention program reduced symptom days and was cost-effective for inner-city children with asthma (Sullivan et al., 2002).

Substance Abuse

Substance abuse, another priority for nursing involvement in health promotion and disease prevention, is a leading cause of death and disability in the United States. Substance abuse involving tobacco, alcohol, and drugs is the primary cause of preventable illness, injury, and death in the United States. Prevention efforts and early intervention are enhanced by the involvement of school health nurses. Nurses in all settings should know how to counsel patients about smoking and about how to refer patients to smoking cessation programs in the community. School-based prevention programs can be very effective when they are developed and implemented with full student, faculty, and staff participation, and they have administrative support (Lowe et al., 2001).

JCAHO Standards

General Considerations

Since 1993, the hospital accreditation standards published by the Joint Commission on the Accreditation of Healthcare Organizations (JCAHO) made patient and family education outcomes a high priority and a focus survey area. Meeting this requirement to achieve accreditation placed heightened emphasis on patient education activities within hospitals and in their relationships with other posthospitalization health care providers. The JCAHO standards and scoring guidelines for education of patient and family have brought renewed

interest, accountability, and leadership for patient education, which has ultimately benefited both nurses and patients.

Staff nurses committed to patient education have long struggled to gain recognition for the skill, time, and resources needed to succeed. Patient education often competes with high-technology nursing skills for recognition. JCAHO supports and requires accountability for all health care providers to show evidence of patient learning outcomes for accreditation. This provides important reinforcement of nursing's long-standing commitment to teach.

The JCAHO upholds the concept of patient-centered care, with patient and family education viewed as a centerpiece for involving patients as members of the health care team. Patient education also is seen as central to processes for quality management. Health care organizations are expected to show evidence of patient learning outcomes, focus on discharge and continuity of care, and coordinate patient teaching across disciplines. The development of patient-centered care guidelines requires renewed attention to the ways patients and families are educated and to innovative approaches to achieve patient outcomes appropriate to the patient's length of stay. Nurses must turn their attention to what the patient and family can do, rather than to what the nurse has taught. Figure 1.1 illustrates how this educational partnership is evaluated and documented in a Neonatal Intensive Care Unit (NICU).

JCAHO Education Function

The JCAHO identifies the goals of patient education outlined in the Comprehensive Accreditation Manual for Hospitals. Patient education improves patient health outcomes by promoting healthy behavior and by involving the patient in care and care decisions. Education supports recovery, a speedy return to function, and enables patients to be involved in decisions about their own care (JCAHO, 2001).

LUCILE PACKARD CHILDREN'S☐
HEALTH SERVICES AT UCSF

UCSF Stanford Health Care

Instructions: Check box when patient understands the content presented. Date and sign at bottom of form. Document problems/issues with learning on the Pediatric Flowsheet or Progress Notes. Patient/Family signs when form complete.

1. Health Management

a. I have received the following printed materials:

- ☐ Your guide to breast feeding
- ☐ Breastfeeding your ICN baby
- ☐ Taking your child's temperature
- ☐ Car seat information
- ☐ Positioning your baby
- ☐ 17 ways to cope with a crying baby
- ☐ Going home with baby booklet
- ☐ RSV precautions
- ☐ CPR booklet
- ☐ Bathing your baby

b. I know how to

	demo/info given	date	pt/caregiver demo	date	needs rein-forcement	independent	date	NA
Taken my baby's temperature/NL range	☐		☐		☐	☐		☐
Give my baby a bath	☐		☐		☐	☐		☐
Feed my baby with a bottle	☐		☐		☐	☐		☐
Breastfeed my baby	☐		☐		☐	☐		☐
Use breast pump and store breast milk	☐		☐		☐	☐		☐
Prepare and store formula	☐		☐		☐	☐		☐
Clean bottles and nipples	☐		☐		☐	☐		☐
Mix higher calorie formula	☐		☐		☐	☐		☐
Care for my baby's circumcision	☐		☐		☐	☐		☐
Comfort, burp, and position my baby	☐		☐		☐	☐		☐
Care for my baby's skin and cord	☐		☐		☐	☐		☐
Use a bulb syringe	☐		☐		☐	☐		☐
Care for my baby if she/he has a fever	☐		☐		☐	☐		☐

2. Activity

I have reviewed special activity guidelines with my: ☐ Occupational Therapist   ☐ Physical Therapist   ☐ Nurse

3. Precautions – I know to call the doctor if my baby:

- ☐ has a fever of 101°F or 38.6°C
- ☐ has a fever of 99.5°F or 37.5°C that lasts over 4 hours
- ☐ has diarrhea and/or vomiting
- ☐ is so sleepy he/she will not wake up to eat
- ☐ is so fussy that he/she will not sleep or eat
- ☐ is breathing very fast or hard and looks pale or bluish
- ☐ has a cough or runny nose lasting over a few days
- ☐ has not wet his/her diapers at least 6 times a day

4. Medications

I know:
- ☐ which medication my child needs and how to give it
- ☐ my baby's medication schedule
- ☐ medication clock
- ☐ what to do if my child vomits or misses a dose
- ☐ what to do if my child gets a dose by mistake

5. Additional information

- ☐ I have a car seat and know how to use it
- ☐ I have seen the CPR video
- ☐ I have received my follow-up Doctor's appointment
- ☐ taken class (date) _____

6. See additional teaching records: ☐ _____   ☐ _____   ☐ _____

7. Other Special Instructions: _____

_____

☐ Translator used for instructions: _____

Patient/Family Signature _____

Instructor Signature:

Name	Title	Date
Name	Title	Date
Name	Title	Date
Name	Title	Date

FIGURE 1.1 Intensive care nursery teaching record.

16

These education standards call for a systematic approach to patient education. Scoring guidelines reflect the expectations that all patients will benefit from appropriate education. The accountability for patient teaching lies within the scope of practice of every nurse. Accountability must also be assumed by management, staff development, and clinical specialists to ensure health care providers develop necessary patient education skills. Many patient educators have not been formally prepared for the complexity, instability, uncertainty, and ambiguity of health promoting practice (Hartrick, 2000).

Nurses frequently struggle with implementing outdated protocols that are nurse-centered and based on outcomes unrealistic for current lengths of stay. Nurse managers and educators need to promote patient education by:

- Helping nurses define and evaluate patient learning outcomes
- Aiding in the identification of critical learning needs and teaching priorities
- Promoting innovative programs that ensure continuity of patient education
- Reflecting the value of patient education in the nursing performance appraisal system
- Suggesting continuing education that aids skill acquisition in patient education based on Benner's (2001) four stages of development: advanced beginner, competent, proficient, and expert.

The JCAHO standards and scoring guidelines and the role of staff development in promoting patient education are more thoroughly discussed in Chapter 5. Also see Box 1.1.

Interdisciplinary Teams

The Pew Health Professions Commission (1998) issued its report Recreating Health Professional Practice for a New Century, calling for interdisciplinary competence in all health professionals. Describing this competency as essential for the future, the Commission cited the current integrated

---

BOX 1.1 JCAHO's Goals of Patient Education

As outlined in the 2001 (JCAHO) Standards, patient education should:

- Promote interactive communication between patients and providers.
- Improve patients' understanding of their health status, options for treatment, and the anticipated risks and benefits of treatment.
- Encourage patient participation in decision-making about care.
- Increase the likelihood that patients will follow their therapeutic plans of care.
- Maximize patient self-care skills.
- Increase the patient's ability to cope with his or her health status.
- Enhance patient participation in continuing care.
- Promote healthy lifestyles.
- Inform patients about their financial responsibilities for treatment when known.

JCAHO defines family as the person(s) who play a significant role in the patient's life. This includes an individual who may or may not be legally related to the patient (JCAHO, 2001).

---

health care delivery systems evolving toward acute care and chronic care management by interdisciplinary teams of providers, including nurses, physicians, and allied health. The interdisciplinary model uses resources in a timely, efficient way, avoids error and duplication of services, and elicits the expertise of all professionals in an environment of collaboration and consultation.

The Pew Commission noted that medical and professional schools must reassess their curricula to ensure that they apply an interdisciplinary vision. Education should be provided in interdisciplinary settings, students should demonstrate interdisciplinary skills, and students should seek work or study experiences that expose them to interdisciplinary care. Incentives for interdisciplinary management of care are found not only in cost reduction but also in patient satisfaction and helping patients better manage chronic diseases. Competencies needed within interdisciplinary teams include:

- Providing integrated health services
- Emphasizing health promotion and disease prevention
- Functioning in managed care environments
- Evaluating the quality and cost of health care

Everyone benefits when an interdisciplinary model of care is used to plan and coordinate patient and family education. Numerous examples offered throughout the text describe nurses who work with other disciplines and the opportunities to provide leadership for the team. The goal is not simply providing more teaching, but also helping to assure that the patient and family are the focus of teaching efforts. Overloading the patient is less likely, outcomes can be measured and tracked, and brainstorming by the larger team leads to innovative approaches to challenging patient teaching situations.

Integrating Patient Education in Nursing Practice Education

How patient education is accomplished varies from setting to setting. In outpatient clinics, nurses have a short time with each patient and must teach throughout the encounter; they must set priorities and rely on educational materials appropriate for the patient. In acute care settings, nurses face shortened lengths of patient stay and thus refine their skills at setting priorities and realistic goals, making referrals, and evaluating a patient's ability to perform survival skills. These nurses also must evaluate the patient's readiness and ability to learn and incorporate patient education literature (Haber, 2001).

In home care settings, nurses share more high-technology care with the family and coordinating community resources in the patient education role. In long-term care, nurses rely on their skilled assessments to set priorities and to develop meaningful plans of care by valuing the input of patients and families; they use patient education to involve the patient and family in restorative care.

The same process for patient education is used by health care providers in all settings and with all types of patients.

We hope that students and experienced clinicians will find the text helpful by applying the principles of patient education described in the following chapters to daily practice. The principles of patient education also are illustrated by case studies throughout this text to provide practical examples of how to perform various steps of the process. According to Benner, much can be learned from the wisdom of nurses who are expert teachers and coaches. Teaching and coaching are embedded in nursing care and vary based on demands, resources, and constraints of the situation. Yet, she cautions us that learning from experts requires attention to the context and avoidance of hasty generalizations (Benner, 2001).

The Patient Education Process

Health care providers teach patients and families through the application of the patient education process, a problem-solving method designed to meet patient needs in a systematic way. The process has four steps:

1. **Medical and nursing diagnoses.** Health care providers gather information about patient needs and formulate a list of medical and nursing diagnoses. Nursing diagnoses are statements of human responses to actual or potential health problems, which the nurse can legally identify and for which the nurse can intervene (Carpenito, 2002). Many nursing diagnoses relate to patient and family learning needs. The nurse focuses on functional

problems and daily management.

2. **Plan for care.** The interdisciplinary team develops the plan for patient care, outlining priorities and patient goals (both short- and long-term). Specific learning objectives are part of the patient care plan.

3. **Implementation.** This step details how the plan will be implemented, including patient teaching targeted to meet mutually established goals.

4. **Evaluation.** Evaluation provides information about how well goals were met. During the process of evaluation, medical and nursing diagnoses are either resolved or referred for continuing care. Thus, implementing the patient education process entails more than a cognitive, four-step procedure.

Clinical Decision-Making and Clinical Judgment

Clinical decision-making based on clinical judgments arises from the expert nurse's grasp of qualitative distinctions in individual cases. The nurse must be attuned to each patient situation, with a sense of what is salient and the confidence to set priorities. Clinical judgment is learned through experience, that is, a combination of hands-on care, mentoring, and continuing education with a case study approach. Expert nurses learn to notice patients and families in new ways and adapt agency patient education resources to culture, beliefs, context, and environment (Benner, Tanner, & Chesla, 1996). A faculty member who teaches BSN students shared with us one of the difficulties of teaching patient education skills in the undergraduate program: "Students see only a small proportion of the hospital episode. They are not prepared to teach patients during the long run." This text offers case studies, quotes from practicing nurses, and study questions to promote clinical relevance, reflection, and the development of critical thinking.

The nurse must recognize significant others, especially the family members, who directly influence the patient. When education (assessment, teaching, or evaluation of understanding) is incorporated into every encounter with the patient and family, it enables them to assume an active role in their care and provides a safer transition on the day of discharge. The patient who can recognize symptoms and ask for help, who can cope effectively with the exacerbations of chronic illness, and who can prevent injury, accident, and illness has an autonomy that will help in negotiating an increasingly complex health care system.

Patient education plans are part of the total plan for patient care and are targeted to priorities for each patient. Patient education begins with early screening on admission to determine what is likely to cause trouble for this patient and to anticipate functional problems rather than with a preset teaching plan for all patients with a common medical diagnosis, such as diabetes. Health care providers must realistically consider the anticipated length of stay and determine how much and when to teach the patient. For example, standardized teaching plans for patients with diabetes need to be modified when a patient's needs vary because of age, complications, experience, presenting problem, and other simultaneous health issues. Thus, patient education cannot be accomplished with a cookbook approach and should not be delegated to inexperienced or unlicensed personnel. Effective patient education requires critical thinking and clinical judgments that allow health care professionals to plan individualized approaches for patient care.

Patient education is not accomplished by simply tucking a list of instructions or a booklet into the patient's hand, or instructing him or her to turn on the television to the patient education channel. Patient education requires a therapeutic relationship, providing an individualized response to patient needs rather than to a broad medical diagnosis, and the introduction of whatever resources are available to meet those needs.

CHALLENGES IN PATIENT EDUCATION

Preparing Content for Teaching

How can nursing students anticipate patient and family learning needs and prepare the content needed for patient teaching?

Knowledge of the nursing process itself does not assure that one is fully prepared to deliver patient education. Nurses must know about the health problems faced by their clients and must anticipate the needs the patient typically exhibits. To be a capable patient teacher, nurses must assess their own learning needs, their patient's needs, and find resources to meet them.

A community health nurse receives the referral of a new patient who was discharged from a nearby medical center with a rare diagnosis. The nurse is unfamiliar with the diagnosis, the prognosis, the functional problems typically affecting the patient, and the learning needs of the patient and family. The nurse goes to the medical center library and asks the librarian to help her choose the most appropriate search terms. The librarian tells her the hospital has purchased subscriptions to several online data bases of journals, and shows her how to access them on the computer. The nurse finds a recent article from a nursing journal describing the disease, epidemiology, clinical characteristics, medical management, and nursing management. Fortunately, the article also outlines nursing diagnoses applicable to patients with this diagnosis, suggests actions, and reviews infection control guidelines. This prepares the nurse to make an individual assessment of the patient and family and to anticipate their needs and priorities. (Chapter 10 provides valuable guidance for nurses who increasingly turn to the Internet for accurate information resources.)

Cultural Sensitivity

Health care providers also understand that cultural factors have a profound effect on patient education. The patient education process must consider the cultural diversity of patients and their families (U.S. Department of Health and Human Services, & The Office of Minority Health, 2001). Patient education for chronic diseases, such as hypertension and diabetes, typically target lifestyle changes, such as dietary habits and daily activities, that may be associated with cultural patterns and traditions. Health care providers recognize the need to learn about religions and cultures and the need to incorporate cultural assessment in the process of patient teaching. To design effective patient teaching interventions, health care providers need skills to work with patients from culturally diverse backgrounds. Clinicians provide culturally relevant care by understanding the cultural context of the patient and family, using culturally sensitive strategies to meet mutual goals, and integrating appropriate community resources (Garity, 2000).

Chapter 3 addresses special challenges involved in teaching patients whose ethnocultural groups are different from that of the clinician.

Health Care Providers as Role Models

How important is it for nurses to "practice what we teach" to be positive role models for our patients?

Many nurses and other health care professionals sacrifice their own health practices because of the multiple demands of families, patients, and work (Jackson et al., 1999). They may smoke, be overweight, exercise poor nutrition and fitness, experience stress-related symptoms, and invite chronic health issues. Also, nursing faculty members and students face academic pressures, late-night reading and writing, demands of caring for children and older parents, and participation in community and church volunteer activities.

One family nurse practitioner described that she has always prided herself in the holistic care she provides to patients and families. Diet, exercise, and stress management are integral to every patient encounter. She coaches her students to make realistic demands of themselves because they often must balance jobs and families in addition to studies. She felt dishonest, giving advice she did not follow, because she struggled with a serious weight problem and an associated depression. She finally decided to make a change. She joined a weight loss program, started walking, and lost 50 pounds. She says, "Now, when I counsel patients, I do not feel like I am giving them the company line. I know what it is like to struggle with hunger and emotional eating. I can talk with them about their food choices, talking about their emotions rather than insulting them" (Gomez, 1999).

Promoting Teamwork

What can nurses do to promote collegiality with other disciplines on the health care team and to help patients reap the benefits of interdisciplinary teaching?

The importance of interdisciplinary involvement by the total health care team is central to effective patient care. The lack of good communication between disciplines often leads nurses to feel they are not valued as patient teachers. Lack of communication can lead to battles about turf and the inability to collaborate, both one-on-one and in team conferences.

Understanding the contributions that other health care professionals can make to patient teaching increases the effectiveness of patient education and improves attempts to develop collegiality and collaboration of the health care team. We have found that members of other health care professions tend to be as involved as nurses are in patient teaching, particularly those nurses who are recent graduates and those who actively pursue continuing education. However, we have also heard nurses assume that because one physician opposed their patient education efforts, most physicians, for example, are not supportive of patient education. Such assumptions thwart collaboration and the delivery of patient education.

During the last three decades, the emphasis of nursing education and practice has reflected an expanded focus for interdisciplinary patient teaching efforts. Furthermore, because of nursing's continuous and visible presence at the patient's side, nurses are in the unique position to provide leadership for patient education and to capitalize on the strengths of each discipline for the patient's ultimate benefit. The need to coordinate teaching efforts is especially critical for patients who are acutely ill and who cannot absorb ambitious teaching activities. Involvement of the patient and family is key to ensuring effective patient education with appropriate learning outcomes to empower rather than to overcome the learner (Aruffo & Gardner, 2001).

Case Management

Case management involves leadership from a nurse or another health professional to oversee the process of providing care, with the goal of improving efficiency, increasing effectiveness of interventions, and containing costs. Critical paths, care maps, and other case management tools incorporate patient and family education consistently across the plan of care. This plan for patient learning involves the input of the health care team and a focus on patient learning outcomes. When nurses assume the role of case manager or care coordinator, they must be especially committed to interdisciplinary planning and team building. Chapter 12 addresses in greater detail how patient education is provided in the context of case management.

Staff Development and Continuing Education

Staff development and continuing education, targeted to helping health care professionals increase skills in patient education, must also address the health care team approach. This is accomplished most effectively when members of the health care team engage in the learning experience together. Chapter 5 explores the role of staff development in patient education and offers suggestions for organizing such continuing education programs.

TABLE 1.1 Comments on Patient Education From Health Care Professionals

PHYSICIANS	DIETITIANS	PHYSICAL THERAPISTS	PHARMACISTS	HOSPITAL SOCIAL WORKERS
What is your involvement in patient education?				
"I teach patients one-on-one. I try to tell them what they want and need to know in language they understand. I want them to understand and agree with the treatment plan, to know what the goals are, and to participate in decision-making." "I try to incorporate patient education into my interaction with the patient. I think you need to be consciously aware of patient education, and you have to have a good feeling that your patients are understanding and doing what you agree is appropriate. I think we assume more than we should."	"We educate patients about the diets they must follow at home. We try to find out what the patient usually eats and how we need to modify this. Sometimes we discuss the diet with the doctor because what he or she orders is inappropriate. We make the necessary changes and teach the patient."	"We inform patients about their disease, about what to expect, and about any procedures that are done. We teach them about ambulation, functional activities, and safety, especially postsurgically. Physical therapists have a large role in educating patients about rheumatic diseases and how to deal with and prevent flareups. We also teach patients about prostheses and help patients with them."	"The pharmacist is often the first person to see patients when they have problems. When patients ask for advice, the pharmacist must know if a referral to other health care providers is needed. The pharmacist also must teach about how a drug works in the body. If the patient knows the reason for taking the drug, he or she is more likely to take it as prescribed. Many patients know nothing about their medication. They don't know what it is or how to store it. Sometimes they don't even take it, depending on how they feel. This is especially true for hypertensive patients."	"Our biggest role is as a hospital, staff, and community liaison. If patients cannot take care of themselves after leaving the hospital, we talk with the patient, doctor, and family about agencies or resources that can help and coordinate the plans. Many families have problems before they even come into the hospital. We help with these too. We give emotional support and answer questions about things patients are really afraid of. Patients tend to tell things to social workers that they are embarrassed to tell doctors and nurses."
How do you see the nurse's role in patient education?				
"I see it as necessary and important. Nurses have a different perspective from mine. The doctor teaches about diagnosis and prognosis; the nurse teaches daily management. There is combined strength. Patients tend to confide different information to nurses. For example, patients are more open about fear of cancer with the nurse,	"Nurses reinforce what the dietitian tells the patient and emphasize the importance of following the diet plan. Nurses tell us what is going on with the patient, and this helps us to evaluate whether the patient understands the diet plan. Nurses also teach medications, treatments, and basic survival skills. They explain what the	"The role of the nurse is educating and orienting the patient about the disease and reinforcing the teaching of other health care personnel. Nurses give patients emotional support, teach them about activities of daily living, and give general instructions about medications. Nurses reinforce precautions in transfer and positioning. This is	"All patients have a right to know what medications they take, how much, and why. Nurses can teach this when they administer medications. There are so many new drugs. For nurses to teach patients, we need to collaborate. The nurse can reinforce the teaching done by the team and communicate with other team members to meet	"The nurses do much patient teaching, especially with surgical patients. They answer questions patients never ask their doctors. I get my best referrals from nurses. There's something about hanging an IV bag, giving a shot, washing hair, giving a bath—patients tell things to nurses at these times. Some nurses are very

and talk with me about stomach pain. Nurses clarify and reinforce what I teach. Nurses teach patients and families, especially in dealing with chronic diseases."

"Patient education is often left to the nurse. Yet, nurses often lack confidence in their ability to teach.

doctor has said to the patient after the doctor leaves."

crucial. They can help to motivate the patient and coordinate pain medications with the treatments."

the patient's learning needs. Nurses have a big job to do, and patients expect a lot of them."

aware of the situation a patient is going home to and they involve us when we are better able to handle certain kinds of crises."

What increases your collaboration with the nurse and other members of the health care team in patient education?

"Personal knowledge and trust. Having time to get to know other members of the health care team. Asking the patient who is teaching him. The patient is the center of the team and can help me work with the team. Writing and reading interdisciplinary progress notes is important. One of the most crucial things you do for the patient is document how you educate him."

"The most important thing is discussion. There has to be a desire on all parts. People can find the time to do it. Take a half hour to discuss a difficult patient and bring in everyone who is involved in the care. You formulate an approach and cross-educate one another. It optimizes patient care for that particular patient, but it also teaches people how to deal with difficult patients."

"We need planning meetings. We need to know what other people are teaching the patient. The patient should not have to hear things repeatedly, in different ways. Protocols for teaching help. You know what other people are teaching, although you don't always know at what level the patient is understanding."

"Documentation! The nurse's assessment of the patient's readiness to learn is especially helpful. For team work people must go out of their way to communicate with one another."

"We should acknowledge that we have the same goal: getting the patient ready to handle discharge. We should plan teaching together and construct teaching programs where we reinforce teaching and give emotional support from admission to discharge."

"Nursing shifts change frequently. Therefore, we often have no consistency and have little interaction. Frequent team meetings and good verbal and written communication would increase collaboration in patient education. This would promote mutual respect among the disciplines, cooperation, and knowing how to use other's expertise in different cases."

"Nurses make valuable assessments about the patient and family and what their supports are like. The nursing assessment should be shared more, especially in the progress notes."

"There should be continuing education for health care professionals. Pharmacists could teach nurses about new drugs, making nurses better able to teach patients. Pharmacists should be more open to nurses' questions and should encourage their calls."

"Nurses need to know their limits. The patient needs follow-up after discharge to learn and to reinforce teaching. Social workers can help by making referrals that go beyond discharge, but we have to work together and focus less narrowly on rescuing."

"Good notes in the patient record are important. I read all the notes, especially the patient's response to the nurses. Details help me assist the family in planning for discharge, such as whether the patient is incontinent or nonambulatory. Notes from the health care team validate what I see. Patient care rounds are also a good opportunity to collaborate."

Nurses gain valuable insights that promote the work of the health care team by talking with other health care professionals who are interested in patient teaching. We have initiated such conversations with physicians, nutritionists, physical therapists, pharmacists, and hospital social workers. We asked them to tell us how they see their patient teaching roles and how they perceive the nurse's role. Each suggested ways to increase collaboration. These interviews were also an opportunity to teach other health care professionals about the nurse's involvement in patient education and to generate ideas for new teaching programs. Table 1.1 (on the previous page) provides some comments from these interviews.

Although the health care team members we interviewed stressed the importance of protocols and organization (eg, development of critical pathways and teaching protocols), they frequently stated that attitudes and skills of people directly influenced the success of teamwork in patient education. They emphasized the following criteria for successful teamwork:

- **Communication.** Verbal and written communication, facilitated by planning meetings, care conferences, telephone consultation, good documentation, and the willingness to go out of your way to communicate with one another.
- **Mutual respect among disciplines.** Including recognizing respective areas of expertise, knowing one's limits, and teaching each other
- **Desire to work as a team** and recognition of a common goal.

SUMMARY

The nursing profession embraces patient education as a central factor in the nursing process and as a dimension of nurse caring. During the past three decades, changing needs and mandates have increased the visibility, involvement, and expertise of nurses as patient teachers. Informed consent, discharge planning, the prevalence of chronic health problems, and patient compliance are issues that require nursing leadership in patient education. Mandates from JCAHO, debate about the need to reform health care delivery, the emergence of managed care, and the growth of the nurse practitioner movement are also directly related to patient education.

Every health care provider, regardless of title, setting, or specialty, is called on to provide patients and families with an opportunity to learn in their health care encounters. Patient education reduces feelings of helplessness, enhances knowledge and skills, and promotes continuity of care.

In providing care that is truly patient centered, nurses acknowledge the importance of a health care team approach. Clinicians must reflect on their roles and the roles of others, and the respective strengths that each brings to patient care. Patient education is built on the foundations of respecting one another, caring, and communicating, not just among the nurse and patient and family, but also among all members of the health care team.

The next chapter reviews several key theoretical frameworks that provide the foundation for teaching and motivating patients.

STRATEGIES FOR CRITICAL ANALYSIS AND APPLICATION

1. Review the nine objectives of patient and family education as stated by JCAHO. Provide examples of how the health care provider might meet these objectives when caring for a patient and family.
2. Identify a patient, friend, or family member who has a chronic health problem. Ask this person to describe what knowledge and skills are needed to care for him or her. What resources has this person found helpful for learning to manage care?
3. Look in the media for examples of innovative patient and family education pro-

grams in the community. Consider how the need was assessed and how patients and families were involved in the design of those programs.

4. Interview members of other health care disciplines about their involvement in patient education. Then summarize what you learn and discuss how health care professionals might promote teamwork in providing patient education. You might pose the following questions to physicians, nutritionists, occupational and physical therapists, pharmacists, dentists, and hospital social workers:
   - How are you involved in patient education?
   - How do you see the role of other health care professionals in patient education?
   - How does your role interact with that of other health care professionals on the team?
   - How can members of the health care team increase their collaboration in patient education?

To find the latest information

Key search terms:
caring, patient education, health care delivery, advanced practice, adherence, interdisciplinary teams, health care reform, informed consent, chronic illness, disease management, substance abuse, JCAHO, clinical decision making, clinical judgment, cultural sensitivity, role model, case management, staff development, continuing education

Websites
- Healthy People 2010 documents online: http://www.health.gov/healthypeople/.
- Joint Commission on Accreditation of Healthcare Organizations (JCAHO). (2003). Weaving the fabric: Strategies for improving our nation's health care: http://www.jcaho.org/about+us/weaving+the+fabric.htm
- Canadian Nurses Association http://www.cna-nurses.ca
- World Health Organization www.who.int

REFERENCES

American Academy of Family Physicians. (2000). Patient Education: Recommended core educational guidelines for family practice residents. *American Family Physician, 62*(7), 1712–1714.

American Nurses Association. (1999). *Nursing-Sensitive Quality Indicators for Acute Care Settings and ANA's Safety & Quality Initiative.* Retrieved July 10, 2004, from http://nursingworld.org/readroom/fssafety.htm.

American Nurses Association. (1991). Nursing's agenda for health care reform. Retrieved 3/16/2003, from http://nursingworld.org/readroom/rnagenda.htm

Aruffo, S., & Gardner, C. (2001). Patient education: a collaborative process. *Case Manager, 12*(4), 74–77.

Balik, B. (1998). The impact of managed care and integrated delivery systems on registered nurse education and practice. In O'Neil, E., and Coffman, J. (Eds.), *Strategies for the Future of Nursing.* San Francisco: Jossey-Bass Publishers.

Bellack, J. (1998). Changing roles, responsibilities, and employment patterns of registered nurses in ambulatory care settings. In O'Neil, E., and Coffman, J. (Eds.), *Strategies for the Future of Nursing.* San Francisco: Jossey-Bass Publishers.

Benner, C., Tanner, C., & Chesla, C. (1996). *Expertise in Nursing Practice: Caring, Clinical Judgement, and Ethics.* New York, NY: Springer Publishing Co.

Benner, P. (2001). *From Novice to Expert: Excellence and Power in Clinical Nursing Practice* (commemorative edition ed.). Upper Saddle River, NJ: Prentice Hall Health.

Boyd, M. D., Graham, B. A., Gleit, C. J., & Whitman, N. I. (1998). *Health Teaching in Nursing Practice: A Professional Model* (3rd ed.). Stamford, CT: Appleton & Lange.

Carpenito, L. (2002). *Nursing Diagnosis: Application to Clinical Practice* (9th ed.). Philadelphia, PA: Lippincott Williams & Wilkins.

Edwards, K. A. (1998, February 22, 1999). *Informed Consent.* Retrieved March 16, 2003, from http://eduserv.hscer.washington.edu/bioethics/topics/consent.html.

Freda, M. C. (2002). *Perinatal Patient Education: A practical guide with education handouts for patients.* Philadelphia, PA: Lippincott Williams & Wilkins, p. 4.

Garity, J. (2000). Cultural competence in patient education. *Caring, 19*(3), 18–20.

Gilliss, C., Mundinger, M. (1998). How is the role of the advanced practice nurse changing? In O'Neil, E., and Coffman, J. (Eds.), *Strategies for the Future of Nursing*. San Francisco: Jossey-Bass Publishers.

Gomez, D. (1999). Caring for others means caring for ourselves. *The American Nurse,* July/August, 31(4), 5.

Haber, D. (2001). Promoting readiness to change behavior through health assessments. *Clinical Gerontologist, 23*(1/2), 152–158.

Hartrick, G. (2000). Developing health-promoting practice with families: one pedagogical experience. *Journal of Advanced Nursing, 31*(1), 27–34.

Henderson, V. (1966). *The Nature of Nursing*. NY: Macmillan.

Jackson, B., Smith, S., Adams, R., Frank, B., & Mateo, M. (1999). Healthy life styles are a challenge for nurses. *Image—The Journal of Nursing Scholarship, 31*(2), 196.

Joint Commission on Accreditation of Healthcare Organizations (JCAHO). (2001). *2001 Hospital Accreditation Standards*. Oakbrook Terrace, IL: Joint Commission on Accreditation of Healthcare Organizations.

Kramer, E. J., Bucher, J. A., Glassman, K. S., & Siu, S. (1999). Strategies for patient teaching: how to seize the teachable moment. In W. B. Bateman, E. J. Kramer & K. S. Glassman (Eds.), *Patient and Family Education in Managed Care and Beyond: Seizing the Teachable Moment* (pp. 19–36). New York, NY: Springer Publishing Company, p. 19.

Lowe, J. M., Knapp, M. L., Meyer, M. A., Gall, G. B., Hampton, J. G., Dillman, J. A., et al. (2001). School-based health centers as a locus for community health improvement. *Quality Management in Health Care, 9*(4), 24–32.

Mundinger, M. (1994). Advanced-practice nursing—good medicine for physicians? *New England Journal of Medicine, 330*(3), 211–214.

Mundinger, M. (1996). New Alliances: Nursing's Bright Future. *Nursing Administration Quarterly, 20*(3), 50–53.

National League for Nursing Education. (1918). *Standard Curriculum for Schools of Nursing*. Baltimore: Waverly Press.

Neal, L. (1999). Neal theory of home health nursing practice. *Image—The Journal of Nursing Scholarship, 31*(3), 251.

Nightingale, F. (1992). *Notes on Nursing: What It Is and What It Is Not* (commemorative ed.). Philadelphia: J. B. Lippincott.

Office for Protection from Research Risks. (1993). Tips on Informed Consent. Retrieved 3/16/2003, from http://ohrp.osophs.dhhs.gov/humansubjects/guidance/ictips.htm.

Pew Health Professions Commission. (1998). Recreating Health Professional Practice for a New Century. Retrieved March 16, 2003, from http://www.futurehealth.ucsf.edu/pewcomm.html.

Resnick, B. (2002). Geriatric rehabilitation: the influence of efficacy beliefs and motivation. *Rehabilitation Nursing, 27*(4), 152–159.

Sanford, R. C. (2000). Caring through relation and dialogue: a nursing perspective for patient education. *Advances in Nursing Science, 22* (3), 1–15.

Shinitzky, H. E., & Kub, J. (2001). The art of motivating behavior change: the use of motivational interviewing to promote health. *Public Health Nursing, 18*(3), 178–185.

Sullivan, S. D., Weiss, K. B., Lynn, H., Mitchell, H., Kattan, M., Gergen, P. J., et al. (2002). The cost-effectiveness of an inner-city asthma intervention for children. *Journal of Allergy and Clinical Immunology, 110*(4), 576–581.

Szabo, V., & Strang, V. (1999). Experiencing control in caregiving. *Image—The Journal of Nursing Scholarship, 31*(1), 71–75.

Tanner, C., Benner, P., Chesla, C., & Gordon, D. (1993). The phenomenology of knowing the patient. *Image—The Journal of Nursing Scholarship, 25*(3), 273–280.

U.S. Department of Health and Human Services. (2000). *Healthy People 2010: Understanding and Improving Health*. Retrieved July 10, 2004 from http://www. health.gov/ healthypeople, http://www. healthypeople. gov/.

U.S. Department of Health and Human Services, & The Office of Minority Health. (2001). *National standards for culturally and linguistically appropriate services in health care* (final report).

Wolf, Z., Giardino, E., Osborne, P., & Ambrose, M. (1994). Dimensions of nurse caring. *Image—The Journal of Nursing Scholarship, 26* (2), 107–111.

Health Promotion: Models and Applications to Patient Education

LEARNING OBJECTIVES

After reading this chapter, the student should be able to:

1. Define the terms health promotion, disease prevention, and health maintenance, and give examples of each.

2. Describe the historical transition from a compliance orientation to a health promotion and disease prevention orientation.

3. List five of the six factors used in the Health Belief Model to determine a person's likelihood of complying with health care recommendations.

4. Compare the Health Belief Model with the Health Promotion Model; describe the difference in the definition of health for each model.

5. Identify a community health education dilemma to which the Precede-Proceed Model might be applied.

6. Compare the Care-Seeking Behavior Theory to the Health Promotion Model.

7. List two benefits that would be obtained in using the Self-Regulation Model to guide patient education.

8. List three criteria for prescribing a screening test.

9. Describe a plan for using the Guide to Clinical Preventive Services and the Clinician's Handbook of Preventive Services in an outpatient family practice setting.

INTRODUCTION

In conjunction with the evolution of highly sophisticated medical and surgical interventions, an appreciation of the importance of promoting healthy lifestyles and reducing risk factors for disease has developed. Health care consumers and providers recognize the importance of promoting healthy lifestyles to prevent the onset of preventable diseases and conditions.

Primary care providers, in particular nurse practitioners, recognize the importance of partnering patient education with health promotion and risk factor reduction to encourage better health outcomes. If patient education were more effectively used to promote health and reduce risk factors, many patient education techniques (discussed in other sections of this book) to intervene with diseases would become unnecessary!

This chapter provides important definitions related to health promotion and risk factor reduction, an overview of health belief and health promotion models, and application of cases to the *Guide to Clinical Preventive Services* and *Clinician's Handbook of Preventive Services*.

HEALTH PROMOTION, DISEASE PREVENTION, AND HEALTH MAINTENANCE

Definitions

The concepts of health promotion, disease prevention, and health maintenance are interrelated; however, it is important to understand the nuances of each.

Health Promotion

Health promotion includes activities that a person undertakes to enjoy life to the fullest. Generally, health promotion is associated with wellness behaviors rather than with disease prevention. For example, a healthy 32-year-old who walks on a treadmill is performing a health-promoting activity that may prevent disease, but she walks primarily to feel self-actualizing and to enhance her health and well-being.

Other activities and lifestyle decisions that are considered health promoting include deciding not to smoke tobacco, controlling or avoiding ingestion of alcohol, using family planning to promote maternal and child health, seeking psychological counseling to promote mental health, and eating nutritious food for enjoyment and health. Many people can tell their health care providers what they do to promote their health; others will be unaware of the concept of health promotion and will focus on disease prevention.

Disease Prevention

Disease prevention is comprised primarily of screening for asymptomatic diseases in children and adults, counseling to prevent diseases and the onset of chronic conditions, and immunizing to prevent diseases. Currently, controversy exists about which screening tests are most essential and which risk factors indicate someone should be screened. The *Guide to Clinical Preventive Services* attempts to answer these questions through a careful review of evidence for and against screening tests. Although there may be overlap between health promotion and disease prevention (and certainly health promotion may aid in disease prevention), the authors generally do not consider disease prevention to reside in the same health-enhancing and self-actualizing arena as health promotion.

Health Maintenance

Health maintenance involves screening for disease prevention and counseling provided by the advanced practice nurse (especially the nurse practitioner). For example, a pediatric or family nurse practitioner performs a Denver Developmental Screening Test on an eight-month-old infant as a health maintenance activity. If the infant does not meet the appropriate developmental milestones, the nurse practitioner will either continue to monitor the infant (depending on the degree of the developmental delay) or refer the infant and parents for further testing or counseling. Health maintenance is always the first part of the plan when the nurse practitioner charts a SOAP note (Subjective, Objective, Assessment, Plan). Making health

maintenance a priority helps the nurse practitioner remember that promoting and maintaining health are a crucial part of his or her role.

Attention has turned to health promotion and disease prevention. Therefore, patient teaching regarding compliance with a medical regimen is still important, but shares the stage with health promotion. Most of the theoretical frameworks of health promotion have evolved from the Health Belief Model.

Understanding Compliance as the Framework for Health Promotion

General Considerations

Before health promotion and health maintenance became well-known concepts in the health care lexicon, most health care providers focused on compliance. Health promotion and disease prevention were not common approaches in health care arenas in the first half of the 20th century; at that time, health care focused on disease. However, the public has become more knowledgeable about disease prevention, and health care providers recognize that preventing major illness is more effective than coping with an established illness. Consequently, there has been a burgeoning of health promotion activities. Nevertheless, it is important to understand that the roots of health promotion are in compliance.

Early Approaches to Compliance

Sackett and Haynes (1976) defined compliance as "the extent to which the patient's behavior (in terms of taking medications, following diets or executing other life-style changes) coincides with the clinical prescriptions" (p. 1). They further state that "the presentation of compliance data has clinical relevance only when it is related to the simultaneous achievement of the treatment goals" (p. 3). This definition influenced compliance research and literature in two major ways. First, it indelibly associated the control of illness with compliance to physician-directed regimens (ie, control resulted from complying with the prescribed treatment.) The physician determined the dose and timing of medication, the specific diet to be followed, and the kind of body monitoring to be completed by the patient. Completing these actions as ordered was assumed to lead directly to control of the illness. Compliance was measured by the extent to which the patient accomplished these activities.

Second, the patient's adherence to the prescribed regimen became the focus of the indices of compliance or noncompliance. Noncompliance describes patient behaviors that deviate from the practitioner's plan, often attributed to a willful disobedience on the part of the patient (Dreger & Tremback, 2002). According to this model, the educator's task involves motivating patients to see the value of treatment plans as a means to attaining health or controlling illness, providing patients with the skills and knowledge needed to manage continuing care without daily professional supervision, and encouraging patients to change behavior patterns to conform with the regimen. The prescriptive or compliance model was the philosophical basis even in the innovative nurse-managed clinics developed by Allison (1973) and Backscheider (1974), in which Orem's nursing theory of self-care was used to organize the clinic practice. The goal of nursing care was to assist the patient in following the prescribed treatment plan; the person's definition of self-care was rarely considered.

Despite prescribed regimens to treat illness and education to inform the patient about the importance of following the medical prescription, the rate of noncompliance is notoriously high. Marinker and Shaw (2003) reported that about half of the medicines prescribed for patients with long-term conditions are not taken as prescribed.

THE HEALTH BELIEF MODEL

General Considerations

To identify factors that influence compliance or noncompliance with a health care regimen, a group of cognitive and social psychologists began a work group that probed many psychological questions that affect health. Among this group were Bandura, Leventhal, Rosenstock, Becker, and Hochbaum, major contributors to health psychology and, indirectly, to patient education.

The Health Belief Model is a framework that arose from this group. The Health Belief Model was originally developed to predict the likelihood of a person taking recommended preventive health action and to understand a person's motivation and decision-making about seeking health services (Hochbaum, 1958). It has been used to explain food-handling behaviors in older adults (Hanson & Benedict, 2002). This model has also been used to identify methods to increase screening for breast and cervical cancer in Hispanic women (Austin et al., 2002).

The Health Belief Model attempts to identify compliers and noncompliers by examining six factors considered important to health care decisions:

1. The patient's perception of the severity of the illness
2. The patient's perception of susceptibility to illness and its consequences
3. Value of the treatment benefits (eg, Does the cost and adverse effects of the treatment outweigh the disease consequences?)
4. Barriers to treatment (eg, degree of social support, expense, regimen complexity, length of treatment, and side effects)
5. Costs of treatment in physical and emotional terms
6. Cues that stimulate taking action toward treatment of illness (eg, illness in family or friends, television or other media coverage, newspaper stories, or health pamphlets)

Variables including nationality, social class, race, employment status, occupation, and behavior patterns have a significant impact on disease and health (Jonas, 2000). They influence a person's perceptions about the seriousness of health conditions and the need to take action for those conditions.

Research Studies

The Health Belief Model has been used in many research studies that cover a wide range of health-related, decision-making situations (Ehiri, 2000; Koch, 2002; Mikhail & Petro-Nustas, 2001; Wallace, 2002).

However, studies using the Health Belief Model have been inconsistent in identifying the differences between those who comply with professional recommendations and those who choose not to comply; similarly, the model has not delivered on its promise to predict those who are likely to engage in health promotion activities.

Studies show various components of the model as effective for prediction, although the model as a whole has not been a consistent predictor of compliance. Janz & Becker (1984) suggest that perceived barriers and costs are the most prominent factors associated with not participating in preventive health practices or maintenance of treatment regimens.

Application of the Health Belief Model

The Health Belief Model demonstrates the complex relationship between motivation, health behavior, and health outcome. For example, Koch (2002) found that aging African-American women with a diagnosis of type 2 diabetes mellitus who maintain a regular exercise regimen possess different health beliefs and benefit from greater glycemic control than those who do not exercise regularly.

Subjects who exercised regularly reported fewer barriers to exercise and perceived greater benefits from adhering to a regular exercise regimen than those who did not

exercise on a regular basis. Non-exercisers found more barriers to, and fewer benefits from, exercising. Although the Health Belief Model acknowledges the importance of a patient's belief in compliance, the assumption is that the variables specified regarding health beliefs are the most significant factors in decision-making about health behaviors.

THE HEALTH PROMOTION MODEL

General Considerations

Nola Pender, a nurse who began her work in the early 1980s, developed another model that attempts to explain how people arrive at decisions about behaviors toward health promotion (Pender, 1982). Pender believed that the Health Belief Model focused on an avoidance orientation related to seeking preventive care to decrease the probability of negative health and illness outcomes.

Pender theorized that the Health Belief Model did not address positive actions taken to sustain or increase a person's level of health. She maintained that the Health Belief Model was tested on preventive actions requiring the performance of a single act of compliance and was insufficient to explain behavior directed toward health promotion. Pender defined health not as the absence of disease, but as self-actualization. She thought that this definition suggested that health was related to self-initiated behaviors directed toward attaining higher levels of health. From her perspective, defining health as adaptation or stability directed a person's behavior toward health protection or toward avoiding illness and disease.

Health-Promoting Behaviors and Health Protection

Health-promoting behaviors are operationalized for purposes of research as activities that are integrated on an ongoing basis into a person's lifestyle. Health promotion behaviors include exercise, obtaining optimum nutrition, stress management, and the development and maintenance of social support systems. These behaviors are directed toward self-actualization and fulfillment; the behaviors serve to increase well-being and actualize human health potential.

However, health protection is described by Pender as the motivation to avoid illness, detect it early, and maintain functioning when ill. Health protection is similar to the concept of health maintenance, a primary focus of the nurse practitioner role. Nurse practitioners and other primary health care providers work to promote health maintenance through the recognition of needed immunizations for adults and children, identification of age-appropriate screening examinations, and clarification of safety issues (eg, seatbelt and child car seat safety, smoking cessation).

The role of the health care professional is to help people overcome barriers to health-promoting activities and support preventive health practices. Assistance by health providers is accomplished by removing genuine barriers (eg, lack of access to care), emphasizing the positive consequences of preferred behaviors, and by reducing the frequency of negative consequences.

Components of the Health Promotion Model

The Health Promotion Model is organized into three categories: (1) individual characteristics and experiences, (2) behavior-specific cognitions and affect, and (3) behavioral outcome.

The components of the Health Promotion Model are based on many features in the Health Belief Model and on a synthesis of health promotion and wellness literature.

The Health Promotion Model is based on a number of assumptions. It assumes people seek to create conditions of living through which they can express their unique human health potential. It assumes people have the capacity for reflective self-awareness, value growth, try to achieve a balance between change and stability and seek to regulate their own behavior. It assumes people interact with their environment, progressively transforming the environment and being transformed over time. The model also assumes health professionals are part of this environment that exerts influence on people throughout their lifespan, and self-initiated changes in this person-environment relationship are essential to behavior change (Pender, Murdaugh, & Parsons, 2002).

Individual Characteristics and Experiences

This category consists of prior-related behavior and characteristics that are inherited and acquired and that influence beliefs, affect, and health-promoting behavior—the habits, skills, and knowledge acquired in the past, as well as biological, psychological, and cultural factors.

Behavior-Specific Cognitions and Affect

The behavior-specific cognitions and affect determining health promotion activities are:

1. Perceived benefits of action in which people engage in behaviors they expect will give them benefits.
2. Perceived barriers to action can prevent people from acting, or committing to act.
3. Perceived competence or self-efficacy to perform a given behavior increases the likelihood of commitment to action and actual performance of the behavior.
4. A greater perceived self-efficacy results in fewer perceived barriers to a specific health behavior.
5. A positive affect toward a behavior results in greater perceived self-efficacy, which can in turn result in increased positive affect.
6. When a behavior is associated with positive emotions or affect, the probability of commitment and action is increased.
7. People are more likely to commit to and engage in health-promoting behaviors

when significant others model the behavior, expect the behavior to occur, and provide assistance and support to enable the behavior.

8. Families, peers, and health care providers are important sources of interpersonal influence that can increase or decrease commitment to, and engagement in, health-promoting behavior.

9. Situational influences in the environment, such as options, can increase or decrease commitment to, or participation in, health-promoting behavior.

Behavioral Outcomes

Factors that influence behavior include:

1. The greater the commitment to a specific plan of action, the more likely health-promoting behaviors are to be maintained over time.

2. Commitment to a plan of action is less likely to result in the desired behavior when competing demands over which persons have little control require immediate attention.

3. Commitment to a plan of action is less likely to result in the desired behavior when other actions are more attractive, and therefore preferred over the target behavior.

4. People can modify cognitions, affect, and the interpersonal and physical environment to create incentives for health actions (Pender, Murdaugh, & Parsons, 2002).

Research Studies

Pender and others have reported the results of studies that demonstrated that perceived self-efficacy, benefits, and barriers have been empirically supported as predictors of health-promoting behaviors (Pender, Murdaugh, & Parsons, 2002). Demographic variables, such as education, occupation, household size, age, religion, and rural versus urban environment, have also been supported

in research related to the Health Promotion Model and generally have a positive relationship with, and are predictive of, health behaviors (Garcia, Pender, Antonakos, & Ronis, 1998).

Other studies have further confirmed the relationships among various components of the Health Promotion Model and health-promoting behaviors. Duffy (1993) reported that subjects who believed that their current health was good, had high self-esteem, and who believed that health was under their own control more frequently practiced the health promotion activities of self-actualization, nutrition, interpersonal support, stress management, and exercise.

Pender's willingness to revise and enhance the model over time is a good example of model respecification, a task that is not frequently assumed by nurse theorists. Pender's contributions to health promotion have been crucial. Although she does not directly address patient education, her model has many implications for understanding a patient's willingness to undertake health protection and health-promoting activities.

OTHER HEALTH PROMOTION FRAMEWORKS

Three additional health promotion frameworks will be mentioned in this chapter: the Precede-Proceed Model, Care-Seeking Behavior Theory, and the Self-Regulation Model. A fourth model, the Transtheoretical Model of Motivation and Change, is covered in Chapter 4, as it relates to motivation and teaching principles.

The Precede-Proceed Model

Developed by Lawrence Green, a leading public health and health education expert, this model was created for use with people and communities to promote health and, as a desired endpoint, to enhance quality of life (Green et al., 1980). The model applies more reasonably to health promotion for aggregates than to individuals because policy and environmental factors are major components of the framework.

The model offers a guide to assuring the comprehensiveness of approaches to change through techniques that enable and reinforce change. Because communities are involved in their own desired changes, the changes are internalized and reinforced rather than created from outside the community. Different from other health promotion models, this model seeks to create change not just through admonitions from health professionals but through the altering of knowledge, attitudes, and beliefs at a macrosystem level, which alters knowledge at the community or family level (Green, 1999).

A unique feature of the model is that instead of planning interventions to bring about desired outcomes, the health care professional starts at the outcome and determines the quality of life of the designated population. The health care professional asks *Why does this group have these health outcomes?* Instead of planning a program to meet the needs of the population, the advanced practice nurse should start with an assessment of the current situation and then try to determine deductively, by working backward, the original cause of the situation. The origin of the problem is referred to as a social diagnosis; it is a type of self-assessment. Once the self-assessment has occurred, an epidemiological diagnosis is made; the epidemiological diagnosis is followed by a behavioral and environmental diagnosis. After the behavioral and environmental diagnoses are made, the educational and organizational structures are considered so that a diagnosis involving these components is made. Last, an administrative and policy diagnosis leads to a plan for health promotion that eventually culminates in methods and strategies to achieve the desired health-promoting behaviors.

Evaluation is a major part of the iterative process involved in the Precede-Proceed model. For example, this model was used in Nepal to identify the factors behind the high incidence of the parasitic zoonosis, *Taenia solium*, which causes a preventable, yet prevalent endemic problem in urban Nepal. The model enabled the authors to define three specific actions that needed to be taken to control the spread of *T. solium*. They identified which standardized law enforcement and meat inspection practices are needed (Joshi et al., 2001).

Care-Seeking Behavior Theory

This theory was developed from Harry Triandis's work related to behavior theory. It was modified by Diane Lauver, a nurse, to represent the reasons that patients seek health care (Lauver, 1992). Lauver posits that psychosocial variables, such as affect or feelings, expectations and values about outcomes, norms, and habits, influence care-seeking behavior. Pre-existing clinical and sociodemographic variables (eg, chest pain or gender) modify the psychosocial variables but do not directly influence care-seeking behavior. Also, facilitating conditions, such as ease of access to health care and insurance, may influence the psychosocial variables.

Lauver's research demonstrates the importance of considering psychosocial variables (eg, anxiety, norms about appropriate actions, and habits) and facilitating conditions (eg, access to health care); these factors appear to influence psychosocial behaviors. The implications are that a nurse would consider the anxiety, mores and norms, habits, and access to care pertaining to a given patient. If the patient represents a particular group for whom preventive action, such as mammography, is feared or not valued—and if this particular patient is also highly anxious, has never participated in preventive screening, and cannot easily access mammography—she is less likely to obtain mammography than is a woman with a different profile.

The care-seeking behavior theory is obviously an outgrowth of the Health Belief Model and the Health Promotion Model. Lauver has reduced the number of variables and simplified the model so that it is easier to test. The emphasis on psychosocial variables seems logical because most realize that people seek health care based on their own past experiences with illness or health-seeking behavior (habits), their own feelings and beliefs, and the feelings and beliefs expressed by significant others (norms). Pender's current Health Promotion Model reflects the importance of psychosocial variables, an example of the cross-fertilization that occurs among nursing theorists.

Self-Regulation Model

Another model that examines decision-making related to health promotion includes the patient's personal meaning of, and responses to, illness. The Self-Regulation Model was developed from studies that considered the

effect of fear-arousing communications on preventive health care actions (Figure 2.1). For example, in the 1950s, attempts were made to promote polio vaccinations through fear-inducing messages to parents. Studies were conducted using the psychological framework of drive theory that suggested a drive, such as fear (eg, fear of polio), would precede performance of an activity (eg, taking children to be vaccinated). Therefore, fear-arousing information could be used to make people comply with health-related activities (Keller, Ward, & Baumann, 1989).

Leventhal, Meyer, and Nerenz (1980) proposed that in illness both cognition (the objective interpretation of a threat) and emotion (the subjective interpretation of a threat) are interactive. The Self-Regulation Model provides a structure for understanding the factors

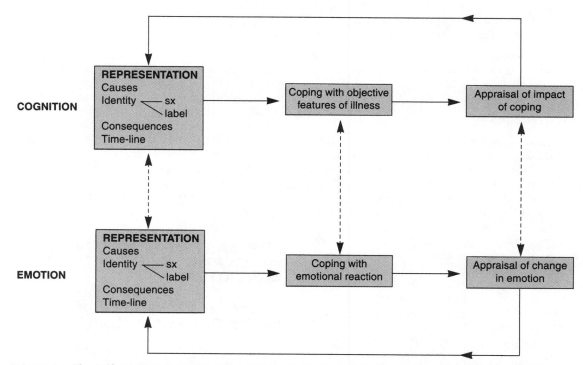

FIGURE 2.1 The Self-Regulation Model. (From: Keller, M. L., Ward, S., & Baumann, L. J. [1989]. Processes of self-care: Monitoring sensations and symptoms. *Advances in Nursing Science, 12*[1], 54–66.) Reprinted with permission.

that influence how a person perceives threats of illness, the relationship between these perceptions and how illness symptoms are reported, and how these personal beliefs influence decisions about self-care (Jayne & Rankin, 2001).

Representations of health threats are constructed from accumulated experience and are an integration of knowledge gathered from the media, personal contacts, health professional input, symptoms and body sensations, and past experience with illness. The model views four factors as the key features of a person's construction of health threats:

1. Identity or identification of concrete symptoms (eg, a headache means a brain tumor is present)
2. Cause (eg, improper food habits or stressful life events)
3. Time line or the perception of how long the illness will last (ie, acute or chronic)
4. The patient's perception of the consequences of the threat

Interpretation and synthesis of these factors will influence how a person copes with illness (see Figure 2.1).

Research Studies

Research studies that use the Self-Regulation Model are an expansion of the medical model's conception of compliance as a result of fixed patient characteristics, situational barriers, and inadequate motivation or education. The concepts developed in the Self-Regulation Model suggest that a person's understanding of an illness may be the critical factor in decisions about continuing treatment.

Furthermore, beliefs about illness will determine what symptoms people choose to monitor in evaluating health status. The interpretation of symptoms as a health threat will have an impact on a person's actions to correct the problem. For example, Jayne & Rankin (2001) applied the Self-Regulation Model to understand how Chinese immigrants understood their type 2 diabetes, so

interventions could be planned to meet their unique situations. They found participants were unclear about the etiology and chronicity of diabetes, and interpreted the illness as stigmatizing. Their coping strategies included wishful thinking, belief in powerful others, keeping diabetes a secret, and avoiding social situations.

The authors concluded the Self-Regulation Model was useful in profiling a vulnerable group whose diabetes management, social environment, and self-image could be improved through thoughtful patient education strategies.

In summary, the Self-Regulation Model focuses on the patient's interpretation of the meaning of the illness as a vehicle for understanding why patients comply with health promotion and disease prevention guidelines and medical treatment. However, the model maintains a purely cognitive approach to illness management and does not address health and illness in the context of everyday life. Environmental factors (eg, home and work stresses) are only acknowledged in research as important in the construction of beliefs about the cause of illness. Unrecognized in the model is how modifications in health definitions affect emotions and social activities. Furthermore, this model fails to address how valued social activities (eg, meals with family members) affect emotional adjustment to illness, health definitions, and health practices. The inability to engage in valued social activities may dissuade patients from adhering to the medical regimen.

SUMMARY OF MODELS AND IMPLICATIONS FOR PATIENT EDUCATION

Historical Background of Health Promotion Models

Historically, the Health Belief Model spawned the Self-Regulation Model, and later the Health Promotion Model. Rosenstock, Hochbaum, Leventhal, and Kegeles worked together in the Public Health Service in the 1950s and 1960s to ascertain why people failed to seek disease prevention or screening tests for the early detection of asymptomatic disease. In addition to the Health Promotion Model, the influence of the Health Belief Model is obvious when one examines the Care-Seeking Behavior Theory. These models attempt to better discern what characteristics best describe people who would or would not comply with prescribed health promotion and treatment plans. Although they are useful heuristics for trying to explain health promotion behaviors, they are difficult to test in toto and are still more useful as philosophical perspectives to try to understand behavior than they are useful at actually predicting it.

The only model that does not have direct origins in the Health Belief Model is the Precede-Proceed Model. Green has also been engaged in public health research; however, his work generally involved aggregates (ie, groups of people or communities) rather than individuals. Although his model is intuitively appealing, it is probably not as useful to clinicians in direct patient care because their focus tends to be more individual and family-oriented, rather than aggregate-based. However, health professionals trying to work with community aggregates may find the Precede-Proceed Model invaluable.

Models in Context of Patient Education

All of the models discussed are useful for planning patient education oriented toward health promotion.

The Health Belief Model

The Health Belief Model was the first to postulate that a patient's belief in his or her personal susceptibility to, and the severity of a health condition, are important variables influencing the decision to take action to prevent health problems. In terms of patient education, the health care provider should consider if the person believes in his or her own personal susceptibility to, and the potential severity of, a health condition. If the health care provider ascertains that the patient has no belief in personal susceptibility to the severity of a condition, the first step in patient education is to provide information and reality orientation that makes the patient more open to preventive screening and risk factor reduction strategies. Likewise, other variables (eg, benefits, barriers and cost to treatment, and cues to stimulate action) are important to consider when attempting patient education.

The Current Health Promotion Model

The current Health Promotion Model makes a unique contribution to patient education through its focus on commitment to a plan of action and immediate competing demands and preferences. Evaluating the patient's commitment to a plan of action is key to planning an educational intervention. If the health care provider determines a great commitment to promoting healthy lifestyles or to seeking preventive screening, then it is logical to draw up a contract with the patient that specifies what the actions should be and that provides some type of reward. (See Chapter 8 for strategies to develop contracts.) Immediate competing demands and preferences are also important for the health care provider to consider before launching patient education. For example, if a young father is worried about losing his job, he is probably less likely to take time off from work to renew a tetanus immunization than would another person whose work situation was more stable.

The Precede-Proceed Model

The Precede-Proceed Model has been used in many different health promotion studies for aggregates or communities with particular needs, such as communities with high rates of child pedestrian injuries. Its contribution to patient education is generally applicable to certain populations with specified health education needs and includes the backward method of assessment; that is, the targeted group participates in determining health-promoting outcomes rather than the community interventionist deciding what's best for the population. Health care providers working in the area of public health, school health, or with other population aggregates may find that this model provides helpful direction in planning health education.

Care-Seeking Behavior Theory

This theory's primary contribution to patient education is its focus on psychosocial variables that influence care-seeking behavior. Not only do psychosocial variables directly influence care-seeking behavior, but they also are indirectly influenced by pre-existing clinical, sociodemographic, and access variables. This theory highlights the necessity to assess psychosocial variables, including feelings and affect, expectations and values, beliefs expressed by significant others (norms), and past experiences with illness (habits). This assessment is critical for determining how to proceed with patient education.

Understanding norms and habits is essential for teaching health-promoting behaviors and for counseling for risk-factor reduction. Patients frequently do not openly express certain norms related to sexual activity or child-rearing (eg, child discipline that includes corporal punishment). The patient's norms may conflict with those of the health care provider, especially if cultural differences between patient and health care provider exist. Therefore, it is important to understand the norms from which different cultural or religious groups operate to help patients engage in health-promoting activities. For example, it is unlikely that counseling will persuade a member of the Jehovah's Witness religious group to use any type of pooled immunoglobulins, such as those given after exposure to hepatitis A, because Jehovah's Witnesses proscribe use of blood products. Although attempts should be made to persuade patients to use desirable interventions, religious beliefs must be respected.

Also, a patient's habits are assessed before beginning health-promoting patient education. If a patient had a negative experience with a health screening, he or she may be unlikely to undertake other health screening procedures. For example, a patient who had a negative experience with a sigmoidoscopy is not as likely to agree to a colonoscopy. This example reiterates the importance of conducting a careful patient education assessment before attempting any health promotion patient education.

The Self-Regulation Model

The Self-Regulation Model is useful for trying to understand the cognitive process by which people make decisions regarding health promotion and disease management. This model's contribution to patient education is its focus on the parallel pathways of emotion and cognition. The model denotes that people do not operate solely on cognitive bases but also process information emotionally. Recognition of the parallel pathways demands that the nurse constantly assess the emotional and cognitive processing. If the emotional pathway is uppermost in priority for the patient, and little cognitive processing occurs, it is unlikely that the patient will undergo health screening or make rational decisions regarding health promotion. Therefore, the nurse should help the patient use both cognition and emotion to derive health-promoting behavior that is consonant with his or her desired self-actualization.

Summary

In sum, all the health screening and promotion models presented in this chapter make important contributions to patient education. Pender's Health Promotion model is the only one that focuses on actualizing healthy outcomes, rather than on disease prevention. However, Pender's model intersects health promotion and disease prevention and can be used successfully in either situation to enhance patient education.

HEALTHY PEOPLE 2010

Healthy People 2010 has been important in guiding the nation toward a health promotion agenda. This document focuses on the prevention of disability and morbidity. It addresses improvements in the health status of populations most at risk for premature death, disease, and disability, and includes screening interventions to detect asymptomatic diseases before disability, chronicity, or death ensues.

It was initiated as Healthy People 2000 in 1979 with the publication of *Healthy People: The Surgeon General's Report on Health Promotion and Disease Prevention*. It was revised and amended in 1995 with the publication of *Promoting Health/Preventing Disease: Objectives for the Nation* (Midcourse Review and 1995 Revisions). The publication in 1990 of Healthy People 2000 was made possible by a consortium of more than 300 organizations, representing all levels of government, professional workers, and people from various sectors of American communities. In 1990, 15 priority areas were established under the headings of preventive services, health protection, and health promotion.

Healthy People 2010 contains 467 objectives in 28 focus (or priority) areas. These focus areas are subsumed under two main goals—to increase quality and years of healthy life and to eliminate health disparities (U.S. Department of Health and Human Services, 2000). Healthy People 2010 provides a set of "leading health indicators," which will help people and communities gauge their progress in meeting the objectives. For example, the focus area of tobacco use has two leading indicators: to reduce cigarette smoking by adolescents from 36% to 16% by the year 2010, and to reduce cigarette smoking in adults from 24% to 12% by 2010. These leading indicators give concrete national goals against which communities and the health care providers serving them can measure their own effectiveness.

The vision for Healthy People 2010 moves beyond hospitals and outpatient settings to communities, schools, workplaces, and homes. Thus, the report has major implications for patient education, charging health care providers to find methods of implementing health promotion, disease prevention, and health maintenance in practice. According to the final review of Healthy People 2000 (National Center for Health Statistics, 2001), 68 objectives (21%) met the year 2000 targets and an additional 129 (41%) showed movement toward the targets. Data for 35 objectives (11%) showed mixed results and 7 (2 %) showed no change from the baseline. Only 47 objectives (15%) showed movement away from the targets. The status of 32 objectives (10%) could not be assessed.

GUIDE TO CLINICAL PREVENTIVE SERVICES AND CLINICIAN'S HANDBOOK OF PREVENTIVE SERVICES

Guide to Clinical Preventive Services

The *Guide to Clinical Preventive Services* (2003) and *Clinician's Handbook of Preventive Services* (1998) are two useful texts developed by the U.S. Preventive Services Task Force, a task force of the Department of Health and Human Services. The first edition of the *Guide to Clinical Preventive Services* was published in 1989 and immediately became an important reference for health care providers concerned about health promotion, health maintenance, and disease prevention.

Nurse practitioners in particular found this text helpful. Divided into screening, counseling and chemoprevention, the Guide provides a summary of the evidence, with recommendations and rationale. It includes topics such as hormone replacement therapy, healthy diet counseling, and screening for diabetes.

Clinician's Handbook of Preventive Services

The *Clinician's Handbook of Preventive Services* is a companion of, and closely related to, the *Guide to Clinical Preventive*

Services. The *Clinician's Handbook of Preventive Services* is the cornerstone of the "Put Prevention Into Practice" (PPIP) campaign, which was initiated in 1994 after the U.S. Preventive Services Task Force did its groundbreaking work. The *Clinician's Handbook of Preventive Services*, now in its second edition (1998), provides clinicians with helpful tools for adopting a systematic approach to screening and counseling. Useful features of this book, which are not available in the *Guide to Clinical Preventive Services*, are a resource list of pamphlets, books, and videotapes for patients, and a resource list of supplemental reading for providers.

CLINICAL RELEVANCE OF HEALTH PROMOTION TO PATIENT EDUCATION

Health promotion has become a buzzword for those involved in primary care. Many have jumped on the health promotion bandwagon, especially those of us who have seen the ravages of unhealthy lifestyles. The better educated, affluent consumer demands health promotion from his or her primary care provider and in his or her workplace. Convincing these people that screening and disease prevention is important is usually not a problem; they may request screening tests before the primary care provider suggests them. However, people who cope with many daily problems and limited discretionary income may be less enthusiastic about spending limited funds for taxicabs to clinics, where they can be screened for diseases about which they are unaware and for which they are asymptomatic. If the exigencies of daily life outweigh the promised rewards from obscure screening tests, it is dubious that these people will seek screening tests. Until all Americans can meet their basic survival needs, it is doubtful that screening will be universally accepted.

Health Screening

Screening for health risks is a form of secondary prevention; it is not primary prevention. Screening has been defined as the detection of disease in asymptomatic, apparently healthy people. Screening is the presumptive identification of an unrecognized disease or defect, with tests or examinations that rapidly sort apparently well persons who probably have a disease from those who probably do not. It does not make conceptual or economic sense to screen for all conditions.

Screening that meets the following criteria can be cost-beneficial:

- The disease is an important health problem (eg, hypertension) in that many people are susceptible.
- Accepted therapy is available.
- Facilities are available for diagnosis and treatment.
- The disease has an asymptomatic (or latent) phase during which detection and treatment decrease morbidity and mortality.
- Treatment in the asymptomatic phase yields a therapeutic result.
- The natural history of the disease is understood.
- The test(s) for the disease is (are) acceptable and available at a reasonable cost.
- An agreed-on policy exists regarding who is to be treated.
- The cost of case finding and treatment is less than the cost if the disease is discovered when it becomes symptomatic.

Patient education is an important adjunct to screening. If the nurse can help the patient understand why screening is important, the patient is more likely to accept screening. Conversely, it is important that nurses understand why some screening exams are not indicated for particular situations. For example, a healthy 28-year-old male who has had no symptoms of heart disease and does not have a positive family history does not need a rest-ing electrocardiogram, even though he may request one. Therefore, the nurse must understand which forms of disease prevention are most important at which ages and for which populations.

Application of Resources: Nutrition and Weight

One sentinel objective of Healthy People 2010 is to reduce the proportion of people who are overweight or obese. Obesity is one of the most significant health problems in westernized countries, and the United States probably has more obese persons than any other country in the world. More than half of the adults in the United States are estimated to be overweight or obese. The proportion of adolescents from poor households who are overweight or obese is twice that of adolescents from middle- and high-income households. Overweight and obesity substantially raise the risk of illness from high blood pressure, high cholesterol, type 2 diabetes, heart disease and stroke, gallbladder disease, arthritis, sleep disturbances and problems breathing, and certain types of cancers. In addition, obese individuals also may suffer from social stigmatization, discrimination, and lowered self-esteem (U.S. Department of Health and Human Services, 2000). Box 2.1 presents formulas for calculating adult body weight.

BOX 2.1 Height-Weight Formula for Calculating Adult Body Weight

Female
Allow 100 lbs for first 5′ of height and then add 5 lbs for each additional inch above 5′.

Male
Allow 106 lbs for first 5′ of height and then add 6 lbs for each additional inch above 5′.

The following case study incorporates information from the *Guide to Clinical Preventive Services* and the *Clinician's Handbook of Preventive Services* to a family that presents to the nurse and nurse practitioner in a midwestern pediatric practice.

CASE STUDY

THE VAN DAMME FAMILY

HISTORY AND PHYSICAL EXAMINATION
The Van Damme family has been part of the Hollander Family Practice for the past 7 years. The Van Dammes have three children: Anna, 7 years of age; Peter, 5 years of age; and Marta, 9 months of age. Mr. Van Damme is a 28-year-old wheat and dairy farmer and Mrs. Van Damme previously worked as an administrative assistant but now stays home with the children.

Mrs. Van Damme, who has recently discovered that she is pregnant with their fourth child, brings Marta in for her second diptheria-tetanus-pertussis (DTP) injection; Marta had to miss the scheduled 6-month injection because of otitis media. When the nursing staff weighs Marta they note that she weighs 24 pounds and is 27 inches long, placing her above the 100th percentile in weight and just below the 50th percentile in height. Anna weighs 72 pounds (above the 100th percentile for weight). Peter's weight is 35 pounds, which is appropriate for a 5-year-old male. Mrs. Van Damme is 5 feet 6 inches and weighs 164 pounds, which is more than 20% above her desired weight. (Box 2.1 provides a quick, easy method of calculating body weight for adults.)

After the physical examination, the nurse practitioner compliments Mrs. Van Damme on the manner in which she relates to Marta and the two older children. She notes that all three children are progressing well developmentally, and that Marta is almost updated on her immunizations. The nurse practitioner conveys to Mrs. Van Damme that Anna and Marta are overweight and that this is a potential health risk factor. Mrs. Van Damme is surprised to hear that being overweight can be a health risk for children. She notes that everyone in her family has been "solid," but she believes they are all healthy. After further data gathering, the nurse practitioner learns that Mrs. Van Damme's mother and maternal grandmother have the "type of diabetes that old people get." Mr. Van Damme's 58-year-old father recently died from a massive heart attack, which Mrs. Van Damme relates to the downturn in farming profits and the stressors involved in farming.

PLAN
The nurse practitioner decides that health maintenance and health promotion are major parts of the plan in the Problem-Oriented Medical Recording that she will enact with the Van Damme family. When the nurse practitioner refers to the *Healthy People 2000 Midcourse Review,* she notes that achievement of the nutrition objective is not being met nationally and that it continues to be an objective in *Healthy People 2010.* More Americans are overweight now than when the objectives were written. A review of the *Guide to Clinical Preventive Services* provides her with helpful patient education and counseling strategies (Box 2.2).

The nurse practitioner reviews Chapter 56 (Counseling to Promote a Healthy Diet) of the *Guide to Clinical Preventive Services.* She learns that reduced intake of dietary fat helps reduce the incidence of coronary artery disease and that intake of dietary fats also may be associated with increased incidence of cancers. Additionally, she notes that increased

intake of dietary fiber improves gastrointestinal function; decreasing sodium may help to decrease sodium-dependent cases of hypertension; intake of complex carbohydrates, rather than simple sugars, improves calorie balance and decreases the incidence of dental caries; and that adolescent girls and women generally need more dietary calcium than they usually ingest.

Remembering that Mrs. Van Damme is pregnant, the nurse practitioner reads about the nutritional needs of women, infants, and children. She is particularly impressed by the findings related to breast-feeding (eg, its health benefits and the lower likelihood of adult obesity in breast-fed infants).

IMPLEMENTATION
Armed with this information, the nurse practitioner covers the basics of the food pyramid with Mrs. Van Damme. Based on findings in the *Guide to Clinical Preventive Services* that counseling by dietitians is probably more likely to bring about changes in dietary patterns than counseling by physicians or nurse practitioners, the nurse practitioner refers Mrs. Van Damme to the clinic nutritionist. Finally, the nurse practitioner refers to the *Clinician's Handbook of Preventive Services* and copies down the patient resources dealing with nutrition.

In the *Guide to Clinical Preventive Services,* Chapter 55 (Counseling to Promote Physical Activity) also provides helpful information related to type 2 diabetes, for which Mrs. Van Damme is at considerable risk based on her family history and her current obesity. The nurse practitioner schedules the Van Damme family for a follow-up visit after the nutritionist appointment. At this time she will cover the guidelines on physical activity and use information from the *Clinician's Handbook of Preventive Services* to make informational materials available to the Van Dammes. The nurse practitioner charts the following SOAP note on Mrs. Van Damme's chart and an appropriate note on Marta's chart.

S: 31-year-old female member of the practice accompanying infant for DPT. Denies concern about her weight or that of her children. Reports positive maternal family history for type 2 diabetes and positive paternal family history (husband's father) for fatal myocardial infarction at age 58. Relates that she is newly pregnant.

O: Height and weight: 5'6" tall, 164 pounds. Pregnancy confirmed with urine test.

A: First trimester pregnancy. Obesity. Health maintenance:
    Appropriate weight loss
    Increased physical activity
  Diagnostic:
    1. Schedule for ultrasound and early pregnancy tests

Patient education:
Refer to nutritionist for dietary counseling for self and children.
Discuss benefits of breast-feeding at the next appointment.
During next appointment discuss benefits of exercise, weight loss, and physical activity for herself and children.
Provide patient handouts on weight loss and physical activity for herself and children.
Note: if the nurse practitioner lived in Canada rather than the United States, she could access similar resources offered by her government (Health Canada, 2003).

Although health care providers should always individualize treatment plans for each patient, the broad objectives in Healthy People 2010 offer an overall approach to working with aggregates in achieving healthy lifestyles. They are useful adjuncts to achieving Healthy People 2010 objectives.

SUMMARY

Chapter 2 provides various frameworks for applying health promotion to patient education. Health promotion was reviewed from its earliest origins in the compliance literature to the more current approach that presumes human beings' desire to improve their health status by engaging in healthy lifestyles, undergoing immunizations, and making other various attempts to self-actualize. The Health Belief Model, Pender's Health Promotion Model, Green's Precede-Proceed Model, Lauver's Care-Seeking Behavior Model, and Leventhal's Self-Regulation were reviewed for their applicability to patient education. The application of Healthy People 2010 to health promotion was examined. One goal with implications for health promotion and patient education, obesity, was used as an example. The *Guide to Clinical Preventive Services* and the *Clinician's Handbook of Preventive Services* counseling guidelines for obesity were applied to demonstrate evidence-based patient education regarding health-promoting lifestyles.

Health promotion is a logical and easy arena in which the health care provider can teach patients and families. Once people understand the reasons for engaging in healthy behaviors, they are frequently amenable to new information. Box 2.2 highlights patient education and counseling strategies.

Motivation to make behavior changes that promote health will be covered in Chapter 4.

The next chapter addresses the assessment and integration of cultural systems and beliefs, to best individualize teaching.

STRATEGIES FOR CRITICAL ANALYSIS AND APPLICATION

1. Suppose that you are working in an inner city neighborhood in an outpatient clinic that serves primarily new immigrants. These immigrants are struggling to learn English, find jobs, and obtain necessary

BOX 2.2 Patient Education and Counseling Strategies

1. Frame the teaching to match the patient's perceptions. Elicit information about the patient's belief system; match teaching with cultural sensitivity.
2. Inform patients of the purposes and expected effects of interventions. Also inform them when to expect these effects. Trace the trajectory of the recovery process and what signifies a recovery or complications.
3. Suggest small changes rather than large ones. Patients need to experience success and are more likely to be successful if recommended changes are not overwhelming.
4. Be specific. Explain the rationale, demonstrate any needed activities, and write down instructions.
5. Add new behaviors. It may be easier to add new behaviors than eliminate old ones. It is usually easier to get patients to add exercise to their daily regimens than to convince them to change their eating patterns.
6. Link new behaviors to old ones. If some activities are performed daily, such as brushing one's teeth, it's easier for patients to remember to take medications at the same time they brush their teeth than at other times.
7. Use the power of the profession. Health care providers serve as powerful influences in the lives of their patients; it is acceptable and useful to say, "Cigarette smoking is the worst thing that you can do for your health. I would like for you to stop now."
8. Get explicit commitments from the patient. Ask patients to describe how they will achieve the recommended health promotion and disease management activities. Obtaining commitments is more likely to result in adherence to the treatment plan.
9. Use a combination of strategies. Multiple strategies are more likely to result in behavior change than a single strategy. Combinations of group teaching, individual, audiovisual, and printed materials are more likely to bring desired changes than only using printed materials.
10. Involve office staff. A team approach facilitates patient education efforts. Some patients may be more attuned to medical assistants or front-office staff in terms of cultural background; thus, their suggestions may be more helpful than those of professional staff. Nurse practitioners and clinical nurse specialists are generally excellent patient educators but at times patients may prefer other professionals.
11. Refer. Although health care providers are responsible for patient education for all patients, it may be preferable at times to refer patients for special teaching activities. There are four major referral sources: community groups and agencies, such as diabetes teaching centers at university hospitals; national voluntary health organizations (eg, American Lung Association or the American Cancer Society); instructional references, such as books and videotapes; and other patients who can serve as role models and peer advisors.
12. Monitor progress through follow-up contact. Progress can be monitored through telephone calls or office visits. Follow-up should occur frequently so that any problems that arise can be solved, successes can be recognized, and instructions can be reinforced.

Source: Guide to Clinical Preventive Services, 1996; http://hstat.nlm.nih.gov/hq/Hquest/action/GetText/hitno/9/query/counseling+strategies/fws/S/lhit/421/searchid/1048450925467/screen/Browse/db/local.gcps.cps/s/46878

health care for themselves and their children. Which health promotion model would be most useful in your work with families in this clinic?

2. Apply Pender's Health Promotion Model to the Van Damme family. What are the interpersonal influences (eg, family, peers, providers), norms, and support that might influence Mrs. Van Damme to engage in health promotion behavior? What do you think some of the immediate competing demands might be in Mrs. Van Damme's life that would interfere with health-promoting behavior?

3. Using the *Guide to Clinical Preventive Services* and the *Clinician's Handbook of Preventive Services*, establish a teaching plan related to health promotion and disease prevention for the following situation: Ms. Mahoney is a 55-year-old patient of yours in a family practice. Her most recent fecal occult blood test series that she performed at home was reported by the lab as positive for one of the smears. Ms. Mahoney has resisted having a colonoscopy in the past. What is your recommendation to Ms. Mahoney? Using the patient counseling strategies in Box 2.2, describe your plan for health maintenance and disease prevention.

To find the latest information

Key search terms
The Health Belief Model, Health Promotion Model, Precede-Proceed Model, Care-Seeking Behavior Model, Self-Regulation, health promotion, community health, illness prevention

Websites
- National Institutes of Health & National Cancer Institute, Theory at a Glance: A Guide for Health Promotion Practice: cancer. gov/cancerinformation/ theory_at_a_glance
- Health Canada. Population Health: http://www.hc-sc.gc.ca/hppb/pphb-dgspsp

- Nola J. Pender, PhD, RN, FAAN, Professor Emeritus: http://www.nursing.umich.edu/faculty/ pender_nola.html

REFERENCES

Agency for Healthcare Research and Quality (AHRQ). (1998). *Clinician's handbook of preventive services: Put prevention into practice.* Retrieved March 18, 2003, from http://www.ahcpr.gov/clinic/ppiphand.htm

Allison, S. D. (1973). A framework for nursing action in a nurse-conducted diabetic management clinic. *Journal of Nursing Administration, 3*(4), 53–60.

Austin, L. T., Ahmad, F., McNally, M. J., & Stewart, D. E. (2002). Breast and cervical cancer screening in Hispanic women: a literature review using the health belief model. *Women's Health Issues, 12*(3), 122–128.

Backscheider, J. E. (1974). Self-care requirements, self-care capabilities, and nursing systems in the diabetic nurse management clinic. *American Journal of Public Health, 64*(12), 1138–1146.

Dreger, V., & Tremback, T. (2002). Optimize patient health by treating literacy and language barriers. *AORN Journal, 75*(2), 278, 280–273, 285, 287, 289–293, 297–300, 303–304.

Duffy, M. E. (1993). Determinants of health-promoting lifestyles in older persons. *Image— The Journal of Nursing Scholarship, 25*(1), 23–28.

Ehiri, B. I. (2000). Improving compliance among hypertensive patients: A reflection on the role of patient education. *International Journal of Health Promotion Education, 38*(3), 104–108.

Garcia, A. W., Pender, N. J., Antonakos, C. L., & Ronis, D. L. (1998). Changes in physical activity beliefs and behaviors of boys and girls across the transition to junior high school. *Journal of Adolescent Health, 22*(5), 394–402.

Green, L. W. (1999). What can we generalize from research on patient education and clinical health promotion to physician counseling on diet. *European Journal of Clinical Nutrition, 53*(Suppl. 12), S9–18.

Green, L. W., Kreuter, M. W., Deeds, S. G., & Partridge, K. B. (1980). *Health education planning: A diagnostic approach.* Palo Alto, CA: Mayfield Publishing.

Hanson, J. A., & Benedict, J. A. (2002). Use of the Health Belief Model to examine older adults' food-handling behaviors. *Journal of Nutrition Education & Behavior, 34*(Suppl 1), S25–30.

Health Canada. *Healthy living.* Retrieved March 23, 2003, from http://www.hc-sc.gc.ca/english/lifestyles/index.html

Hochbaum, G. M. (1958). Public participation in medical screening programs: A sociopsychological study. (Public Health Service Publication No. 572). Washington, DC: U.S. Government Printing Office.

Janz, N. K., & Becker, M. H. (1984). The health belief model, a decade later. *Health Education Quarterly, 11*, 1–47.

Jayne, R. L., & Rankin, S. H. (2001). Application of Leventhal's Self-Regulation Model to Chinese immigrants with type 2 diabetes. *Journal of Nursing Scholarship, 33*(1), 53–59.

Jonas, S. (2000). *Talking about health and wellness with patients: Integrating health promotion and disease prevention into your practice.* New York: Springer Publishing Company.

Joshi, D. D., Poudal, P. M., Jimba, M., Mishra, P. N., Neave, L. A., & Maharjan, M. (2001). Controlling *Taenia solium* in Nepal using the Precede-Procede model. *Southeast Asian Journal of Tropical Medicine and Public Health, 32*(Suppl 2), 94–97.

Keller, M. L., Ward, S., & Baumann, L. J. (1989). Processes of self-care: Monitoring sensations and symptoms. *Advances in Nursing Science, 12*(1), 54–66.

Koch, J. (2002). The role of exercise in the African-American woman with type 2 diabetes mellitus: Application of the health belief model. *Journal of the American Academy of Nurse Practitioners, 14*(3), 126–129.

Lauver, D. (1992). A theory of care-seeking behavior. *Image—The Journal of Nursing Scholarship, 24*(4), 281–287.

Leventhal, H., Meyer, D., & Nerenz, D. (1980). The common sense representation of illness danger. In S. Rachman (Ed.), *Contributions to medical psychology* (pp. 7–30). New York: Permagon Press.

Marinker, M., & Shaw, J. (2003). Not to be taken as directed: Putting concordance for taking medicines into practice. *BMJ, 326*, 348–349.

Mikhail, B. I., & Petro-Nustas, W. I. (2001). Transcultural adaptation of Champion's Health Belief Model Scales. *Journal of Nursing Scholarship, 33*(2), 159–165.

National Center for Health Statistics. (2001). *Healthy People 2000 final review.* Retrieved March 20, 2003, from http://www.cdc.gov/nchs/products/pubs/pubd/hp2k/review/highlightshp2000.htm

Pender, N. J. (1982). *Health promotion in nursing practice.* East Norwalk, CT: Appleton-Century-Crofts.

Pender, N. J., Murdaugh, C., & Parsons, M. A. (2002). *Health promotion in nursing practice* (4th ed.). Upper Saddle River, NJ: Prentice-Hall Health, Inc.

Sackett, D. L., & Haynes, R. B. (1976). *Compliance with therapeutic regimens.* Baltimore: The Johns Hopkins University Press.

U.S. Department of Health and Human Services. (2000). *Healthy People 2010: Understanding and improving health.* Retrieved July 10, 2004, from http://www.health.gov/healthypeople; http://www.healthypeople.gov/

U.S. Department of Health and Human Services. (2000). *Leading health indicator: Overweight and obesity.* Retrieved March 23, 2003, from http://www.healthypeople.gov/Document/html/uih/uih_bw/uih_4.htm#overandobese

U.S Preventive Services Task Force. *Put prevention into practice (PPIP).* Retrieved March 18, 2003, from http://hstat.nlm.nih.gov/hq/Hquest/db/local.ppip/screen/ColTitle/s/40020

U.S. Preventive Services Task Force. (1996). *Guide to clinical preventive services* (2nd ed.). Retrieved July 11, 2004, from www.ncbi.nlm.nih.gov/books/bv.fcgi?call=bv.view..Show Second & rid=hstat3.chapter.10062.

U.S. Preventive Services Task Force. (2003). *Guide to clinical preventive services* (3rd ed., 2000–2003). Retrieved March 19, 2003, from http://www.ahcpr.gov/clinic/cps3dix.htm

Wallace, L. S. (2002). Osteoporosis prevention in college women: Application of the expanded health belief model. *American Journal of Health Behavior, 26*(3), 163–172.

Integration of Cultural Systems and Beliefs

Barbara Hollinger

LEARNING OBJECTIVES

After reading this chapter, the student should be able to:

1. Apply the Cultural Assessment Framework to better understand the similarities and differences between the mainstream culture and the ethnic or cultural group targeted for patient education.

2. Develop a patient teaching plan for a patient who is a migrant farm worker.

3. Using the Kleinman model as part of the assessment, plan a teaching program for a Native American man with diabetes.

4. Plan a culturally sensitive prenatal teaching plan for a Mexican-American adolescent.

5. Assess the acculturation level of various members of a three-generation Vietnamese family.

6. Create a teaching plan for the parents of a Hmong toddler with otitis media, using a medical interpreter as a cultural broker.

7. Analyze the stressors facing a hypertensive African American grandmother, who is raising her 2-year-old twin grandsons who have asthma, and identify sources of cultural support that might be available to her.

INTRODUCTION

The Hmong Family: A Case of Cross-Cultural Challenges

Anne Fadiman's 1997 book, *The Spirit Catches You and You Fall Down,* recounts the experience of a Hmong family in Merced, California, in the health care system. Lia Lee is 3 months old when she experiences her first seizure. Her American doctors believe she has a disorder caused by damaged cells in the cerebral cortex, transmitting neural impulses simultaneously and chaotically. The Lees believe their daughter's condition is caused by a "spirit catching her and making her fall down." The parents' belief is consistent with their belief that soul-stealing spirits are often the cause of illness. The physicians involved are considered the most caring, compassionate, and well-trained pediatricians in the area.

This case history spans several years and, despite many changes in medication, several hospitalizations, and the removal of the child from parental custody for several months, the child's seizures are never adequately controlled and she suffers irreversible brain damage. Misunderstandings abound throughout the multiple encounters regarding procedures (such as spinal taps and blood tests), the lifetime use of medication for a chronic condition, and the roles and responsibilities of the parents and the physicians.

Ethnic Diversity and the Health Care System

The Lee family's story illustrates the complexity of cross-cultural challenges facing all medical professionals. According to the United States Department of the Census in 2000, 75.1% of the U.S. population was white. In this census, people could report themselves as being members of more than one race. This leaves 24.9% of the population as being, at least partially, non-white (U.S. Census Bureau, 2000). This figure is expected to approach 50% by the year 2050. This ethnically diverse population includes an increasing number of foreign-born persons; currently 1 of 13 persons (or 19 million Americans) is foreign-born.

The foreign-born population is not only ethnically diverse, but also, its attitudes toward its adopted and native countries vary considerably. Some immigrants chose to establish a new life in the United States. Others, such as traumatized refugees fleeing war, ethnic cleansing, or the socioeconomic upheaval after a natural or manmade disaster, may dream of returning to their native country. Some migrant workers have homes and families in their native country and come to the United States to work for a limited time and return home. Even longtime United States residents, whether foreign born or U.S. born, vary tremendously in their level of acculturation. The health professions have begun to acknowledge that the melting pot has become more of an ethnic stew, with each element retaining its own flavor and characteristics.

Because ethnically diverse persons are underrepresented in the health care professions, it can be assumed that other health care providers will increasingly care for persons that are ethnically and culturally different from them. Likewise, culturally diverse health care providers will care for the full spectrum of patient clientele and will also work cross-culturally. Communication patterns are integrated into culture. Each cultural group has codes, symbols, language, and values that are meaningful. It is important to consider culture when providing patient education, because the teaching process can only be successful if there is clear communication between learner and provider (Wilson et al., 2003).

This chapter presents the Cultural Assessment Framework that is useful for understanding factors that affect patient education in the cross-cultural exchange. Although an in-depth understanding of all ethnocultural groups in the United States is not possible, we hope that health care providers will study the characteristics of those cultural groups with whom they regularly interact. In many health care settings, one or two diverse cultural groups form most of the ethnic patient population. All providers are capable of learning a deeper understanding of one or two ethnocultural groups different from their own. Because tremendous diversity exists within each cultural group, any framework is only a blueprint; the details of diversity are clarified during individual patient encounters.

At some time, even culturally prepared health care providers find themselves teaching patients with cultural backgrounds with which they are not familiar. To most effectively assess individual beliefs, Kleinman's model is presented. Having a broader idea of the complexity of issues that influence cross-cultural exchanges can add meaning to the individualized exploration. The clinical relevance of the Cultural Assessment Framework in patient education is presented, along with

some factors the health care provider should consider when working with special populations within a cultural group, such as pediatric patients and older people.

In this chapter, *culture* is defined as the sum total of ways of living by a group of human beings (ie, concepts, habits, beliefs, skills, and art), which is transmitted from one generation to another. An *ethnic group* is a group of people—racially, linguistically, or historically related—having a common and distinctive culture. Again, as much diversity exists within ethnic groups as exists between them. Hispanics, or Latinos, are often stereotyped as one ethnic group; however, Latinos vary between countries and within the same country, despite sharing Hispanic surnames.

THE CULTURAL ASSESSMENT FRAMEWORK

The framework of Huff and Kline (1999) is presented in their book, *Promoting Health in Multicultural Populations*. The framework is designed for use in individual patient encounters and health promotion and disease prevention education activities with small groups or in the community. The Cultural Assessment Framework explores five areas through the following assessment categories as illustrated in Box 3.1.

1. Culture-specific demographic factors
2. Culture-specific epidemiological and environmental factors
3. Cultural characteristics
4. Health care beliefs and practices
5. Western health care organization and service delivery variables

Culture-Specific Demographic Factors

This assessment category evaluates the culture or ethnic group in relation to age, gender, social class or status, education and literacy, language and dialect, religious preferences, occupation and income, patterns of residence,

---

BOX 3.1 Cultural Assessment Framework

Factors Pertaining to the Cultural or Ethnic Group Demographic Factors
- Age profile
- Gender roles
- Social class/Status
- Education/Literacy
- Languages/Dialects
- Religion
- Occupation/Income
- Residence
- Acculturation

Epidemiological and Environmental Factors
- Morbidity rates
- Mortality rates
- Disability rates
- Environmental exposures
- Other environmental risk factors

Group Characteristics
- Cultural/Ethnic
- Cosmology
- Time orientation
- Self-perception
- Community perception
- Social norms, identity values, customs
- Communication patterns

Health Care Beliefs and Practices
- Explanatory models
- Response to illness
- Western health care use
- Health promotion use
- Health behavior practices

Factors Pertaining to the Health Care Provider Western Health Care Organization and Service Delivery Variables
- Cultural competence/Sensitivity
- Organizational policy and mission
- Facilities and program preparation
- Evaluation of culturally competent services

Source: From Huff, R. M., & Kline, M. V. (Eds.) (1999). *Promoting health in multicultural populations: A handbook for practitioners.* Thousand Oaks, CA: Sage Publications. Adapted with permission.

---

living conditions, and acculturation and assimilation. *Acculturation* is the process of cultural change in people, leading them to adopt elements of one or more cultural groups different from their own. The term is commonly used to indicate the degree to which a person has given up traits of his or her native culture in exchange for elements of the dominant culture. *Assimilation* is defined as cultural and group integration into the political, social, and economic mainstream of the dominant culture. Assimilation is an essential factor in evaluating how to present patient education.

Age

Age can affect a given population in terms of demographics or culture. Age may determine who makes decisions in a family. Age is often a factor in terms of acculturation and language acquisition; younger people are associated with more rapid language acquisition and with faster acculturation.

Gender

In cultural groups, gender is often a factor that affects specific role expectations within a family, decision-making, and patient comfort with physical examinations by opposite-gender health care providers.

For example, Latinas who are neither in school nor part of the workforce may be less assimilated or acculturated than Latino children or men (Diaz Jr., 2002). Certain health care situations, like childbirth, are culturally shaped and socially constructed (Ottani, 2002). Cultural competency is especially important for the provision of care that is individualized to the needs of the patient.

Social Class and Status

Each social class has its own world view and driving force, and hidden rules about family structure, money, and possessions (Payne, 2001). It is helpful to know which persons in the ethnic community are held in the highest esteem (eg, clan elders, teachers, or a grandmother). These people often help a patient to make difficult health-related decisions.

The social class and status of an individual is often closely associated with educational level, occupation, and income. English proficiency and greater acculturation are often associated with high educational achievement in the United States. Many professionally trained immigrants experience a decrease in social status and occupation on arrival in this country.

In every group, some people have great influence among their peers. Making a favorable impression with the cultural broker within the community can greatly affect the entire group's acceptance of a health care provider.

Literacy and Education

Literacy and educational levels are important factors in all aspects of patient education. Among immigrants, rural or urban status in their native country or political upheavals may have affected their educational attainment. Throughout the 1980s and early 1990s, the civil war in El Salvador left many rural Salvadorans in war-conflicted zones with no schools. Those who were literate taught their children what they knew, but rural refugees who fled to the United States often have a much lower educational level than their urban counterparts.

Symbols are often designed for teaching low literacy populations; however, they need to be tested to ensure they convey the desired message. A safety study (Grieshop, Stiles, & Domingo, 1995) to determine universal understanding of sketches indicating pain, danger, poison, or death was conducted in California among Mixtec Indian farm workers from Oaxaca, Mexico. The study subjects almost always interpreted the symbols differently from other Mexican farm workers. In Figure 3.1, which was used in this study, *1c* was meant to indicate pain, yet it brought comments, such as "I don't understand what he has on his back." Drawing *8a*, intended to convey "Danger—no entry for 48 hours," was also confusing. Interpretations included, "Maybe it is dangerous to enter when it is too bright or too dark," and "The intense light from the sun can make you blind."

Language

Language is an important assessment tool. The person's command of the English language is often closely related to his or her level of acculturation. A person's reading and writing proficiency in his or her native language may affect how quickly he or she learns English and is closely related to educational level. A language that is spoken throughout a large geographic area (such as Spanish) typically has many local dialects; words can have different meanings, depending on the region. Paying close attention to nonverbal cues can help bilingual health care providers understand when they may have used a word or phrase with several meanings.

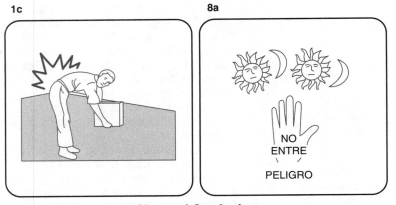

Signs of Confusion

FIGURE 3.1 Pictorial teaching symbols understood differently by Mixtec Indians and Spanish-speaking Mexican American farm workers.

Religious Beliefs

Religious beliefs often affect health care beliefs. Praying for oneself or for others who are experiencing problems is an important spiritual belief. Among the Amish, religion is central to their maintenance of a lifestyle apart from the dominant culture. A recent adolescent study listed church affiliation as a protective factor for youths at high risk. The church has played an integral role in the development and survival of African American communities.

Occupation and Income

Occupation, income, and place of residence are socioeconomic indicators that may place patients at greater risk for accidents, exposures, or health problems. New immigrants and refugees are more likely to be employed in unskilled, low-wage jobs. Many Mexican immigrants are employed as seasonal agricultural workers. Farming is one of the most dangerous occupations in the United States. Over 700 farmers and ranchers die in work-related accidents every year (National Education Center for Agricultural Safety, 2003). Many new immigrants and refugees work as janitors, gardeners, cooks, housekeepers, child-care workers, and home health aides. Low income directly affects residency.

Synthesis: Farm Worker Population

For this chapter, the Cultural Assessment Framework is applied to the U.S. farm worker population. The assessment begins with evaluation of the cultural or ethnic group–specific demographic factors. According to the United States Department of Labor National Agricultural Workers Survey (Mines, Gabbard, & Steirman, 1997), this population is a young population (two-thirds are younger than 35 years of age), male (approximately 80%), and approximately 70% foreign-born. Ninety-four percent of foreign-born farm workers were born in Mexico, with an additional 5% coming from other Latin countries. Their occupation is comprised of various agricultural tasks. Income for a worker averaged from $5,000 to $7,500 in the survey conducted from 1994 to 1995, with median household incomes between $7,500 and $10,000 annually. Although the majority (60%) of male farm workers are married and although 50% of them have children younger than 18 years of age, many live apart from their families while employed as farm workers. The living pattern showed approximately 50% living with a family member and 50% of all farm workers surveyed living with nonrelatives. Many live in shared living arrangements with five or more people per unit. Most households were in poverty.

Although not addressed in the survey, previous studies have indicated these workers typically have a fifth- or sixth-grade education level. Because 20% of the survey population were in their first year of U.S. farm work and had immediate family in Mexico, it can be assumed that acculturation is low. The language preference is Spanish, but among workers from Oaxaca, Mexico, Mixteco may be the first language, with varying degrees of Spanish fluency. The dominant religion is Roman Catholic, but an increasing number of people adopt Pentecostal, Mormon, or Jehovah's Witness denominations.

Patient Education Implications

For the farm worker population, written, verbal, or video materials must be in Spanish (or Mixteco if available) and geared to a fifth- or sixth-grade reading level. Health care providers should reinforce written or symbolic educational materials with verbal explanations and ask for return demonstration of new procedures.

Workers who live in crowded, low-income housing may have inadequate toilet, bathing, refrigeration, and cooking facilities that may further increase health risks. Patient education regarding food preparation for patients with diabetes should assess cooking arrangements and food storage availability. Risk reduction for pesticide exposure requires daily bathing and clothing changes. Health care providers must assess if workers bathe and wash clothes at home, in the river, or in the local irrigation ditch.

Culture-Specific Epidemiological and Environmental Influences

This second category of the Cultural Assessment Framework has two subcategories:

1. Morbidity, mortality, and disability rates
2. Environmental influences

Despite the difficulty in separating health care access and socioeconomic factors, the morbidity, mortality, and disability subcategory recognizes some specific physical, biologic, and physiologic variations in ethnic and racial groups. For example, the U.S. Department of Health and Human Services (2002) reports in 1999 the rates of death from cardiovascular disease were about 30% higher among African American adults than white adults. The prevalence of diabetes in African Americans is 70% higher than that of whites. The prevalence of diabetes in Hispanics is nearly 100% more than that of whites.

Environmental racism refers to the tendency for hazardous waste disposal sites to locate in neighborhoods in which people are poor and less politically able to defend their own interests. Environmental racism often occurs in ethnic neighborhoods, increasing the inhabitants' risks for toxic exposures. Inner city environments may expose residents to increased violence, drug dealing, and alcohol abuse.

Synthesis: Farm Worker Population

The second Cultural Assessment Framework category is also applied to the farm worker population. Among Mexican-American migrant workers, infections and communicable and parasitic diseases continue to be major health risks. Tuberculosis rates are increasing among this population; many people acquire the disease after entering the United States. Hepatitis B, amoebic dysentery, shigella, and intestinal parasites are common. A higher incidence of sexually transmitted diseases (eg, syphilis, gonorrhea, chlamydia, and human immunodeficiency virus [HIV]) exists among these workers than in the general population.

Although this population is young, diabetes is a significant risk. The Mexican-American population experiences five times higher the incidence of diabetes along with an increased risk of diabetes-related complications than the non-Hispanic white population. Chemical dependency, especially alcoholism, is also increased in Mexican Americans.

Environmental influences consist of physical, biological, and chemical agents. Farm workers are exposed to extremes of hot and cold temperatures, dust, wind, vibration, and noise for those working with farm equipment. Biological exposures include insects, snakes, animals (wild and domestic), and toxic plants. Poison oak is one of the most common dermatological complaints among farm workers. Chemical exposures include fertilizers, cleaning or degreasing compounds, and many classes of pesticides. Farm worker families, including children, also suffer environmental exposures.

This population is at risk for some of the communicable and parasitic infections. Family is an important cultural value to this population, and this can be used in patient education to address some of these issues. For workers who travel without family or relatives, ask how often they hear from family members and ask about how they cope with the isolation and separation. This may be a natural opening for discussing safe sex or alcohol use by focusing on being responsible for the family by not bringing home sexually transmitted diseases or by not mixing drinking with driving. If a patient is thought to have a problem with alcoholism, the health care provider might suggest an organization, such as Alcoholics Anonymous, that has Spanish language groups. Some think that the most effective groups for this population are those in which the participants have a similar acculturation level.

The family can also be used when teaching patients about the importance of work safety practices. Many workers dislike wearing cumbersome protective equipment; however, wearing proper equipment might be encouraged by emphasizing to the person how the family depends on the hardworking provider; therefore, he should protect himself for the family's sake.

Patient education regarding child safety must include discussion about the risks of open irrigation canals, the hazards of children riding and playing on tractors and other farm equipment, and the risk of poisoning from chemicals. A coloring book with this information has been developed with bilingual captions and reinforces the message for children. For families that migrate together, older children often help with child care for younger siblings or cousins. Teaching the older children and the parents about safety is another way to prevent accidents.

Cultural Characteristics

The third category of the Cultural Assessment Framework includes general and specific cultural characteristics. These characteristics include how the person or group identifies self, general concepts regarding how natural and supernatural forces interact in the universe, time orientations, communication patterns, social norms, values, and customs. This category also includes the relative priority that the cultural community places on the needs of the person versus the needs of the group.

Among the African American population, age may determine how a person identifies himself or herself. Older people may still use terms, such as Negro or Colored, whereas the 1960s generation may prefer the term Black. African American is the expression more commonly preferred by younger people. African Americans with West Indian heritage may self-identify more with this cultural group.

Views of the Universe

Cultural and ethnic groups view the universe in diverse ways. Some Hmong people believe that those who suffer much in this life may have an easier time in a future life. One woman reported she thought this was her third life and she was blessed with 14 children because of great hardship in her previous life. Some Mixtec Indians believe people have spirit animals to assist them in this world. The animal is determined by leaving an infant at a crossroads while the family watches at some distance. The first bird or animal that approaches the child is believed to be that child's spirit animal.

Time Orientation

Time orientation varies among cultures. Many Latin cultures are oriented in the present. The European-American culture is future-oriented; investing for later security is encouraged. People living in poverty consider the present most important. They make decisions for the moment based on feelings or survival. People in the middle class tend to make decisions based on future ramifications. Wealthy people place value on traditions and history, making decisions at least partially based on tradition and decorum (Payne, 2001)

Perceptions, Social Norms, Values, and Customs

In the European American culture, self-actualization and competition among peers to achieve are common perceptions. In many cultures, community or family goals take precedence over individual desires. Mixtecs have a strong sense of community and even those who have immigrated to California raise funds to support projects that meet the needs of the home community in Mexico.

Social norms, values, and customs describe accepted and expected behavior among a particular group. Practices regarding birth, marriage, pregnancy, and death are described here. Many East Indians residing in the United States have arranged marriages with women from India. Jewish male infants are circumcised on the eighth day after birth, in a religious ceremony. In Peru and many Latin countries, a cross is placed on the road at the site of a fatal accident.

Communication patterns, including verbal and nonverbal expressions, may vary among cultures. Filipino communication strives to maintain a smooth interpersonal relationship and to avoid confrontation. A hospital director in a San Joaquin Valley community in

California had many Filipino employees. An open-door policy was established and the staff was invited to visit him with any concerns or problems that might arise. However, none of the staff members came to the hospital director. When the communication pattern was better understood, employees were encouraged to come together in pairs and each could present the concern of the other; this was a less direct, but more culturally accepted means of communication.

Synthesis: Farm Worker Population

Cultural characteristics can be applied to the seasonal agricultural worker. Mexican-born farm workers, with family living in Mexico, identify strongly with their Mexican heritage. Many have a fatalistic view of the universe, and health is regarded as a result of good luck, reward for good behavior, or a gift from God not to be taken for granted. These families typically take an active role in caring for a family member who is ill. This population has a present-focused time orientation, and its sense of time is relaxed. Newer immigrants from rural areas may not own a clock or may not know how to tell time. The family is generally considered more important than the individual member. Communication is characterized by *personalismo* or asking about the children or family before discussing the business at hand. Greeting people by name and shaking hands on initial meeting builds an atmosphere of trust. Because education levels are low among this population, television and radio are primary sources of information; written materials may be largely pictorial.

Important cultural values include the importance of family, with children being valued. Men and women have established roles; the man is the head of, and is responsible for, the family. The woman cares for the children and is considered the primary purveyor of the culture. Courtesy and respect for adults, elders, teachers, doctors, and authority figures is another important cultural value. Although touching, hugging, and kissing are common forms of expression, this is a modest and private culture in areas of sexuality. Religion is important to most Mexican Americans, and most life events are celebrated with a religious ceremony. An isolated patient who wears a religious symbol might be encouraged to visit a church with a large Spanish-speaking population.

Patient Education Implications

Emphasizing the importance of responsibility for the family and being a good role model can be a useful teaching tactic with Mexican farm worker men. When you are discussing smoking cessation or second-hand smoke, one approach might be to discuss how children are most affected by smoking and the role model this behavior creates if the patient smokes. Respect can be shown by acknowledging the physically demanding nature of farm work and the financial insecurity that comes with poorly paid temporary employment. Coming to the clinic for an appointment usually translates into missing a day of work, so caring for as many issues as possible in one visit and trying to accommodate walk-ins on rainy days when patients cannot work are ways of showing respect for the farm worker patient.

A study of low-income Mexican-American women in rural Oregon showed that virtually all families had radios and many families subscribed to cable television with a Spanish language channel (Thompson, Curry, & Burton, 1998). Local radio and television programs are important venues for disseminating health information. Many communities have only one or two minority language stations, so public interest programming reaches a wider audience than a similar English-language program.

Health Beliefs and Practices

This fourth category encompasses explanatory models of disease and how the culture responds to illness. It also assesses the person's or group's attitude toward Western medicine and preventive medicine. Specific health behavior practices are also examined. Every culture uses some explanatory model for the origins of disease. Beliefs regarding disease causality tend to be consistent with cultural and personal values and behaviors, and social training. Flores, Rabke-Verani, Pine, & Sabharwal (2002) provide charts summarizing conditions, symptoms, and treatments found in a wide variety of cultures. In addition to culture, education and socioeconomic factors influence beliefs.

In some belief systems, disease causality may be linked to an action of a family member, something happening in the community, or to a supernatural agent. For example, one Peruvian family reported their child has Down syndrome because the mother of the child had spoken ill of her mother-in-law during her pregnancy. Health care providers can best individualize care when they understand how the patient and family explain health and illness.

The Hmong View of Illness

The Hmong categorize illness in two ways: illnesses caused by spirits and requiring a spirit healer (a shaman) and illnesses curable by the use of herbs. According to the Hmong, spirit illnesses may be caused by the good shaman spirit, your own body spirits, a spirit from the dead, or an evil spirit. The good spirit of the *txiv neeb* (or shaman) may cause illness by coming to test someone to see if he or she is strong enough to become a shaman. Body spirits could be frightened or stolen away. Illness would result when a few left and death would result when all the spirits left or did not come back. A spirit from the dead could be the spirit of an animal that you mistreated or of a dead person wanting to take you with him or her.

The Hmong's response to illness is consistent with their beliefs. An herbalist would be sought for a nonspirit illness and a shaman for a spirit illness. Because many medicinal herbs available in Laos are not available in the United States, Hmong patients in the study were willing to see Western health care providers for these problems. If a patient saw a medical doctor, did not respond to treatment and became sicker, the family would decide maybe this was a spirit illness. A shaman would be consulted. The shaman would go into a trance state and contact the spirit world, then recommend rituals and ceremonies that would placate, bring back, or pay back the offended spirit. When promoting health with this population, it is important to follow customs, such as observing postpartum practices, since the failure to do so is believed to result in poor health outcomes.

Explanatory Models of Disease: A Peruvian Culture

In the community of Santa Lucia de Pacaraos, Peru, the village's shoe repairman was lame. He used a cane and always carried his right leg at a fixed angle. He believed in and practiced the traditional medicine of this region of Peru and one day recounted how his leg was injured. When he was 9 years old, he went to the reservoir with two friends. They found some dynamite, and began to play with it. The dynamite exploded and the boy suffered a severe case of susto (fright). His fear was so great that his soul left his body. The prescribed treatment required to regain his lost soul consisted of gathering many food items, the national flower cantuta, other herbs, and a horseshoe. A ceremony using these items was to be performed three times: at midnight, 6:00 AM, and 6:00 PM. The man said he became lame because his family only carried out the ritual twice, thus causing his injury to become permanent. He adamantly believed that the susto, not the dynamite, resulted in his injuries.

Hot and Cold Theory

The hot and cold theory is a belief shared by Mexican Americans and some other Latin cultures. According to this theory, health is maintained when the body maintains proper equilibrium—specifically, a balance between hot and cold elements. Each disease entity is categorized as being caused by hot or cold and must be treated with an opposite remedy to achieve equilibrium of the body. Here, hot and cold do not reflect actual temperatures, but rather the symbolic power given to foods, herbs, and medicines. For example, in Peru, rheumatism is a cold ailment and is treated with a stinging nettle heated with a small amount of rum and applied to the inflamed joint. Nettles cause a burning sensation when touched and are heated before application; thus, a hot remedy for a cold ailment. A health care provider can apply this concept by treating a hot fever by drinking cold liquids.

Synthesis: Farm Worker Population

Many Mexican-American farm workers believe illness is caused by the body being out of balance. Cold entering the body may cause an illness and must be treated with a hot element. The definition of which illnesses or treatment remedies are hot or cold varies among regions, but the concept is consistent. Illness may be caused by dislocation of a body part (such as *caida de mollera*, which is a sunken fontanel in infants) or something in the body (such as *empacho*, in which food or saliva gets stuck in the stomach, causing stomach pain, vomiting, or diarrhea).

Also, certain external events perceived to be magical or supernatural, such as an eclipse of the sun, are believed to cause an illness or defect, such as cleft lip or palate. Some believe strong emotional states (such as fright, rage, jealousy, or nervousness) can cause illness.

Treatments generally correspond to the explanatory model of the illness. For example, a sunken fontanel is treated by holding the infant upside down and pressing up on the palate while someone sucks on the fontanel. Illnesses may be prevented through praying, wearing religious medals, or keeping a small altar of religious relics in the home. Many illnesses are first treated at home by the family with herbs, teas, or medications found in the home or purchased.

Patient Education Implications

Ask patients what they believe is the cause of the illness. Perhaps medication could be taken with cold water or a hot herbal tea to balance the perceived cause of illness. Assess if a strong emotion such as rage, fright, or nervousness may be a contributing factor to a mental health problem. Present a mental health worker as a person who can try to help one get his or her life back into balance.

Western Health Care Organization and Service Variables

The fifth and final category of the Cultural Assessment Framework includes the Western health care organization and service variables. This category, which is not included in many assessments, evaluates the cultural competency and sensitivity of the health care provider and the organization that provides services.

Campinha-Bacote and Purnell have established four stages of cultural competency (Figure 3.2): (1) unconscious incompetence; (2) conscious incompetence; (3) conscious competence; and (4) unconscious competence. Health care providers should identify their placement on the continuum and strive toward unconscious competence. Even the most culturally competent provider will experience difficulty providing optimal care if his or her employer has little interest in promoting these services. One should know if the service organization (such as hospital, long-term care facility, or office-based primary care practice) has a policy or mission statement that includes providing culturally competent care. The pictures or décor of a waiting area can be tailored to present a comfortable atmosphere to a multiethnic population. Many clinics and hospitals provide regularly scheduled in-service educational programs to promote cultural training. Some clinics sponsor outreach programs to specific ethnic enclaves and use public service radio and television spots to promote healthy and safe lifestyles.

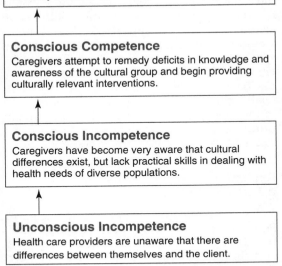

Unconscious Competence
Health care providers are able to automatically provide culturally sensitive care to clients of diverse populations.

Conscious Competence
Caregivers attempt to remedy deficits in knowledge and awareness of the cultural group and begin providing culturally relevant interventions.

Conscious Incompetence
Caregivers have become very aware that cultural differences exist, but lack practical skills in dealing with health needs of diverse populations.

Unconscious Incompetence
Health care providers are unaware that there are differences between themselves and the client.

FIGURE 3.2 Stages of cultural competency.

Ideally, a service organization also should have an ongoing evaluation process to measure progress in meeting cultural competency goals. Evaluation should include assessment of management, staff, the facility, and ongoing feedback from the target group.

Synthesis: Farm Worker Population

The fifth category deals with the U.S. health care system's response to the farm worker cultural group. Clinics that target this population should have bilingual signs and educational materials, bilingual and bicultural staff, and professionally trained interpreters, if possible. Culturally-appropriate art and posters can provide a welcoming atmosphere.

Because this culture prizes children, a child-friendly waiting area with toys and Spanish or bilingual books presents a family-friendly environment. Some clinics insist that only children with appointments should come with a parent to the clinic, but child care for siblings without appointments can be expensive and difficult to find. Although it may be chaotic to have the whole family present for a visit, it also can be an opportunity to observe family functioning. Often, evaluating family interactions reveals opportunities for patient education, such as safety guidance, appropriate discipline, or parenting skills. The agency can be instrumental in setting the climate for clinicians to achieve culturally competent care. Clinics can sponsor outreach programs, such as diabetes classes to a migrant camp, or participation in cultural fairs. Health care workers and service agencies can learn to effectively use public service announcements on public radio and television.

THE KLEINMAN MODEL

General Considerations

When a health care provider has regular contact with a cultural or ethnic group that is unfamiliar, an in-depth study of the culture is ideal. However, due to time constraints, or an unanticipated encounter with a member of a new-to-you cultural group, a briefer model is often necessary.

Application of the Kleinman model is the most direct way to ensure appropriate individualization of care when a health care provider is faced with a patient and family from an unfamiliar culture. Even when familiar with a population, the health care provider needs to assess the specific cultural beliefs of the individual patient. Through time, experience, and cultural blending, a patient could be anywhere on the continuum of acculturation.

Arthur Kleinman, a psychiatrist and anthropologist, makes a distinction between illness and disease: *Illness* is the uniquely personal experience that a sick person has of what is happening to him or her. *Disease* is the health care professional's biomedical understanding of the same problem. Thus, people with the same medical diagnosis may experience illness in distinct ways.

Kleinman has developed eight questions to reveal a patient's illness perspective (Box 3.2) (Kleinman, Eisenberg, & Good, 1978). The first question—*What do you think has caused your problem?*—may be very helpful in revealing differences between professional and lay explanations. A frustrated clinician, baffled by a confusing clinical presentation, finally asked this question of her patient and was told: "In my country they call this Malta Fever" (brucellosis). Patients may be more familiar than the clinician with infectious or tropical diseases common in their country. Typically, the Kleinman questions clarify the patient's explanatory health model and ideas of how this condition would be treated in the patient's culture. By asking the patient and the family these questions in the assessment, the health care provider can learn how to present information in a way the learner can understand and accept (George, 2001).

To best individualize teaching, it is important to use Kleinman's questions to

---

BOX 3.2 Kleinman's Questions

The Kleinman model can be used to assess a patient's own perspective of his or her illness.

1. What do you call the problem?
2. What do you think has caused the problem?
3. Why do you think it started as it did?
4. What do you think the sickness does? How does it work?
5. How severe is the sickness? Will it have a short or a long course?
6. What kind of treatment do you think you should receive? What are the most important results you hope to receive from the treatment?
7. What are the chief problems the sickness has caused?
8. What do you fear most about the sickness?

assess the degree of acculturation. For example, Acevedo (2000) identified the need to consider acculturation in the development of preventive interventions in order to appropriately target the specific needs of different subpopulations of Mexican Americans. Comparing a range of low-income Mexican-American and European-American women, she found ethnic differences in cigarette smoking and parenting beliefs during pregnancy were concentrated on the less acculturated, low-income, and primarily unmarried Spanish-speaking Mexican-American women. Acculturation was differently related to cigarette smoking and parenting beliefs.

Domains of Influence

Kleinman made another important contribution by recognizing the various domains of influence on a person's beliefs and actions regarding disease and illness. These domains comprise professional, popular, and complementary/alternative areas of influence. The professional domain is the one in which the health care professional operates. The popular domain includes the immediate and extended family and the community. The complementary/alternative domain may include *curanderos,* a Chinese herbalist, a shaman or medicine man, or a wise elder believed to have healing powers. To some patients, traditional healers are often much more appealing than professional health care providers. They usually are unhurried and make home visits. They know the patient, the family, and understand the culture and language. They offer free or low-cost services, and do not perform invasive physical examinations. They typically do not perform blood or other laboratory tests. They can offer a definite diagnosis without waiting for test results. The health care provider should ask about the patient's use of services in the popular and complementary/alternative domains. The health care provider may find opportunities to work with these other healers.

CULTURAL RELEVANCE

General Principles for Designing and Implementing Culturally Competent Care

Recognizing the need, the American Academy of Nursing (AAN) convened an Expert Panel on Culturally Competent Nursing Care to present a set of recommendations to the AAN for consideration, adoption, and action (Box 3.3). The consequences of implementing the recommendations are far-reaching, increasing the knowledge base for providing culturally competent care and widening institutional support at all levels for this increasingly important area. As a result of these recommendations, the need for culturally competent patient education will be routinely considered. With the expanded and available knowledge base, providers can better furnish patient education in an informed, skilled, and culturally sensitive way.

Glenn-Vega (2002) offers ten tips for improving relationships with culturally diverse patient populations:

1. Recruit and hire minority physicians and staff.
2. Provide interpretation and translation services.
3. Choose patient education materials carefully.
4. Offer accessible hours.
5. Do your cultural research.
6. Participate in cultural diversity training.
7. Recognize special events and observances.
8. Use good communication skills.
9. Take advantage of resources for minority health initiatives.
10. Remember what we have in common.

Research shows that effective patient and family education programs can be designed when cultural groups are directly involved in planning them. Programs work best when the community identifies its most urgent priorities, preferences, strengths, and resources. Focus

---

BOX 3.3 Overview of the Recommendations of the American Academy of Nursing Expert Panel for Culturally Competent Care*

The Academy explicitly commits to high quality, culturally competent care that is equitable and accessible.

The Academy will foster research, develop, and maintain expertise and a knowledge base that will:

- examine theories, frameworks, and methods
- be interdisciplinary
- reflect heterogeneous health care practices
- identify effective health care delivery models
- identify how organizations are supportive and successful in fostering increased expertise in this area
- identify how organizations attract and retain minority, stigmatized, and disenfranchised students, faculty, and clinicians.

The Academy will promote changes in the U.S. health care system, reflecting effective delivery models.

The Academy will collaborate with other organizations in establishing ways to teach health care professionals to provide culturally competent care.

The Academy will collaborate with racial/ethnic nursing organizations to develop models of recruitment, education, and retention of health care providers from racial/ethnic minority groups.

In collaboration with other organizations, the Academy will develop a document fostering the inclusion of diversity content in curricula, continuing education, state board examinations, etc.

---

*Culturally competent care pertains to that of racial, ethnic, stigmatized, or disenfranchised populations.

---

groups have been used to effectively design educational videotapes for African Americans (Primm et al, 2002) and culturally diverse HIV-positive women (Murdaugh, Russell, & Sowell, 2000), to develop multicultural cancer pain education materials (Lasch et al., 2000), and to customize care for Chinese and Vietnamese immigrants (Ngo-Metzger et al., 2003).

Cultural Brokering

Sometimes it is helpful to use a middleman to connect diverse subcultures, a process called cultural brokering. In relation to health care, brokering is between the patient and the Western health care system. This broker may be needed even if the health care provider speaks the native language of the speaker. Someone perceived as outside the system may do best in this role, such as a skilled medical interpreter. Cultural brokers might also be other members of the culture, such as a health professional, community spokesperson, or respected elder.

Health care providers should also consider forming trusting relationships with cultural insiders who may fill the role of a cultural guide. Even informed, culturally competent health care providers have experiences in which they sense something went wrong with a particular patient encounter. Recounting the situation to a cultural broker can provide insights that are helpful for future encounters.

Patient Negotiation

Patient negotiation is helpful when a health care provider reaches an impasse with the patient about some aspect of patient education. The first step is to listen to the patient's perception of the issues, using Kleinman's eight questions. After clearly identifying the areas of conflict, select areas that are non-negotiable to have the desired patient outcome. Then the health care provider should present the information from the Western medical perspective, in the learner's context. Patients often will go to extraordinary lengths to please the provider if they sense negotiation is coming from a sense of mutual respect. The following example that occurred in an Andean community in Peru illustrates this concept:

A 2-year-old girl sustained second degree burns over most of her right foot. The physician and nurse visited the family, who lived in a sturdy adobe home with a dirt floor. The burn was dressed with a Silvadene ointment and bandaged. The next day, the clinicians saw that the child's bandage had been removed and the wound left open to the air. The clinicians reapplied the ointment and bandage and explained their concern about infection and the need to keep the wound clean.

The clinicians came back on the third day and found the bandage off again. Eventually, a better understanding of the mother's concerns led to compromises. From the mother's perspective, health would be restored when a proper balance between hot and cold elements was accomplished. Burns are caused by heat. The ointment was felt to be cool. However, the bandage kept heat in, adding to heat a heat condition, further disrupting the delicate balance. The mother was happy to use the cream and, despite a busy schedule, chose to carry her daughter everywhere for the time needed to heal, but without the bandage. The foot healed well. In this case, it was important to identify the patient's con-

cept of what caused the condition and how the therapeutic agents were viewed, to negotiate a balance for healing.

Health care providers should look for opportunities to encourage patients to identify their own health care problems and assist with solutions that use the strengths and resources within the community. By using principles of cultural brokering and negotiating compromises with patients, health care providers can work with diverse patients with respectful open communication.

Acculturation and Assimilation

Acculturation is an important consideration factor when planning patient education. Planning postoperative teaching for a third-generation Japanese American would be different from teaching the same content to a recent Cambodian immigrant. Researchers have described various levels of acculturation. The least acculturated immigrants maintain most of their traditional language and belief systems. The most acculturated immigrants have adopted English, forgotten their native language, and accepted the values and belief system of the dominant culture. A bicultural person can operate comfortably in both the traditional and dominant cultural settings. In another, marginal level, the person seems to lack any real contact with norms and values from either culture.

Many factors affect acculturation. Among immigrants, the reason for leaving the native country and the attitude toward the departure is a factor. Immigrants making a considered choice to enter the United States in hopes of improved economic opportunities or a better future for their children will generally acculturate willingly. Persons fleeing natural disasters or war zones may suffer from post-traumatic stress disorder. Some have been tortured. Many hope to return to the country of origin when the crises resolve. Dealing with personal trauma may be a barrier to acculturation. Some persons enter the country to work for a limited period and do not intend to reside permanently. Farm workers with material and family ties in Mexico do not perceive the need to acculturate.

Country of birth and age on entry into the United States affect a person's level of acculturation. Those immigrating at a young age and obtaining some education in American schools usually acquire language and social skills more rapidly than their seniors. Each succeeding generation is usually more acculturated than the one before it.

Language acquisition is often viewed as the dominant factor in acculturation, and many variables have an impact on language skills. People who join family members or settle into ethnic enclaves have an immediate support group on arrival. Old-timers can significantly buffer the initial culture shock for newcomers. Many newcomers attend English as a Second Language (ESL) classes, but if the newcomer's social group consists primarily of the cultural group, little opportunity exists to practice English outside of the classroom. Women who work within the home or immigrants who work with family or relatives may not need to use English to function day-to-day. Even if spoken English is learned, reading and writing skills often lag far behind. One argument for bilingual ballots was based on the difficulties new citizens have in deciphering complex English on the ballots, and in exercising the right to vote.

Ethnic pride is also a factor in acculturation. Native Americans were here long before European Americans and see no reason to adopt some of the cultural values of the dominant society that are disrespectful of maintaining harmony with nature. Some groups have been more successful in encouraging a bicultural accommodation. Acculturation need not be a specific goal for patients, but in planning patient education, the health care provider must understand where on the acculturation scale the patient resides.

Patient Education for Families with Children

Many cross-cultural health care encounters involve young immigrant children or refugee families. Pediatric medical problems are common and often can be avoided.

Most areas of the world use the metric rather than the English scale for measuring liquids and body temperature. Patients are often unfamiliar with pounds, teaspoons, and Fahrenheit measurements. Many families do not own measuring spoons or cups because they prepare recipes by adding a handful of or a pinch of an ingredient. Asking a parent to give a teaspoon of medication to a small child may be interpreted to mean a baby-sized spoon of medication. It is safer to always supply a syringe or measuring cup and indicate the exact amount to be given with each dose.

Many pediatric medications come in liquid form and require refrigeration. Homeless and farm worker families may not own or have access to refrigerators. Some antibiotics must be kept cold and some, such as Septra, are stable even in hot conditions (Box 3.4).

Skin assessment of dark-skinned children can be confusing for clinicians without prior experience. Mongolian spots (dark-bluish areas over the lower back and buttocks) are normal and are present in most Asian, Hispanic, and African American infants. Rashes in African American children must be palpated for heat, edema, tightness, or induration. Jaundice is best noted in the sclera of the eyes or palms and soles of the hands and feet.

Common Vietnamese health care practices leave bruises on the skin and should not be mistaken for child abuse. With coining, hot oil is spread over the back, chest, or shoulders and then rubbed with a coin, leaving ecchymotic stripes. Another practice, cupping, involves heating small cups and placing the open side on the skin. As it cools, suction is created that contracts the skin, leaving bruises. Both practices are used to balance the hot or cold element believed to have caused the illness.

Breast-feeding may be abandoned after arriving in the United States. Some Asian mothers see formula as a way to ensure babies will grow to be physically larger, and more like American males. Previous experiences in

---

BOX 3.4 Some Common Pediatric Antibiotics and Refrigeration Requirements

Septra
Stable up to 1 month without refrigeration

Amoxicillin
Stable 14 days without refrigeration

Ceclor
Stable 4 days without refrigeration

Pediazole
Stable up to 14 days with refrigeration

Ampicillin
Requires refrigeration

Augmentin
Requires refrigeration

Cambodia or Vietnam may lead parents to view infant fatness as an important health criterion, since they have seen that fat babies are more likely to survive (Riordan & Gill-Hople, 2001).

Young children may work in fields or factories in the United States. This is especially true of farm worker children who may work alongside their parents in the fields, because they cannot afford a caretaker at home and because the parents' low wages can be augmented by the children's efforts. Children may be exposed to pesticide residue or drift, or pesticide-contaminated water. Migrant housing is often located adjacent to the fields, so exposures may continue day and night.

Patient Education for Families with Adolescents

Among immigrant and refugee families, adolescence is often a time of intergenerational conflict. As teenagers strive to fit in with their peers in the United States, they may question the values of their country of origin. Young people usually acculturate faster than the older generation, which may disrupt the family roles. Conflicts may revolve around acceptable dating behavior or early marriage expectations. Some young Hmong women have marriages arranged at an early age.

Adolescents may balance school with working expectations. Families may have different expectations for daughters and sons. It is especially important to do a HEADSS assessment, which means assess for information about **H**ome, **E**ducation, **A**lcohol and other drugs, **D**epression, **S**ex, and **S**uicide. These teenagers are often overwhelmed young people.

Patient Education for Women

The time devoted to patient education of women affects both the female patient and the entire family. In many cultures, women are considered the chief source of cultural knowledge and the primary teacher of that culture to the next generation. Women can be a great source of cultural information, if asked respectfully.

In many cultures, the wife, mother, or grandmother is the primary caretaker when a family member becomes ill, and therefore must be included in health care instructions. Usually women prepare food throughout the world, and this role often continues after immigration. Always include the women of the family when teaching about nutrition or special diets.

In planning patient education for a woman, consider the woman's role within her culture. An 80-year-old great-grandmother esteemed for her wisdom and family stories may come to appointments accompanied by extended family with whom she lives. She is in a different situation than an elder living in an extended care facility with infrequent family encounters, despite her children living nearby.

Understanding the role of the woman in her ethnic community can highlight important patient education areas. In some cultures, early marriage is expected, and a 20-year-old who is not pregnant after five years of marriage may cause great concern for her family. Other immigrant families encourage young women to postpone childbearing, so they can focus on their education and learn skills.

Pregnancy, Birth, and the Postpartum Period

Beliefs regarding pregnancy, birth, and the expected behavior during the postpartum period vary among cultures and ethnic groups. It is important to understand beliefs about food cravings, appropriate weight gain, the postpartum diet, and when to resume sexual activity when teaching childbearing patients. For example, for one month after giving birth Hmong women avoid anything cold, avoid hard work, and eat a limited diet, primarily of chicken and rice. All food and liquids must be hot or warm, and no cold water should be used for bathing. These diet and bathing practices can be accommodated in the hospital, and beliefs about work should be kept in mind when teaching about resumption of activities.

Family Planning

Family planning is another area in which cross-cultural sensitivity is especially important. Some minority groups view limiting family size as an attempt to limit the size of their particular population. Refugee populations, who have lost large numbers of their populace to war, may feel a need to replace those killed in the war. Persons migrating from countries with a large infant mortality rate may expect to have larger families to ensure the survival of a few healthy children. One possible approach is to promote the health of the mother and infant by emphasizing family spacing, rather than family planning. For recent immigrant groups that are striving to improve their economic status in the United States, the cost of raising and educating children in this country may be an incentive for spacing births.

Cultural factors also may play an important role in the choice of a family planning method. For example, some groups think it improper to touch one's genitals, and methods that require insertion, such as the diaphragm, are less acceptable than methods like oral contraceptives or Depo-Provera injections.

Cancer Screening

Minority women and women with low-income levels are significantly less likely to practice appropriate mammography and Pap test screening. Southeast Asian women have higher invasive cervical cancer incidence rates and lower Pap testing frequencies than most other ethnic groups in the US. Factors related to higher mortality among Latinas are most certainly due to the underutilization of Pap smear screening in this population. Only 38% of Hispanic women aged 40 and older have regular screening mammograms, a simple procedure that can detect breast cancer at its earliest stage, before clinical symptoms develop. Only 25% of Filipino and 38% of Korean women receive adequate and timely colorectal cancer screening. When colon and rectal cancer among African Americans is detected at a localized stage, the survival rate is 84%; however, only one-third of their cancers are detected at this stage (Intercultural Cancer Council, 2003).

One way to reach these populations, as described in *Patient Education Management* (Better cancer education..., 2002), is to conduct focus groups with the target population to assess how best to connect the message to the learner's reality. For example, a focus group of African Americans emphasized the importance of religion, prayer, and spirituality. Since pastors were very respected in the community, researchers created a video showing a pastor at a church delivering the cancer prevention message.

Domestic Violence

Domestic violence is an area of concern across every ethnic and socioeconomic group. Among many immigrant groups, additional issues include fear of authorities for undocumented women, inability to speak English, and the vulnerability and isolation that occurs due to the women's family and support group being located in her country of origin. Shelters for battered women may be seen as places that help women leave their husbands and break up the family rather than as centers that help victimized women.

Health care providers must educate patients that no person deserves to be mistreated by a domestic partner. However, each culture perceives women's rights differently, and it is often helpful to learn how women of the culture in question address this issue. Women are more likely to follow the examples of other women they identify with, who overcame the same cultural barriers. One such group is called *Lideres Campesinas,* Women Farm Worker Leaders. This group has programs regarding domestic violence and sexual assault, HIV, acquired immune deficiency syndrome (AIDS), a pesticides and work sanitation program, and an economic development program. Fifteen groups currently provide education, often through humorous skits within the community and support groups for women. Many of these groups may have culturally specific videos or literature that health care providers can use to teach diverse patient populations.

Patient Education for Senior Citizens

Patient education with older adults from different cultural groups carries rewards and challenges. Younger nurses caring for post–World War II immigrants may have the opportunity to hear first-person accounts of how the war both disrupted and mobilized people from throughout the world. The perspectives of Japanese interned in the United States will differ from personal histories of Eastern European Jews who fled Nazi Germany, or Filipinos who supported the United States effort and are still waiting to be recognized and compensated for their contributions. Newer immigrants are often less fluent in English, have suffered a tremendous disruption in their role within the ethnic community, and may or may not have legal status in the United States.

Assessment

Planning patient education for seniors involves several factors. First, the health care provider must determine the person's length of stay in the new country, legal status, and general level of acculturation. A patient's legal status can have a significant impact on his or her willingness to venture outside of an ethnic enclave or to participate in any program or intervention that might make him or her more visible to immigration officials. It is also important to assess the older man or woman's role in the culture or country of origin and how this role may have changed since immigrating. Respect for elders is an important cultural value in many cultures and one that is often disrupted because seniors must rely on children or even grandchildren to translate, assist with transportation, and make sense of the new culture.

Health care providers must also evaluate the losses the older adult has experienced. All seniors should be assessed for depression, especially those who have lost family, suffered physical injury, and lost prestigious employment, status, and country of origin. Inability to sleep or problems with recurrent nightmares may be clues to underlying depression. The ability to absorb the health education needed for coping with a current health condition may be compromised if mental health issues are not dealt with first.

Also, one must evaluate the health care role the older adult plays in the family. In many cultures, grandmothers are the primary care providers in the extended family when someone is ill or has just given birth. It is important to know if health beliefs, medicines, or herbs are being used and if they support or interfere with the desired treatment the health care provider wishes to propose. Trying to understand the grandmother's perspective and including her in patient teaching can result in a more harmonious and cooperative relationship.

Death and Dying

Practices around death and dying are often culturally defined. Some ethnic groups believe that a seriously ill person must always have hope and should never be told the status of a terminal illness. The Hmong believe that if a person is told he or she is dying, the medical person essentially condemns him or her to death by encouraging the spirit that takes one's soul away to come closer. According to Fadiman (1997), it would be a great insult for a Hmong to say to one's aged grandparent, "After you are dead," but would express one's death by, "when your children are 120 years old." In some cultures, assessing a patient's feelings about heroic measures can be done by presenting a third-person scenario such as, "What would you want done for an ill person who had a medical condition that the doctors had no more treatments that could make the person better?" When issues arise about what to tell the patient regarding a long-term prognosis for a chronic or terminal condition, it is best to discuss with the family what they want shared, and who should be the person to share that information.

Parenting Grandchildren

Many older adults parent grandchildren or great-grandchildren when the children's own parents cannot provide care. This issue is common in many minorities, especially African American communities. Among immigrant families, the extended family lives in the same household, and seniors provide child care while the parents work or attend school. Because many senior citizens have chronic health conditions, health care providers must assess what psychosocial stressors they may have that may affect their health condition.

Intergenerational parenting often keeps an at-risk family intact in a stable and caring environment. Unfortunately, the older caregiver may be placed in a precarious financial situation at a time when he or she faces a fixed income after retirement. Often, informal kinship placement families are not eligible for the same financial aid as are foster care families. Because the most common reason for out-of-home placement for grandchildren is parental abuse or neglect, secondary to substance abuse, children often exhibit special emotional needs and problems at the time of removal from parental custody. Some parenting seniors feel cut off from peers because they lack the time to participate in social activities that might alleviate some of their stress. Health care providers working with these families can help the grandparents identify resources that might provide support, enabling them to better meet the needs of the children, and improve their health.

Sometimes respite services can be arranged through ethnic social or religious organizations. Many communities now have support groups available for senior citizens. One source for locating grandparent services can be found through the American Association of Retired Persons (AARP), which has a Grandparent Information Center. Their website is http://www.aarp.org, e-mail: gic@aarp.org, address: AARP Grandparent Information Center, 601 E Street, NW, Washington, DC 20049, Telephone: 202-434-2296, and Fax: 202-434-6470.

Working with Interpreters

In many situations, health care providers and other health care professionals do not speak the language of the patient. In these cases, the provider will need to use the services of an interpreter. An interpreter is a person fluent in two or more languages, who has been professionally trained to translate oral or written communication. In many clinics and hospitals, untrained staff, family members, or only partially bilingual persons are asked to interpret complex medical procedures, obtain informed consents, or explain culturally sensitive emotional information. Although professional interpreters are not always available, they should be used whenever possible.

When less-prepared translators are used, look for nonverbal cues from the patient or request a return demonstration to be sure the correct message has been conveyed. When health care providers are asked to interpret, it means they will not perform their other responsibilities during this time. This can lead to resentment from coworkers, who must pick up additional work, or disgruntled patients who must wait longer for services. Many agencies do not list interpreting as part of the job description and do not compensate workers for these skills. Many bilingual persons competent to interpret ordinary conversation may be concerned with liability issues when asked to translate informed consent documents or complex medical procedures. Health care providers also should be aware that in small communities or small ethnic enclaves, confidentiality might be an issue.

Family members often are asked to serve as translators in medical settings. Because children often learn English more rapidly than their elders, they often are placed in this role. This scenario can cause many problems. In many parts of the world, authority rests with the senior members of the family. In much of rural culture, men have authority over women, and younger Hispanic adults defer to older adults. Having children serve as interpreters places them in a position of control and disrupts the social order. Children are sometimes requested to translate emotional information inappropriate for their age. Women are often reluctant to discuss concerns regarding gynecologic or family planning issues when children (especially sons) are translators. Even when a professional interpreter is used, some patients will hesitate to divulge information regarding sexual or other sensitive issues to an interpreter of the opposite sex. Other issues may arise when more acculturated adults translate for parents. Sometimes they feel reluctant to directly translate information regarding traditional health beliefs or practices, thinking the Western health care provider might react negatively to such information.

Language barriers can arise even when proper translation has occurred, because patients may understand instructions more literally then intended. Although this can occur in English-to-English exchanges, it seems to be more common in cross-cultural situations. A call from a Hispanic patient to the Firebaugh Health Center, a clinic in the Central San Joaquin Valley of California, illustrates this concept. The patient had been taking her antibiotic for 3 days and was so hungry she didn't feel she could complete a full 7 days of medication on an empty stomach. She had taken only liquids since beginning the medication; this type of compliance could have serious medical complications for some patients.

Optimizing the Use of an Interpreter

There are several ways to optimize a patient encounter that includes a medical interpreter. Before seeing the patient, have a preconference with the translator. After reviewing the chart and deciding on the goals of the patient encounter, share the goals and any particular concerns you might have with the interpreter. If you are teaching about diabetes, the interpreter may serve as a cultural broker. Perhaps some cultural-belief information regarding this disease can be shared before the interview. The health care provider should face and interact directly with the patient rather than with the interpreter. This places the clinician in a better position to observe any nonverbal communication with the patient. Use short, clear sentences and pause after two to three sentences to allow for translation. The interpreter is more likely to leave out information if too much material is covered between phrases. Always try to allow time for the patient to ask you questions. When teaching a new procedure, such as insulin administration, allow time for a return demonstration. Having the patient recount what he or she understood of the discussion can help clear up any misunderstandings. Finally, to maintain an amicable working relationship with the medical interpreter, respect his or her time. Interpreters often are needed in many areas at once. Jotting down notes to make sure that all pertinent information is covered is much more efficient than having to recall the interpreter later for an essential item overlooked.

SUMMARY

Health care providers often are presented with cross-cultural patient education situations. The health care provider who works on an ongoing basis with a particular ethnic population is encouraged to acquire an indepth understanding of that cultural group by exploring the five levels of the Cultural Assessment Framework. During patient education encounters, factors such as specific demographic data, specific risk factors, and the groups' world view and health care beliefs can be incorporated into the teaching and teaching methodology. For each cross-cultural patient encounter, the Kleinman model provides essential information for individualization of teaching.

Culturally competent care is an essential element of patient care. Cultural brokering and patient-provider negotiation are important elements of culturally competent patient care. The levels of acculturation and assimilation of individuals and families also are major factors to consider in planning patient education.

This chapter introduced some of the challenges health care providers face when trying to understand the unique point of view of the patient, and how to go about negotiating a common ground. The next chapter will address the educational theories for teaching and motivating patients.

STRATEGIES FOR CRITICAL ANALYSIS AND APPLICATION

1. Interview a farm worker family. Determine who in the family works and what types of work each member does. Gather information about sanitation in the fields; determine any work-related, chronic or acute health problems that exist, and problems the family has in getting health care. Determine culturally specific illnesses and learn who provides health care for the family (professional, popular, or folk). Plan an educational program designed to reduce the family's risk for injury, pesticide exposure, and overuse syndrome based on the information gathered.

2. Spend an evening watching a commercial non-English television station. Make a list of the commercial products advertised and for what ages they are targeted. Evaluate food or health products listed for health benefit or deficit, such as fat, salt, or sugar content for food, and toy safety. How might this information aid you in patient education for this population?

3. Read about the principles of yin and yang and plan a diabetes teaching plan for Mr. Chin, a 65-year-old immigrant from China. Base the teaching plan on the concepts of balance between the yin and yang elements.

4. Read the first four chapters of *The Spirit Catches You and You Fall Down*. Imagine you are a nurse caring for Lia, the patient in the book. How could you teach this family to give Lia her medication for the seizure disorder consistently?

To find the latest information

Key search terms

culture, culturally competent, culturally sensitive, translated materials, interpreters, outreach, community involvement

Websites

- Diversity Rx:
  http://www.diversityrx.org/HTML/MAP.htm
- Ethnomed: http://ethnomed.org/
- National Center for Cultural Competence:
  http://gucchd.georgetown.edu/nccc
- ANA on Cultural Diversity in Nursing Practice: http://www.nursingworld.org/readroom/position/ethics/etcldv.htm
- Culture Clues Tip Sheets: http://depts.washington.edu/pfes/cultureclues.html
- Culture, Health and Literacy Materials:
  http://www.worlded.org/us/health/docs/culture/matl_websites.html
- Racial and ethnic differences in the health of older Americans:
  http://www.nap.edu/books/0309054893/html/index.html

REFERENCES

Acevedo, M. C. (2000). The role of acculturation in explaining ethnic differences in the prenatal health-risk behaviors, mental health, and parenting beliefs of Mexican American and European American at-risk women. *Child Abuse & Neglect, 24*(1), 111–127.

Better cancer education through focused research: Design focus groups to determine point of view. (2002). *Patient Education Management, 9*(10), 117–118.

Diaz, V. A., Jr. (2002). Cultural factors in preventive care. *Primary Care, 29*(3).

Fadiman, A. (1997). *The sprit catches you and you fall down: A Hmong child, her American doctors, and the collision of two cultures.* New York: Noonday Press.

Flores, G., Rabke-Verani, J., Pine, W., & Sabharwal, A. (2002). The importance of cultural and linguistic issues in the emergency care of children. *Pediatric Emergency Care, 18*(4), 271–284.

George, M. (2001). The challenge of culturally competent health care: Applications for asthma. *Heart and Lung: The Journal of Acute and Critical Care, 30*(5), 392–400.

Glenn-Vega, A. (2002). Achieving a more minority-friendly practice. *Family Practice Management,* (June), 39–43.

Grieshop, J. I., Stiles, M. C., & Domingo, I. V. (1995). Drawing from experience: Mexican-origin workers' evaluation of farm safety illustrations. *Journal of Agricultural Safety and Health, 1*(2), 117–133.

Huff, R. M., & Kline, M. V. (Eds.) (1999). *Promoting health in multicultural populations: A handbook for practitioners.* Thousand Oaks, CA: Sage Publications.

Intercultural Cancer Council. (2003). *Cancer fact sheets.* Retrieved April 16, 2003, from http://iccnetwork.org/cancerfacts/

Kleinman, A., Eisenberg, L., & Good, B. (1978). Culture, illness, and care: Clinical lessons from anthropologic and cross-cultural research. *Annals of Internal Medicine, 88*(2), 251–258.

Lasch, K. E., Wiles, G., Montuori, L. M., Chew, P., Leonard, C., & Hilton, S. (2000). Using focus group methods to develop multicultural cancer pain education materials. *Pain Management Nursing, 1*(4), 129–138.

Mines, R., Gabbard, S., & Steirman, A. (1997). *A profile of US farm workers: Based on data from the National Agricultural Workers survey.* Retrieved July 11, 2004, from http://www.dol.gov/asp/programs/agworker/report/main.htm

Murdaugh, C., Russell, R. B., & Sowell, R. (2000). Using focus groups to develop a culturally sensitive videotape intervention for HIV-positive women. *Journal of Advanced Nursing, 32*(6), 1507–1513.

National Education Center for Agricultural Safety (NECAS). (2003). *The plain facts about the agricultural industry.* Retrieved April 9, 2003, from http://www.nsc.org/necas/agindus.htm

Ngo-Metzger, Q., Massagli, M. P., Clarridge, B. R., Manocchia, M., Davis, R. B., Lezzoni, L. I., et al. (2003). Linguistic and cultural barriers to care. *Journal of General Internal Medicine, 18*(1), 44–52.

Ottani, P. A. (2002). Embracing global similarities: A framework for cross-cultural obstetric care. *JOGNN Journal of Obstetric, Gynecologic, & Neonatal Nursing, 31*(1), 33–38.

Payne, R. K. (2001). *A framework for understanding poverty.* Highlands, TX: aha! Process, Inc.

Primm, A. B., Cabot, D., Pettis, J., Vu, H. T., & Cooper, L. A. (2002). The acceptability of a culturally-tailored depression education videotape to African Americans. *Journal of the National Medical Association, 94*(11), 1007–1016.

Riordan, J., & Gill-Hople, K. (2001). Breastfeeding in multicultural populations. *JOGNN Journal of Obstetric, Gynecologic, & Neonatal Nursing, 30*(2), 216–223.

Thompson, M., Curry, M. & Burton, D. (1998). The effects of nursing case management on the utilization of prenatal care by Mexican-Americans in rural Oregon. *Public Health Nursing 15*(2), 82–90.

U.S. Census Bureau. (2000). *DP-1. Profile of general demographic characteristics: 2000 data set: Census 2000 summary file 1 (SF 1) 100-percent data.* Retrieved April 7, 2003, from http://factfinder.census.gov/servlet/QTTable?ds_name=DEC_2000_SF1_U&geo_id=01000US&qr_name=DEC_2000_SF1_U_DP1

U.S. Department of Health and Human Services. (2002, September 24, 2002). *Protecting the health of minority communities.* Retrieved March 19, 2003, from http://www.hhs.gov/news/press/2002pres/02minorityhealth.html

Wilson, F. L., Racine, E., Tekieli, V., & Williams, B. (2003). Literacy, readability and cultural barriers: Critical factors to consider when educating older African Americans about anticoagulation therapy. *Journal of Clinical Nursing, 12*(2), 275–282.

Educational Theories for Teaching and Motivating Patients

LEARNING OBJECTIVES

After reading this chapter, the student should be able to:

1. Distinguish between compliance and cooperation as desirable outcomes for patient education.

2. Define the concept of empowerment and apply it to a patient education situation.

3. Compare and contrast the developmental models, self-efficacy theory, and stress and coping theory as useful bases of patient education.

4. Describe Prochaska's stages of change and apply them to smoking cessation.

5. Describe the sequence of events in learning and recount examples of the events as applied to patient education.

INTRODUCTION

Many chapters in this book examine patient education issues from the perspective of health care providers. The authors focus on issues that arise, based on system constraints to effective patient teaching, and contextual and environmental influences that condition the learning situation. This chapter considers the issues the patient faces as a result of various factors, including attitudes, beliefs, and motivational influences. Other influencing factors include teaching and learning theories and their impact on individual patient learning. In addition, developmental models are discussed to show unique approaches to understanding patients within their biophysical, psychosocial, historical, and environmental contexts.

Factors, such as self-efficacy and motivation, cause each patient to approach the health care system in a unique way and influence the person's decision-making as a consumer of health care services. For example, patients who are highly motivated to learn healthy behaviors reinforce patient education efforts. This chapter discusses situations in which the patient's values are in conflict with those of the health care provider and patient education does not result in the behavioral changes suggested by the provider. Effective patient education includes the contextual and developmental status of individuals; therefore, lifespan development and an ecological systems approach to development are presented to focus on the patient's individual situation. Finally, both classic and contemporary learning theories are presented, so students can understand the theoretical underpinnings of patient education.

PATIENT EDUCATION: A PROCESS OF INFLUENCING BEHAVIOR

General Considerations

Patient education is defined as the process of influencing patient behavior and producing the changes in knowledge, attitudes, and skills necessary to maintain or improve health (American Academy of Family Physicians, 2000). This definition seems particularly applicable to the focus of this chapter. Patient education is a holistic process with the goal of changing a patient's behavior to benefit his or her health status. The process of patient education begins with assessment of the patient's needs and concerns; then the educator and patient collaboratively set goals for desired outcomes. Patient teaching refers to only one component of the patient education process—giving the patient information. Patient education is more than imparting information. The skilled patient educator assists the patient to interpret, integrate, and apply the information. Patient education ends with an evaluation of the patient's learning, its usefulness, and the degree to which he or she has integrated it into self-care practices.

Patient education is a process that occurs over time, requiring an ongoing assessment of the patient's knowledge, attitudes, and skills. The patient's readiness or motivation to change behaviors and the obstacles the patient faces to make a behavioral change are important consideration factors during assessment. (Chapter 7 offers an in-depth discussion of assessment for patient education.)

Most practitioners involved in patient education recognize the impact of the family on the patient's behavior. A close, supportive family may facilitate the integration of new health behaviors; a family that faces conflict or that lacks understanding often poses barriers to behavioral change. Strong religious, ethnic, or cultural beliefs may also influence or prevent desired change. The potency of sociocultural belief systems in influencing patient education is discussed in Chapter 3. A Patient and Family Education Assessment Guide, introduced in Chapter 7, identifies the factors that may promote or impede the process of patient education. The practitioner can then offer the patient and the family assistance in overcoming obstacles to behavioral change.

Compliance Orientation

Compliance and Noncompliance

The authors asked physicians and nurses to share what they consider to be obstacles in their experiences with patient education. Each one identified problems with either motivating patients or with achieving patient compliance. When asked to elaborate, they saw these two issues as closely related. The implication was that a sufficiently motivated patient would comply with the health care provider's instructions.

Many of us have justified our involvement in patient education by asserting that it would increase patient compliance, that is, convince patients to follow our suggestions. As research in health education expands, it becomes apparent that, despite teaching, patients frequently do not make the choices recommended to them by health professionals. This situation used to be called noncompliance.

Many health care providers are now uneasy with the terms compliance and noncompliance. They imply that health care professionals dictate to the patient what is to be done or changed, and the patient is to obey, and follow instructions. Further soul-searching makes us realize our discomfort stems from the patient's right to choose not to follow our advice, despite the fact that we believe we know what is best for him or her. It is natural for health professionals to want patients to choose the recommended course of action; however, what we really should strive to enlist is their partnership or cooperation. We want them to choose what we suggest.

Cooperation and Collaboration

An orientation toward cooperation and collaboration, rather than compliance, can help a health care provider examine his or her own effectiveness in patient education in a different light. Patient education successes have more to do with preparing a patient to make informed choices than with a patient obeying our instructions. If, in fact, we acknowledge the patient's free will to make choices, we must understand the importance of his or her values, wishes, and ability to participate in decision-making. If we assess the learner well, and individualize our recommendations in a way that accommodates to the patient's understanding, values, and wishes, our chances for successful patient education outcomes increase.

All health care providers have had experiences with uncooperative patients. These experiences teach us we need to better understand the factors that influence patient decision-making: values, beliefs, attitudes, current life stresses, religion, previous experiences with the health care system, and life goals. These experiences also illustrate that patient education involves not just teaching and learning, but also behavioral changes. Patient educators may begin with giving information and demonstrating skills. However, if the teacher and learner do not collaboratively determine the goals of patient education, and the patient is not included in deciding how learning will be applied, then behavioral changes usually will not occur.

Health professionals tend to view cooperation with a medical regimen as a single choice; however, the patient's cooperation with a regimen involves many choices every day. For example, choosing to follow an appropriate diet to manage diabetes requires constant decisions, often inconvenient and anguishing, throughout each day. The health professional may expect the patient to do this every day for the rest of his or her life, despite no guarantee of freedom from neuropathy, retinopathy, or other complications. Health professionals can offer the patient guidance and support, but we must also respect the patient's right to make choices, even if we disagree with the choices they make. However, we reserve the right to keep trying. Despite poor cooperation, a health care provider can remain hopeful that the patient will be more open to patient education messages during future encounters. As the health care provider learns more about the patient's point of view, collaboration can be better negotiated. The health care provider must also respect the patient's right to change his or her mind. The patient may choose to take the course of action suggested, or disregard the actions if the perceived cost or hardship outweighs the benefit. For example, a terminally ill patient may initially decide to take the treatment, but later decide to discontinue chemotherapy because the costly and uncomfortable side effects outweigh the benefits.

THE AGENDA OF EDUCATION

Health care providers bring their own agenda, or purpose, to the educational setting. Agendas tend to fall into one of four categories:

1. To maintain the status quo, with the health care providers dominant.
2. To prepare patients to be compliant, orderly, and obedient.
3. To improve relationships between patients and health care providers.
4. To provide liberating knowledge, so patients can control their own care.

As patients evolve from being health care recipients to health care consumers, they will choose health care providers whose agendas move away from the first and second choices, toward the third and fourth.

Empowerment in Patient Education

The term empowerment describes a participatory educational process, in which people can identify their own problems and solutions, and through this process, transform themselves and their communities. Empowerment theory views patients as having an inherent, but sometimes unrealized, capacity to make choices about solving problems relating to their own health and wellbeing. However, as Vella (1994) noted, teachers do not actually give power to adult learn-

ers; they encourage the use of the power that learners were born with.

Individual or Psychological Empowerment

Individual or psychological empowerment concerns the patient's ability to have control over his or her own life. Parkin (2001) views empowerment as effective because adults are more likely to make and maintain behavior changes when those changes are personally meaningful and freely chosen. The empowerment approach uses an interactive, four-step counseling model:

1. Identify the problem or issue (past)
2. Explore feelings and meaning (present)
3. Identify goals and choices (plan for the future)
4. Commit to action (future)

When applied to patient education, the health care professional provides a framework for creative thinking. The counseling dialogue helps the patient raise questions of why, how, and who. The health care provider guides the patient through identifying and exploring the problem, considering the choices, choosing a plan of action, and evaluating the results.

For example, apply this model to a patient with hypertension. The nurse ascertains the patient's explanatory model about hypertension and gives the patient all the information necessary to make an informed decision about management of hypertension, including nonpharmacologic (diet, exercise, herbs) and pharmacologic (side effects of medications). The patient is informed of possible complications if high blood pressure is not controlled. The nurse informs the patient of costs of various treatment options and encourages patient to read about hypertension and to talk with friends and relatives. On the next encounter, the nurse meets with the patient to discuss treatment options and asks the patient for a decision regarding treatment. The patient chooses to use a nonpharmacologic approach. The nurse teaches the patient how to monitor his or her own blood pressure at home and asks the patient to call with weekly readings for 6 weeks. When blood pressure does not respond to the non-pharmacologic approach, nurse suggests other nonpharmacologic therapies, such as biofeedback. The nurse monitors the patient's blood pressure by telephone and continues to support patient in an attempt to achieve blood pressure control without drugs.

Many health care providers may not consider this strategy to be a reasonable option. However, a significant percentage of hypertensive patients never take their medication, in which case this approach is at least as likely to achieve a reduction in blood pressure as the more traditional patient education approach. In addition, with the patient's continued participation in self-monitoring, the patient may recognize that medicine is necessary to achieve the desired reduction in blood pressure, and may choose to switch to the pharmacologic approach.

PATIENT DECISION-MAKING

Not following the treatment plan is a serious therapeutic deficit with massive personal, societal, and economic cost. Lack of cooperation is common among patients of all economic and educational backgrounds. This lack of cooperation may be involuntary or intentional. It may be related to the quality of information given, the impact of the regimen on daily life, physical or mental incapacity, social isolation, rationalization, denial, anxiety, depression, or anger. Less than 10% of patients told by a health care provider to lose weight or stop smoking do so (Haynes, McDonald, & Garg, 2002). Half of medicines prescribed for patients with chronic illnesses are not taken as prescribed (Marinker & Shaw, 2003).

To effectively help patients change behaviors through patient education, health professionals must discover the variables that influence each patient's choices. Working through, rather than around, patient issues helps health care providers address the barriers that prevent patients from cooperating. Patient education requires skills in assessing patient issues and problems, and in setting goals with patients. Chapters 7 and 8 address assessment and planning in detail.

MODELS AND THEORIES AS THE RESEARCH AND PRACTICE FOUNDATION OF PATIENT EDUCATION

Various theories and models have been used as the conceptual basis of patient education practice and research. Patient education is complex, and a variety of models are needed to take into account the environment, the patient's needs, and other factors. The theories used in research and practice should be chosen carefully to match all situational contingencies. Most patient education research in the past has not been based on theory, which is characteristic of many disciplines new to research. The following section presents several useful theoretical approaches for patient education.

The Health Belief Model

The Health Belief Model has been the most frequently used theoretical basis for research that examines the efficacy of patient education. The traditional Health Belief Model, also discussed in Chapter 2, was constructed in the 1950s by a group of social psychologists at the United States Public Health Service to predict health behaviors. Built on the earlier work of Kurt Lewin, an influential social psychologist, it provides a tool for understanding the patient's perception of the disease and his or her decision-making process in the consumption of health care services. This model is often applied to research to predict compliance, and it is also useful for gaining a better understanding of the patient's motivation for seeking and obtaining services.

The Health Promotion Model and Self-Regulation Model are also discussed in depth in Chapter 2. These are both based on the Health Belief Model.

Interpersonal Models of Health Behavior

The Health Belief Model is considered a model of individual health behavior, whereas the theories of self-efficacy and stress and coping are characterized as interpersonal models of health behavior. Interpersonal models of health behavior offer promise for health care providers because they enable us to view our roles as a possible instrument of change in our patients' lives.

Self-Efficacy Theory

Self-efficacy theory, also called social learning theory, accounts for learner characteristics and gives direction to the teacher for managing the physical and social environment in which learning occurs. A concept developed by Bandura (1986, 1997), self-efficacy is the confidence that one can carry out a behavior necessary to reach a desired goal. To succeed, the person needs to perceive the action is possible. People tend to take on tasks and situations they believe they can do and avoid challenges they believe exceed their abilities. This theory proposes there are four ways health care providers can help the patient believe behavior change is possible: personal mastery, vicarious experiences, verbal persuasion, and physiologic feedback. Application of this theory is illustrated in Box 4.1.

BOX 4.1 Clinical Application of Self-Efficacy Theory: Breast-feeding

Personal Mastery

The first-time mother learning to breast-feed her newborn is a good example of the need to develop personal mastery. If the new mother has a difficult time getting her newborn to successfully "latch on," she may begin to feel diminished as a mother. Teaching this new mother may become more difficult for the nurse, because each time she attempts to breast-feed, she may become more stressed and tense. Her newborn, sensing her tension, may become more resistant to feeding at the breast, further diminishing the mother's sense of personal mastery.

Vicarious Experiences

Vicarious experiences may help the first-time mother who is learning how to breast-feed. For example, if the mother watched her own mother successfully breast-feed, she had a significant role model available to her. Likewise, watching friends breast-feed, and viewing educational videos of different women who are breast-feeding provides vicarious experiences and gives the first-time mother an opportunity to develop self-confidence.

Verbal Persuasion

Verbal persuasion from lactation consultants is an important source of information for the first-time mother. Lactation consultants can assist with breast-feeding through telephone or in person consultation and encouragement. Breast-feeding groups (eg, La Leche League) also provide an important source of verbal persuasion. The sources of verbal persuasion are important to first-time mothers because they provide answers to questions and, more importantly, provide encouragement, support, and alternate methods of successful breast-feeding.

Physiologic Feedback

Physiologic feedback as a form of information leading to self confidence is provided by the infant's weight gains. The first-time mother usually discovers that her infant has gained weight during the second follow-up visit to the pediatric nurse practitioner or physician. This weight gain, a form of physiologic feedback, reinforces the first-time mother's confidence in her abilities to successfully breast-feed her baby.

Personal mastery is the most important of the four sources of information, and refers to the patient's perceived confidence that he or she can perform the desired behavior. An example of personal mastery is the patient newly diagnosed with diabetes. If the patient had experienced many unsuccessful attempts to draw blood and read the glucometer, the sense of personal mastery, or self-efficacy, would be diminished, and learning would become more difficult.

The vicarious experiences that patients gain from observing role models, such as other patients, health professionals, and family members, are especially important for the new learner. For example, a patient with a new ostomy frequently learns better and more quickly how to manage an ostomy if he or she is taught by another person who has also had an ostomy who can role model successful management. Vicarious experiences are most effective when the role model has similar characteristics to the learner, including age, gender, and ability.

Verbal persuasion reinforces the patient's competence in enacting new behaviors. Blyth and colleagues (2002) describe how breast-feeding self-efficacy can increase with encouragement from friends, family, and lactation consultants.

Elders can serve as peer advisors to other elders when they have both experienced an acute myocardial infarction (MI) (Whittemore, Rankin, Callahan, Leder, & Carroll, 2000). The peer advisors were found to have intervened in situations that involved congestive heart failure, management of physical energy demands, recurrent angina, depression, and obtaining visiting nurse services. They helped older participants by problem solving, and by sharing the common experiences of recovery from an MI.

Physiologic feedback refers to the necessary physical cues patients receive that the behavior they have undertaken is either appropriate or inappropriate, or that alternative actions should be sought. For example, a decreased cholesterol reading tells the patient the dietary changes and increased exercise are working.

Self-efficacy is specific to a task or situation; it does not generalize to all tasks and situations. Ask the patient how confident he or she is to complete a specific task. If the topic is climbing steps, ask about confidence to climb three steps, one flight of steps, two flights of steps, and so on. Ask the patient to quantify this confidence on a scale of not at all confident (0%) to completely confident (100%). The higher the confidence, the more likely the patient will succeed.

Self-efficacy theory specifies mechanisms that enhance learning and increase motivation. It has been criticized for its generality and lack of refinement. In terms of deriving interventions for practice, however, the four discrete sources of information that can result in desired behavior change provide a useful heuristic for designing programs. Application of this theory with a 9-year-old child is illustrated in Box 4.2.

The following interpersonal theories of health behavior are useful in understanding patient responses to threatening situations involving illness.

Stress, Coping, and Social Support

Stress, coping, and social support theories comprise a group of theoretical perspectives derived by various social scientists. The cognitive appraisal approach of Lazarus and the sociologic approach of Pearlin both include social support as an important modifier of stress.

Historically, stress research was given impetus by the work of two physiologists, Walter Bradford Cannon and Hans Selye. They proposed the response of the organism is more important than the nature of the stimulus provoking the response. On the other hand, epidemiologists and sociologists are more concerned with the source of stress, or stressors. Both perspectives are important to understanding the patient during patient education.

BOX 4.2 Clinical Application of Self-Efficacy Theory: Teaching Insulin Injection to a 9-Year-Old Child Newly Diagnosed with Insulin-Dependent Diabetes

Personal Mastery
- Participant modeling; successful injection of insulin by fearful, newly diagnosed, child with diabetes
- Performance desensitization: loss of fear of self-injections
- Performance exposure: continued successful practice of insulin injection

Vicarious Experiences
- Live modeling: demonstration by another child with diabetes performing insulin injection procedures
- Symbolic modeling: successful insulin demonstration by an age- and gender-matched child with diabetes

Verbal Persuasion
- Suggestion: teaching the child insulin injection techniques, and methods to decrease anxiety surrounding the process
- Exhortation: persuasive coaching by parents and nurse to perform successful insulin injection
- Self-instruction: child uses doll to learn insulin injection with persuasion from nurse

Physiologic Feedback
- Attribution: modification of the threat of injection by attributing the fear to something, or someone, else
- Relaxation, biofeedback: modifying threat by deep-breathing exercises before injection

---

The cognitive appraisal approach assists the health care provider in understanding that the patient's response to a stimulus is unique, and that the evaluation of the stimulus is influenced by factors within the person and from the stimulus itself. Lazarus (1999) proposes that psychological stress is thus the relationship between the person and the environment that is perceived as exceeding the available personal resources. Cognitive appraisal is an evaluation of the situation and includes primary appraisal: Am I in trouble? Does this situation threaten me?; and secondary appraisal: What can I do about it? Figure 4.1 illustrates how stress is generated by a mismatch between the person and the environment.

Lazarus (1999) also proposes coping is an ongoing process. Coping does not occur in stages; it is constantly being reworked. Coping consists of cognitive and behavioral efforts to manage specific demands that are appraised by the patient as straining or exceeding personal resources. Lazarus identifies six coping resources:

Health and energy
Positive beliefs
Problem-solving skills
Social skills
Social support
Material resources

Health care providers usually help patients develop problem-solving skills, because this type of coping is most appropriate when something can be done about a situation. A nurse will offer information to enhance problem solving and will mobilize socially supportive resources by helping the family understand how it can be most supportive during periods of stress. By referring the patient and family to a hospital social worker or to a case manager, the nurse mobilizes material resources. Application of this theory with a 36-year-old woman with breast cancer is illustrated in Box 4.3.

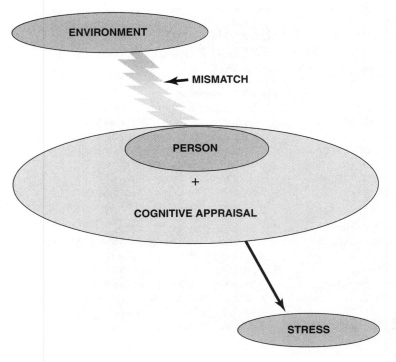

FIGURE 4.1 Depiction of the person—environment mismatch that generates stress.

The sociologic view of stress postulates that the sources and mediators of stress are located within the social environment of people. Sources of stress are those stressors in the biologic or social environment that lead to the experience of stress. Stressors consist of life events and persistent life strains that can be physiologic or psychosocial in origin (Pearlin & Skaff, 1996).

In the case of a woman with an acute MI, stressors may consist of physiologic risk factors, such as diabetes mellitus or hypertension, and problems of a psychosocial origin, such as overeating, smoking, or inactivity. Stress mediators are those social resources that help the patient adjust and adapt to the stressors. Stress assumes various physiologic and psychosocial manifestations. After an acute MI, stress may be manifested by depression, anxiety, arrhythmias, and pain.

Social support is a primary stress mediator and a resource in protecting well-being (Pearlin & Skaff, 1996). Thus, for the woman with an acute MI, stress mediators may include a supportive spouse and family. Mastery is a global sense of control that contributes to well-being. Mastery regulates the impact of stressors and may be elevated or lowered by exposure to stressor conditions.

Adaptation is the dynamic process of adjusting to stress. Although not part of Pearlin's original stress model, it is consistent with his work to view adaptation as the logical outcome of the stress process. Adaptation includes the patient's adjustment to the MI and ongoing coronary artery disease, her perceived quality of life, her assessment of her general health, and her cardiac functional capacity. The health care provider who applies a sociologic view of stress when providing patient education will give more attention to enhancing social resources and decreasing stressors in the social environment than will the health care provider who

---

BOX 4.3 Clinical Application of Stress and Coping Theory: Enhance Coping Resources in a 36-year-old Woman with Breast Cancer

Physical Resources: Health and Energy
- Teach importance of diet to maintain strength and decrease cachectic effects.

Psychological Resource: Positive Beliefs
- Reinforce positive attitudes related to treatment and cure; decrease negative attitudes.

Psychological Resource: Problem-Solving
- Assist patient in finding solutions to problems within her purview to solve; limit scope of problem-solving to those problems in which the patient can realistically intervene.

Social Resource: Social Skills
- Refer to American Cancer Society "I Can Cope" groups, Reach to Recovery; reinforce previously developed social skills.

Social Resource: Social Support
- Mobilize family and friends as support. If family and friends are not supportive, refer for counseling if the patient concurs.

Material Resource: Money, Goods, and Services
- Refer to hospital social services, discharge planning, and other community agency if the patient concurs. Give information about available services.

---

applies a cognitive appraisal view of stress. Both the psychological and sociologic approaches to viewing the stress process are useful for patient education.

DEVELOPMENTAL FRAMEWORKS: THE BASES FOR PATIENT EDUCATION

Developmental frameworks, such as those of Erikson, Piaget, and Duvall, are frequently included in nursing education programs because they offer a theoretical basis to nursing assessment and interventions. Health care professionals use the concepts of Erikson's developmental theory when they prepare the young adult for surgery related to repair of a congenital heart anomaly, remembering that the primary task at this developmental stage is to engender intimacy versus despair. They teach a 6-year-old child to administer insulin, recalling Piaget's stage referred to as preoperational development (see Chapter 5). Likewise, the nurse who pre-

pares a family for the birth of a second child recalls that the tasks of the family with preschool children concern integration of the new family member and ways to cope with sibling jealousy. Although these developmental frameworks are useful, they are limited because they do not consider the multiple determinants that influence individual and family development. Therefore, the following two sections discuss two useful theories, Bronfenbrenner's Ecological Systems Theory and the Lifespan Development Theory, for understanding the dynamic nature of development and its influence on patient education.

Ecological Systems Theory

General Considerations

The 1979 publication of *Ecology of Human Development* by Urie Bronfenbrenner, a child developmental psychologist, highlighted the importance of considering the context of individual development. Bronfenbrenner argues it is impossible to understand the developing person unless you also understand the ecological niches that govern favorable or unfavorable maturation. An ecological niche is formed by a combination of personal attributes and demographic characteristics. Not only is the concept of ecological niche important to understanding development, but it also influences the process of patient education.

An ecological niche for an adolescent, newly diagnosed with diabetes, might consist of a family that is white, urban, upper middle class, with two parents who both work, three children, and the children attending a private school. The ecological niche for this adolescent may be favorable to patient education and to learning necessary self-care management skills. Contrast this ecological niche and its influence on patient education with an adolescent with diabetes who is a high school dropout and lives with a single, unemployed parent, and who has six siblings in a rural, southern U.S. household.

Bronfenbrenner contends that the patient is an actor in this process of development, which is influenced by the environmental context and the reciprocity of the organism. Therefore, in the example above, until more information is available, one cannot assume that the second adolescent is incapable of developing diabetes self-management skills, although at first glance his or her ecological niche appears less favorable.

Bronfenbrenner's Ecological Framework: Interactive Systems

Bronfenbrenner's ecological systems theory includes four levels of nested concentric structures that form a model for interactive systems that influence, and are influenced by, the developing person (Figure 4.2). These interactive systems are microsystems, mesosystems, exosystems, and macrosystems (Huitt, 2002). Microsystems are the patterns of activities, roles, interpersonal relationships, and material characteristics with which the developing person interacts. Important microsystems with which the child interacts are the family, peer group, and school. Microsystems are the most basic level of system influencing development. Regarding patient education and its intersec-

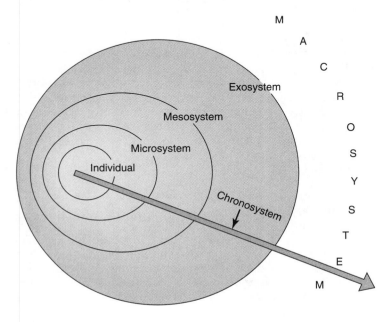

FIGURE 4.2 Bronfenbrenner's ecological framework.

tion with microsystems, the health care professional who works with a child should consider the quality of family, peer, and school life and how these might influence the child's ability to accept patient teaching.

Mesosystems are social systems or interrelated microsystems, such as the interrelationships that occur between a child's family and the school. These interrelationships have an impact on the development of the child. An example of the significance of mesosystems in patient education would be a school that creates a private environment for children to monitor their blood glucose levels, when a child's family wishes to conceal the child's diabetes. When the family and school have limited understanding of each other or if they interact negatively, the child will not have the environmental supports to maintain the self-care activities taught by the health care professional.

Exosystems are environments and conditions external to the child that indirectly affect the child's development. Examples of exosystems are parental occupational environments and parental friendships. Exosystems are systems the child infrequently enters, but they are structures that can have major effects on the child's maturation. The implications of exosystems for patient education include the influence of parental friendships on the way parents interpret health teaching. Parents who are encouraged by their friends to send their child to diabetes camp may open new avenues of patient education for the child who has never been exposed to other children with diabetes. The hospital and health care community are also examples of important exosystems.

Macrosystems are the broadest and most indirect system influences on the child. Macrosystems include the impact of culture, subculture, and embedded belief patterns on the developing child. Macrosystems affect the child through their relationships to the micro-, meso-, and exosystems.

Chronosystems, the dimension of time, were added by Bronfenbrenner in 1986 to expand the theory so the effects of change, and continuities, on the developing person could be bet-

ter understood (Bronfenbrenner, 1986). Chronosystems are typically conceived as life transitions. The chronosystem is an important thrust that intersects the other systems.

The importance of understanding chronosystems as related to patient education and children entails a constant attendance to the transitions that children and adolescents encounter during the first 20 years of life. For example, the 12-year-old youth who is diagnosed with insulin-dependent diabetes mellitus (IDDM) is most likely entering the tumultuous years associated with adolescence; peer relationships and being part of the crowd are more important than euglycemia. However, a 3-year-old child diagnosed with IDDM is still within a parentally controlled orbit in which peer relationships are secondary to the family sphere. Thus, the life transitions, or chronosystem effects, encountered by the 12-year-old can be postulated as making adjustment to diabetes more difficult than for a 3-year-old child.

A poignant example of the power of the chronosystem and life transitions was seen when one of the authors facilitated a support group for parents with a child who has diabetes. One mother told the story of her 12-year-old son who had been relatively compliant in terms of insulin injections, diet, and self blood glucose monitoring (SBGM). She related that as he began spending more time after school in the company of friends, she began noticing candy wrappers in his pants pockets. At first he denied he had been eating candy and then he showed her his SBGM log book, indicating his blood glucose levels were within acceptable guidelines. Finally, after an upper respiratory infection, he was hospitalized in diabetic ketoacidosis. When he began SBGM again, the nurse noted that he was incorrectly performing the process so that he fooled his blood glucose monitor, resulting in false low readings. When confronted with his SBGM technique, he readily admitted what he had done but told his parents it was more important to him that he be part of the gang than to have acceptable blood glucose readings. Health care providers should realize that chronosystem influences are frequently more significant than long-term health outcomes to patients. Understanding patients from the perspective of life transitions can add greater clarity and direction to patient teaching.

In summary, Bronfenbrenner's Ecological Systems Theory can sensitize the health care professional who works with children and adolescents to the various dimensions that influence development not commonly considered in traditional approaches. Although the theory is encumbered by the jargon, the importance of considering people in the broadest context of development is an important contribution of Bronfenbrenner's work.

Lifespan Development Frameworks

General Considerations

Lifespan Development Frameworks, also referred to as Life Course Perspective, evolved in the 1960s and 1970s. It was developed by lifespan developmental psychologists and life course perspective sociologists. Their research looked at the interrelated effects of age, cohort experience, and non-normative life events on development.

Unlike Bronfenbrenner, who added the concept of chronosystem almost as an afterthought, the lifespan developmental psychologists had long been involved in longitudinal studies of various U.S. cohorts. Their work also was influenced by the stage developmentalists, Erikson and Duvall. However, like Bronfenbrenner, they realized there was more to development than simply an orderly progression through stages.

Although Ecological Systems Theory is a useful device for considering the many influences on development and their influence on patient education, it pertains primarily to children and adolescents. The life course approach recognizes that adults and children influence each other's behavior and development and emphasizes that developmental growth continues through adulthood into old age.

Components of the Lifespan Developmental Framework

The Lifespan Developmental Framework is a useful conceptual approach for considering the dynamic, integrated aspects of human functioning (Figure 4.3). This model assumes that biological, environmental, and behavioral determinants, in conjunction with specified developmental influences, shape the lifespan of individuals and families (Baltes, Staudinger, & Lindenberger, 1999).

Important developmental influences that should be considered by health care professionals appraising the effects of adult development on patient education include:

Normative age-graded factors are biological and environmental variables that exhibit a high correlation with chronological age.
Normative history-graded factors are the historical events that influence particular birth cohorts.
Non-normative factors are life events that occur asynchronously with the life course or are not experienced by the population at large.

Normative age-graded factors overlap with the psychological and cognitive stages outlined by developmental theorists, such as Erikson and Piaget; they also coincide with normative physical development. Although normative age-graded factors are frequently taken for granted when planning patient education, the importance of considering the effects of age on patient education is illustrated in the case of women with coronary heart disease (CHD). Women are usually older than men when they experience an acute MI, which has implications for recovery and rehabilitation from MI. Older women are likely to have pre-existing comorbidities that may limit participation in cardiac rehabilitation programs and exercise regimens. For example, limited mobility as a result of osteoarthritis and rheumatoid arthritis, peripheral vascular disease, and orthopedic impairments are comorbid conditions that may impinge on the ability of older women to participate in cardiac reha-

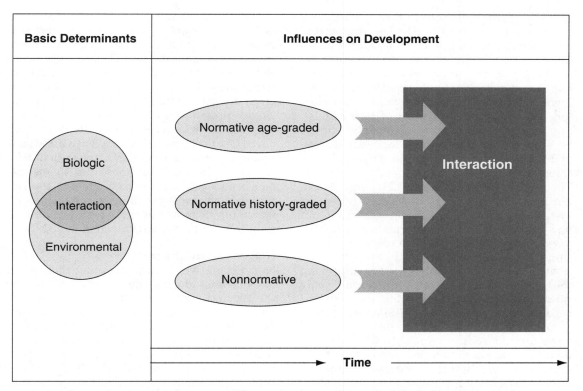

Basic Determinants	Influences on Development

FIGURE 4.3 Determinants and influences on lifespan development: a methodological and theoretical approach. From Life-span Developmental Psychology by Baltes, P. D., Reese, H. W., and Lipsitt, L. P. Used with permission, from the *Annual Review of Psychology*, Volume 31 ©1980 by Annual Reviews www.AnnualReviews.org.

bilitation programs. Thus, any attempts to effectively educate the older woman post-MI must contemplate pre-existing comorbidities and plan methods of exercise that consider them.

Clinical Relevance

NORMATIVE AGE-GRADED FACTORS

A meta-analysis of diabetes patient education research, examining the effectiveness of diabetes patient teaching interventions found that across 73 studies, normative age-graded factors were especially important (Brown, 1992). Brown's meta-analysis revealed that diabetes teaching interventions were less effective for older patients; for patients older than 55 years, glycosylated hemoglobin levels were only minimally improved by teaching interventions. Brown surmises that older patients with diabetes may need more individualized instruction than younger patients. Also, Brown surmises that instead of mixing diabetes management regimen (insulin, oral hypoglycemic, or diet) across group participants, it might be better to segregate by diabetes type and regimen.

NORMATIVE HISTORY GRADED FACTORS

Continuing with the example of older women and acute MI, important normative history graded influences can be identified as attitudes toward promotion, restoration, and maintenance of health. Health promotion, restoration, and maintenance activities relating to CHD include cessation of cigarette smoking, implementation of a proper diet, and regular exercise. Cigarette smoking has been identified as the most prominent risk factor for heart disease in women (Hines, 2001). Smoking appears to have synergistic effects, because it increases the risk for heart disease and MI if used in conjunction with oral contraceptives and if hyperlipidemia is present. The women who experience CHD and MI did not know tobacco harmed the cardiovascular system when they began smoking, and did not have the benefit of the information available to younger women who currently make decisions regarding smoking. Patient education strategies must be oriented toward improving the quality of life in one's remaining years rather than toward preventing the onset of coronary artery and other vascular diseases.

Other prominent health promotion and restoration activities related to CHD include dietary intake and exercise. Similar to information on the harmful effects of smoking, dietary information was not available to older women when they were young and establishing health promotion activities. Today's women over 65 years old with CHD and MI may have amended their current eating patterns, but previous behaviors may have already established irreversible atherosclerosis. The use of exercise to establish adequate cardiovascular health promotes and restores health. However, the women who are experiencing CHD and MI currently were less likely to engage in vigorous exercise when they were younger than are young women today. In addition, only a small percentage of women who experience MI are likely to engage in structured cardiac rehabilitative exercise to restore health (Thomas et al., 1996). Therefore, health care professionals who seek to provide cardiac rehabilitation to older women must consider these history graded factors and amend cardiac rehabilitation programs so they appeal to older women since they are based on their own life experience.

Health maintenance history graded effects include the belief by most women that they were not at risk for CHD and MI because it was considered a male disease. These beliefs, which also have been prominent in the health care community, have resulted in less attention given to the clinical symptoms with which women present with CHD and MI; thus, fewer diagnostic procedures and laboratory tests have been performed that may have assisted in earlier identification of CHD. The patient education implications for these health maintenance history graded effects include the fact that women across the lifespan need education informing them of their risk for CHD and the symptoms that may indicate angina or MI.

Non-normative Factors

Non-normative factors (events that occur unexpectedly during the lifespan) often offer the greatest challenge to the health care professional who conducts patient education. These factors include the onset of acute or chronic illnesses at times they are not normally found. For example, most women are unprepared for the diagnosis of MI at the age of 40 years; indeed, 40-year-old men are equally unprepared. Unexpected and severe illnesses are generally unexpected in young children, and challenge the health care professional who must educate the parents and help the family cope. The family that has an 18-month-old child diagnosed with IDDM, and that faces the challenge of managing the child's illness, is faced with a non-normative event of monumental proportions. The parents will probably require additional teaching time and additional support in managing potential future losses. During the assessment process, health care providers should recognize non-normative factors as conceivably requiring more time and greater resources for patient education.

Implications of the Lifespan Framework for Patient Education

At times, health care professionals do not consider the many factors that influence a patient's receptivity to patient teaching. If the patient is assessed in the context of the multiple constraints of lifespan development, health care providers can better individualize patient education. Examples using the lifespan approach were cited above for older women with CHD. At different ages, people approach learning from distinct vantage points. Remembering that patients are products of the historical eras in which they matured helps health care providers shape appropriate patient education for different birth cohorts.

For example, women born during the Baby Boom Era (1946 to 1964) have willingly embraced physical exercise in many different forms. Their mothers, on the other hand, were less likely to exercise to the point of maximal cardiovascular capacity. The female Baby Boomers who have MIs will probably be open to cardiac rehabilitation, whereas their mothers are less likely to become involved. Attitudinal differences toward sexuality, reproductive health, and raising children are major cohort effects found in these two generations of women. The health care provider must constantly consider history graded factors, or cohort effects, when planning patient education. Lastly, non-normative factors challenge the health care provider to individualize patient education efforts so the patient's own experience is viewed from an appropriate perspective.

The next section of this chapter reviews the process of teaching and learning. The theories presented up to this point have been primarily macroanalytical theories of patient and health education. That is, they are useful to understand the broader aspects of patient education. The actual learning process includes microanalytical theories that pertain to how information is actually learned and processed. This section of the chapter also includes a discussion of motivation.

THE PROCESS OF TEACHING AND LEARNING

Definition of Learning

Learning has been defined as a process involving interaction with the external environment (Gagne & Driscoll, 1988) and as a change in behavior resulting from reinforced practice (Huckabay, 1980). The definition by Huckabay, a noted nurse educator, seems especially pertinent to learning psychomotor skills. (Chapter 9 discusses psychomotor learning in depth.) For this chapter's purpose, the authors define psychomotor learning as pertaining to learning of skills and performance. Learning that requires a change in feelings or belief (affective learning) and learning that requires thinking (cognitive learning) may be more difficult to promote and measure.

Sequence of Events in Learning

Learning and remembering are generally thought of as orderly sequences of events that occur in all learners (Figure 4.4). Educational psychologists (Gagne & Driscoll, 1988; Huckabay, 1980) delineate an eight-phase sequence of learning and remembering:

1. Motivation
2. Apprehending
3. Acquisition
4. Retention
5. Recall
6. Generalization
7. Performance
8. Feedback

Motivation

Motivation can be either intrinsic or extrinsic. Intrinsic motivation factors, such as the patient's anxiety level, success in past educational settings, and openness to learning, are internally integrated into the patient's personality and modus operandi. Extrinsic motivation factors include the learning environment, the pleasure of acquiring new knowledge, and the type of interaction in the learning process. Resnick (2002) found older adults were motivated to participate in a rehabilitation program through both intrinsic and extrinsic factors: personal expectations, per-

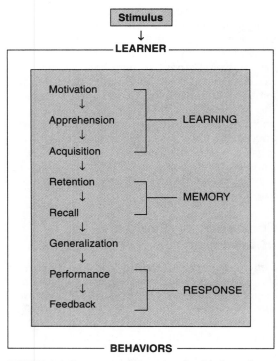

FIGURE 4.4 Sequence of steps involved in learning.

sonality, role models, verbal encouragement, progress, past experiences, spirituality, physical sensations, individualized care, social supports, and goals.

Patient educators can only control extrinsic motivation factors. When they establish a climate of mutual trust and safety, the learning environment can be a positive motivator. Likewise, by injecting fun and levity into the learning situation, health care providers can make the pleasure of learning become a positive force.

Another extrinsic motivating factor the educator can control is the type of interaction in the learning process. Transactional analysis provides a vocabulary useful to describing the desired interaction. Adult learners are poorly motivated when the interaction is structured in a manner in which the adult learner has the role of the child in an adult–child or parent–child situation. The adult learner will profit most from an adult–adult type of interaction. An example of an adult–adult type of interaction would be a group for ostomy patients, in which one patient would share with the group his or her experiences in coping with the ostomy. Adult–adult interactions require the patient to take responsibility for his or her own learning. A patient educator who encourages the patient to set his own agenda for learning the management of heart disease is another example of an adult–adult type of interaction.

Because motivation also has social and task mastery components, health care providers can use them to enhance a patient's motivation to learn. For example, adolescents have a strong need to belong (affiliative needs). These affiliative needs, and related self-esteem and social approval needs, can be used to enhance internal motivating forces when adolescents learn how to stop smoking or how to manage contraception. The use of peers who role model desired behaviors is an exceptionally strong motivator for adolescents.

The health care provider can help the patient to recognize the gap between what his or her situation is and what he or she wants it to be. For example, a young couple recognized they did not want to use corporal punishment with their 3-year-old daughter, but they did not know how else to achieve necessary obedience. Once the care providers helped the couple recognize the gap, they eagerly asked for and then applied other discipline techniques.

Once patients recognize a need for learning, they can be effectively motivated by using written contracts. (The formulation of learning contracts is covered in Chapter 8.) If motivational techniques do not seem to work, the health care provider should reassess the patient. Perhaps something has changed in the patient's situation that makes previous motivators ineffective. For example, a low-to-moderate level of anxiety is an intrinsic motivator and may be used effectively to motivate the patient with coronary artery disease to learn about necessary diet, medication, and lifestyle changes. However, if this patient has a successful coronary artery bypass graft operation, he or she may feel cured and out of danger; therefore, anxiety may no longer be an effective motivator. The health care provider must now reassess the patient to identify other motivators.

Motivation is also determined by the patient's sense of responsibility to learn. The patient ultimately decides whether to accept the health care provider's teachings, selectively accept parts, or ignore all teaching. Health care providers are not responsible for a patient's behavior. They do their best to enhance the learning situation and to use extrinsic motivation factors, but motivation is essentially an inner drive. If a patient does not have this inner drive and sense of personal responsibility, health professionals can do little to foster these motivators. Health care providers should encourage patients to advocate for themselves and to expect patient education services from each of their health care providers, in every setting.

However, some patients will refuse to accept the responsibility to learn. All health care providers can do is to make every effort to provide individualized patient education. If all efforts fail, the patient has chosen not to learn.

Apprehending

During the apprehending phase of learning, learners are exposed to a stimulus, which is then absorbed and processed in a manner that requires discriminative abilities. Patients who are mildly or moderately anxious are often good subjects for patient teaching because they attend to the stimulus with greater care than those who are not anxious. For example, most coronary artery bypass graft surgery patients and their family members are moderately anxious the day before surgery. Their discriminative abilities are

heightened, and patient teaching can be extremely effective.

Acquisition

The acquisition phase of learning includes the changes that occur in the central nervous system (CNS) and make the new material concrete. If the learner has a CNS dysfunction, the new material may not be acquired. For example, a patient with a cerebrovascular accident may apprehend new information, but because of CNS damage, may not perform the desired behavior.

Retention

During the retention phase, the material that was previously apprehended is stored as memories. Age may be an intervening factor, because older people have more problems with short-term memory than with long-term memory.

Recall

Recall is retrieval. During recall, the learner can retrieve his or her new abilities for an external observer or teacher. For example, when parents of an infant with respiratory problems are asked to demonstrate endotracheal suctioning, they recall the basics of suctioning technique, organize the procedure systematically, and then perform the skill safely and correctly.

Generalization

Generalization, the sixth phase in the learning process, is sometimes referred to as the transfer of learning. During generalization, the patient can retrieve something he has learned and apply it within a different situation or context. For example, the parent who has learned the principles of sterile technique in the context of sterile suctioning should be able to apply sterile technique to dressing changes.

Performance and Feedback

Performance and feedback are the seventh and eighth phases of learning. Performance is the observable behavior that demonstrates a change has occurred. Performance is relatively easy to observe in situations of psychomotor learning. However, in situations of affective and cognitive learning, performance frequently must be obtained through verbal methods.

Feedback is the last phase of learning and occurs through reinforcement. In situations of psychomotor learning, successful performance of the newly learned information serves as feedback. In situations of affective or cognitive learning, however, feedback is frequently a function of the instructor who encourages the learner by saying, "That's correct" or "Good job."

Health care providers must frequently educate children or adults with learning disabilities. Their learning styles may be different, and different approaches may be needed. Box 4.4 suggests approaches to match teaching with specific disabilities.

CLINICAL RELEVANCE: PATIENT ADVOCACY AND PROMOTION OF CHANGE

Anyone who has ever tried to stop smoking, lose weight, or exercise regularly knows how difficult it is to change old behaviors. It may seem at times that patients truly cannot be motivated to change their behaviors. There are times when, given all available information, and after engaging in a fully participatory encounter, patients will still choose not to embrace healthy behaviors.

Patient Advocacy

The concept of patient advocacy further elaborates this view of motivation. Patient advocacy addresses how health care providers partner with the patient, meet the patient where he or she is, and assist in whatever manner possible in coming to a decision about assuming certain behaviors. Baldwin (2003) analyzed the literature and concluded that advocacy is only possible when three essential components are present:

1. Valuing: a therapeutic relationship that secures the patient's freedom and self-determination.
2. Apprising: promoting and protecting the patient's rights to be involved in decision-making and informed consent.
3. Interceding: acting as an intermediary between patients and family, significant others, health care providers, or health care systems.

The second attribute, apprising, is a combination of informing, advising, and educating. This ensures the patient is knowledgeable, before making the decision, about the implications, consequences, and alternatives. Patient education is, therefore, an essential component of advocacy.

Patient advocacy is different from consumerism and paternalism. A consumerist view presents the patient with all the treatment options, with little regard for the patient's personal values and beliefs. A paternalistic view makes decisions for the patient and tells him or her what to do. In contrast, patient advocacy values the patient's right to choose, promotes and protects patient involvement in decisions, ensures informed consent, and actively helps patients overcome barriers to meet their needs.

Prochaska's Stages of Change

One of the most appealing aspects of Prochaska's work is that his stages of change have been applied successfully to some of the most hazardous and unhealthy behaviors, with moderate success. The Transtheoretical Model of Behavior Change explains why some people do not modify risky behaviors, despite adequate information. It has been used to study behaviors most resistant to change, including

---

BOX 4.4 Meeting the Needs of Children and Adults with Learning Disabilities

Points to remember

1. **Children with learning disorders** (eg, attention deficit disorder, dyslexia) may learn better using sensory systems—auditory, visual, or tactile—that are different from those used by the patient educator. Also, their learning abilities may be affected by problems affecting memory, language, and motor, and integrative process problems.

2. **Auditory learners** are thought to have visual perceptual disabilities (eg, dyslexia). These children and adults learn best through auditory modes; therefore, the nurse should not rely on written teaching materials, but instead use auditory materials, such as tapes, records, and verbal instruction.

3. **Visual learners** often have an auditory perceptual disability. These learners usually have difficulties distinguishing subtle differences in sounds and may have problems picking up cues that they are being spoken to, especially when others are in the same room. These learners do well with films, written materials, and charts. Group instruction may be confusing to these learners.

4. **Tactile learners** are children with learning disabilities that are most amenable to learning that includes hands-on, tactile experience. If they do not have other sensory learning disabilities, they may be good candidates for group games and learning experiences that involve movement.

5. **Integrative process disabilities** usually involve the inability to sequence visual, auditory, or tactile input correctly. Children with these learning disabilities may read words backward, may not correctly process words, or may hear words or sentences improperly, or may not understand the meaning. The most effective learning strategies involve simple instructions with the opportunity for immediate return demonstration.

6. **Short- or long-term memory disabilities** are manifested as the inability to remember information presented recently or in the past. These disabilities often accompany other learning disabilities, adding to the problems involved in achieving effective patient education. Adults or children with memory disabilities need the opportunity for short and frequent teaching sessions.

7. **Language disabilities** are manifested as the inability to answer when some type of response is demanded. The most important response of the nurse educator is to provide sufficient time for the individual to organize his or her thoughts so that a coherent answer can be given. These learners are not good candidates for learning activities that require quick verbal responses (eg, spelling bees).

8. **Motor disabilities** can be exhibited in two different ways—gross and fine motor disabilities. Fine motor disabilities are evident in children or adults who cannot write or draw but possibly can use a computer or paint. Gross motor disabilities frequently result in clumsiness and poor performance in sports activities.

---

addictive behaviors, diet and weight control, smoking cessation, sexual behavior related to HIV infection, and other life-endangering behaviors (DiClemente & Prochaska, 1998).

Prochaska and colleagues propose that the stages of change are a developmental sequence of motivational readiness that includes precontemplation, contemplation, preparation, action, and maintenance (Prochaska, Redding, Harlow, Rossi, & Velicer, 1994, p. 473). They note that the stages of change are not necessarily linear and that people may revert to previous risk-taking behaviors. They suggest that interventions to motivate people must be tailored for each stage. (See example in Table 4.1.) The theory is complex and includes the concept of self-efficacy, which was discussed earlier in this chapter. The Transtheoretical Model of Behavior Change is especially useful for staging advanced practice nursing counseling interventions (Bastable, 2003).

THEORIES OF LEARNING

Before 1950, comprehensive theories of learning were proposed that asserted an explana-tion for all types of learning. However, as educational psychologists learned more about the nature of learning, it became clear that no one theory could explain the entire realm of teaching and learning. Therefore, theories emerged that attempted to explain certain facets of teaching and learning, such as concept learning, problem solving, and skill mastery.

Tables 4.2 and 4.3 present various theories on teaching and learning. The first three theories (mental discipline, natural unfoldment, and apperception) belong to the pre-1950s generation of theoretical precepts that pertain to the process of teaching and learning. The theories in Table 4.3 have emanated from the various schools of educational psychology that evolved during the 20th century.

TABLE 4.1	Prochaska's Transtheoretical Model of Motivation and Change as Applied to Weight Loss	
STAGE OF CHANGE	**PERIOD OF TIME ASSOCIATED WITH STAGE AND CHARACTERISTICS OF STAGE**	**INTERVENTION**
Precontemplation	• 6 mos • Little intent to change • Resistant to change • Defensiveness regarding obesity	Consciousness raising—providing information about health risks related to obesity. Increase awareness of various approaches to weight loss.
Contemplation	• Time in this stage is variable but has been reported from 6 mos to yrs • More serious about changing behavior • Ambivalent about the costs and benefits of changing behavior	Self-reevaluation—thoughtful attention to one's self and problems may provide an opportunity for health care professionals to influence decisions about healthy eating.
Preparation	• Variable period of time • Preliminary healthy behavior attempts, such as brief attempts to eat less	Self-liberation—belief in one's ability and commitment to change. Health care provider can reinforce belief in self through provision of support.
Action	• Usually lasts up to 6 mos • Periods of weight loss interspersed with recidivism and relapse	Helping relationships—need for open, caring, honest relationships can be fulfilled by health care provider.
Maintenance	• Begins 6 mos after successful behavior change in the action stage; may last for years if behavior change was successful • Relapse may occur but is less common than during the action stage	Counterconditioning—substitution of positive behaviors for negative ones. Health care provider can assist with planning meals, suggesting alternative rewards to food. Stimulus control—through restructuring of the environment, access to food can be controlled.

Source: Adapted from Prochaska, J. O., Redding, C. A., Harlow, L. L., Rossi, J. S., & Velicer, W. F. (1994). The transtheoretical model of change and HIV: prevention: A review. *Health Education Quarterly, 21*, 471–476.

TABLE 4.2 Important Early Teaching and Learning Theories and Their Application to Patient Education

LEARNING THEORY AND KEY PERSONS	ATTRIBUTES OF THE TEACHING/LEARNING PROCESS	NATURE OF LEARNING	APPLICATION TO PATIENT EDUCATION
Mental Discipline			
Plato, Aristotle—early developers M. J. Adler, R. M. Hutchings—contemporary proponents	Teacher trains intrinsic mental power. Learner maintains strict discipline to strengthen mental faculty of attention, memory, will, and perseverance. Rote memory, repetitive drill. Teacher centered with active learners.	Disciplined mind and memorization of factual material.	Helpful when teaching exchange diet and basic pathophysiology. Should be used with oral drills.
Natural Unfoldment			
F. Froebel, J. J. Rousseau—early developers A. H. Maslow—contemporary proponents	Learner discovers that which nature or a creator has put within him. Teacher waits until learner expresses desire to learn before attempting to teach him or her. Promotes intuitive awareness of self. Learner's feelings are authority for truth. Student centered with active learners.	Self-directed active unfolding of knowledge with intuitive awareness expressed.	Applicable to clients interested in self-care, prenatal clients, well-child care.
Apperception			
J. F. Herbart, E. B. Titchener—original proponents	New ideas are associated with ideas that already exist in the learner's mind. Teacher explains and learner grasps generalizations, relationships, rules, or principles. Teacher centered with passive learners.	Recognition, explanation, or use of understandings, insights, principles, relationships, concepts, theories, or laws.	Applicable to clients who have previous knowledge or experience on which to build (ie, previous surgical experiences, knowledge of medications).

Source: Adapted from Bigge, M. L. (1976, 1998). *Learning theories for teachers* (3rd and 4th ed.). New York: Harper & Row.

TABLE 4.3 Important Twentieth Century Teaching and Learning Theories and Their Application to Patient Education

LEARNING THEORY AND KEY PERSONS	ATTRIBUTES OF THE TEACHING/LEARNING PROCESS	NATURE OF LEARNING	APPLICATION TO PATIENT EDUCATION
Individual Learning Theories			
Conditioning—Behavioristic			
C. L. Hull, E. L. Thorndike—early developers E. R. Guthrie, B. F. Skinner, R. Gagne—later proponents	Involves conditioning or behavior modification. Formation of stimulus—response linkages or response—stimulus reinforcements. Teacher centered with passive learners.	Increased probability of desired response.	Useful for reinforcing desired behaviors in children.
Cognitive-Gestalt Information Processing (IP)			
M. Montessori, J. Dewey, K. Lewin, G. W. Allport, E. C. Tolman—early developers	Gains or changes insights, outlooks, or thought patterns. Reorganizes perceptual or cognitive fields. Purposive involvement, problem-solving, and problem-raising.	Purposefully acquired insights, principles, relationships, concepts, generalizations, rules, theories, or laws with enhanced scientific outlook and instrumental thinking. Diagnostic reasoning.	Applicable to affective learning (ie, working with parents on child-rearing issues). Useful when working with groups with common problems (ie, parents of handicapped children, myocardial infarction spouse groups).
J. S. Bruner, M. L. Bigge, M. Deutsch, S. Koch, Newell and Simon. W. Kohler—later proponents	Teacher-student centered with cooperative and interactive inquiry. Information processing model consists of short- & long-term memory. Long-term memory is banked and can be retrieved later for use by short-term memory.		IP is useful for building and connecting information.

Mastery-Learning

B. Bloom, J. Block	Breaks down complex units of instruction into smaller learning units that build on each other. Strives for many (90%) learners, able to achieve or master tasks. Encourages self-development.	Increased self-esteem from learning results in changed perception of self and external world.	Helpful when the information to be taught requires mastery of many skills (ie, patients with diabetes who are insulin-dependent).

Interpersonal Learning Theories

Social Learning

A. Bandura, W. Mischel	Process of learning is influenced by four sources of information: personal mastery, vicarious experiences, verbal persuasion, and physiologic feedback. Learner centered. Teachers can be family members or other learners.	Increased belief that one is capable of performing desired behavior and that the performance will lead to expected outcome.	Enhancement of self-confidence and self-efficacy can lead to desired health behavior changes and maintenance of desired behavior.

Source: From Bigge, M. C. & Shermis, S. S. (1982, 1992). *Learning theories for teachers* (3rd and 5th eds.) New York: Harper Collins; Bandura, A. (1982). Self-efficacy mechanism in human agency. *American Psychologist, 37,* 122; Glanz, K., Lewis, F. M. & Rimer, B. K. (Eds.). (1990). *Health behavior and health education. Theory, research, and practice.* San Francisco: Jossey-Bass. Adapted with permission.

Generally, there are individual and interpersonal learning theories. The individual learning theories include the conditioning-behavioristic family, the cognitive–Gestalt–information processing family, and mastery learning. Interpersonal learning theory includes social learning theory, developmental theories, and stress and coping theories. The last two are not included in the table, but were discussed earlier in this chapter.

Learning theories help provide approaches to patient teaching and learning, using different theories used at different times, depending on the situation. An eclectic approach probably serves patients best. The examples provided showing application of theories to various patient education situations are merely illustrations. They do not imply such situations should always be guided by those specific theories.

The following case study demonstrates the application of behavioristic, cognitive–Gestalt, and social learning theory principles.

CASE STUDY 4-1

DIABETES MELLITUS

HISTORY

Claire Patterson is a 25-year-old white woman with IDDM; onset was at age 16. She is 5', 4" tall and weighs 125 lb. (4.4 lb. above desired weight). She attended a comprehensive diabetes education program 5 years ago and subsequently controlled her blood glucose levels with multidose insulin therapy. Her glycosylated hemoglobin level recently dropped from 13% to 7%, a desired level.

After marriage and relocation to Los Angeles, she changed physicians and insulin therapy. Her new physician prescribed 28 U of Lente (insulin zinc suspension USP) and 8 U of regular human insulin. She began having seizures in the middle of the night and was hospitalized several times during the month of October. In December, she returned to the comprehensive diabetes teaching program to gain better blood glucose control.

FAMILY SETTING

Claire Patterson lived at home with her parents before her marriage. Her mother, a registered nurse, was a primary participant in her daughter's diabetes management. Claire feels that she can openly express her feelings and concerns to her parents. Her mother hesitates between allowing her daughter to be more independent in managing her diabetes and taking control of diabetes management for her daughter because, she says, it "breaks my heart" to see her having convulsions. Claire requested that her mother accompany her to another week-long session at the diabetes teaching center.

Claire's husband is in military service out of state, and portions of the program were audiotaped for his benefit because he could not attend. Both Claire and her husband are motivated to get the diabetes under control so that they can have children.

IDENTIFIED PROBLEMS

Contradicting attitudes about diabetes control resulted from Claire's insulin reactions. The family recognized that long-term complications frequently resulted from high blood glucose levels, but they believed that high blood glucose levels were safer than the threat of short-term hypoglycemic reactions. Additionally, their experiences with normal, or euglycemic, blood glucose levels led them to believe they were the antecedents of low blood glucose levels.

GOALS AND RECOMMENDED INTERVENTIONS: APPROPRIATE TEACHING AND LEARNING THEORIES

First, Claire and her family implement an insulin regimen better suited for euglycemia. This goal presumed an understanding of multiple-dose, split-mix insulin therapy. The type of learning is cognitive-Gestalt, in which the process of gaining or changing insights is critical. A reorganization of the family's cognitive field and problem-solving abilities is required, one of the attributes of this type of teaching and learning theory. Additionally, insights, concepts, and principles are needed to enhance the Pattersons' scientific thinking because the previous type of learning related to insulin resulted from a stimulus-response or behavioristic-conditioning learning process. In other words, the stimulus of hypoglycemia and convulsions resulted in a response that reinforced high blood glucose levels to diminish the undesired stimulus.

The recommended interventions teach Claire and her mother about her insulin requirements and the need to split the doses into four different injections, so that early morning high blood glucose levels can be accommodated and finer blood glucose control can be maintained. Claire's understanding about the link between high blood glucose levels and diet is reinforced by performing her own glucose monitoring, logging the results at different times during the day, and associating these levels with her food intake. The nurse instructors use a student/teacher-centered, individualized learning situation for Claire, so that she can understand the necessary relationships among diet, insulin, and exercise and then make decisions about adjusting them to maintain euglycemia.

Second, Claire demonstrates the ability to manage her diabetes independently by telephoning the nurse instructors 2 weeks after attendance at the course to report blood glucose levels and insulin dosages. This goal presumes that Claire has learned the principles of insulin, diet, and exercise and their effects on blood glucose levels as outlined in the first goal. An appropriate type of teaching and learning theory for this type of learning situation is social learning.

The recommended interventions include enhancing Claire's perceived self-efficacy or self-confidence that she can manage her diabetes without her mother's intercession.

The four discrete sources of information leading to perceived self-efficacy include personal mastery, vicarious experiences, verbal persuasion, and physiologic feedback. Claire develops personal mastery through her ability to interpret her blood glucose levels, based on her intake of food during the past 48 hours. Vicarious experiences are an important aspect of teaching and learning theory as applied in the diabetes teaching program. Claire's observation of one of the staff nurses in the program is paramount to her learning. This nurse had diabetes and yet maintained perfect metabolic control during her pregnancy. The nurse who shared this experience contributed to Claire's self-confidence. Additionally, the sharing of experiences by other patients who had managed to artfully wrest regulation from family members is an important vicarious learning experience for Claire. Another recommendation made to Claire by the center staff is that she attend a support group sponsored by the American Diabetes Association in Los Angeles.

SUMMARY

It may be difficult to accept the patient's prerogative to make a decision contrary to the suggestions offered by the health care provider. A broader understanding of the patient's choice can be gained from the applications of the Health Belief Model, models of stress and coping, social learning theory, and developmental theories. Learning why these issues arise and how to deal with patient decisions helps the health care provider remain committed to patient education. The ultimate role of the health care provider is to encourage patients to make informed choices about health, rather than to guarantee compliance or obedience. Strategies to help patients advocate for their own health education needs include empowerment theory and patient advocacy.

Understanding the theory related to teaching and learning helps the health professional understand the relationship between knowledge and action. Simply knowing or understanding is insufficient to bring about change in a patient's life; action must follow understanding. The health care provider who understands the principles of teaching and learning can better help the patient achieve desired health behaviors.

The theoretical foundation for teaching patients and families has now been defined. The next chapter will address how to help health care providers apply these principles to practice.

STRATEGIES FOR CRITICAL ANALYSIS AND APPLICATION

1. Using the concept of individual or psychological empowerment, design a program to increase adolescents' ability to withstand peer pressure to smoke.
2. Using Bandura's principles of personal mastery, vicarious experiences, verbal persuasion, and physiologic feedback, design a program to encourage men who are at risk to participate in prostate cancer screening. Which of these principles is the most difficult to incorporate in such a screening program?
3. Which stress and coping model would be most useful in understanding the teaching needs of a second-generation, unemployed, Chinese American with NIDDM? Why? In what type of situation would the other stress and coping model be most useful?
4. Using a lifespan developmental perspective, develop an individualized cardiac rehabilitation program for a 75-year-old woman 2 weeks after an acute MI. What are the cohort influences that may mitigate against her participation in cardiac rehabilitation at the YMCA?

To find the latest information

Key search terms
compliance, cooperation, alliance, learning theories, health behavior model, self-efficacy theory, stress, coping, ecological systems theory, lifespan development, lifespan psychology, learning, teaching, motivation, stages of change

Websites
- Stress and Deprivation: http://www.nlm.nih.gov/hmd/emotions/stress.html
- Urie Bronfenbrenner: http://www.psy.pdx.edu/PsiCafe/KeyTheorists/Bronfenbrenner.htm

REFERENCES

American Academy of Family Physicians. (2000). Patient education: Recommended core educational guidelines for family practice residents. *American Family Physician, 62*(7), 1712–1714.

Baldwin, M. A. (2003). Patient advocacy: A concept analysis. *Nursing Standard, 17*(21), 33–39.

Baltes, P. B., Staudinger, U. M., & Lindenberger, U. (1999). Lifespan psychology: Theory and application to intellectual functioning. *Annual Review of Psychology, 50,* 471–507.

Bandura, A. (1986). *Social foundations of thought and action: A social cognitive theory.* Englewood Cliffs, NJ: Prentice-Hall.

Bandura, A. (1997). *Self-efficacy: The exercise of control.* New York: W. H. Freeman.

Bastable, S. (2003). *Nurse as educator: Principles of teaching and learning for nursing practice* (2nd ed.). Sudbury, MA: Jones and Bartlett Publishers.

Bigge, M. L., & Shermis, S. S. (1998). *Learning theories for teachers* (6th ed.). New York: Harper Collins.

Blyth, R., Creedy, D. K., Dennis, C. L., Moyle, W., Pratt, J., & DeVries, S. M. (2002). Effect of maternal confidence on breastfeeding duration: An application of breastfeeding self-efficacy theory. *Birth, 29*(4), 278–284.

Bronefenbrenner, U. (1979). *The ecology of human development.* Cambridge, MA: Harvard University Press.

Bronefenbrenner, U. (1986). Ecology of the family as a context for human development. *Developmental Psychology, 22*(6), 723–742.

Brown, S. A. (1992). Meta-analysis of diabetes patient education research: Variations in intervention effects across studies. *Research in Nursing and Health, 15,* 409–419.

DiClemente, C. C., & Prochaska, J. O. (1998). Toward a comprehensive transtheoretical model of change: Stages of change and addictive behaviors. In W. R. Miller & N. Heather (Eds.), *Treating addictive behaviors* (2nd ed., pp, 3–24). New York: Plenum Press.

Gagne, R. M., & Driscoll, M. P. (1988). *Essentials of learning for instruction* (2nd ed.). Englewood Cliffs, NJ: Prentice Hall.

Haynes, R. B., McDonald, H. P., & Garg, A. X. (2002). Helping patients follow prescribed treatment. *JAMA, 288,* 2880–2883.

Hines, S. E. (2001). Heart disease in older women. *Patient Care for the Nurse Practitioner, 4*(5), 28–44.

Huckabay, L. (1980). *Conditions of learning and instruction in nursing.* St. Louis: C. V. Mosby.

Huitt, W. (December 2002). *A systems model of human behavior: The context of development.* Retrieved April 21, 2003, from http://chiron.valdosta.edu/whuitt/materials/sysmdlc.html

Lazarus, R. S. (1999). *Stress and emotion: A new synthesis.* New York: Springer.

Marinker, M., & Shaw, J. (2003). Not to be taken as directed: Putting concordance for taking medicines into practice. *BMJ, 326,* 348–349.

Parkin, T. (2001). An audit of the theoretical basis of education during dietetic consultations with diabetic patients. *Journal of Human Nutrition & Dietetics, 14*(1), 33–42.

Pearlin, L. I., & Skaff, M. M. (1996). Stress and the life course: A paradigmatic alliance. *The Gerontologist, 36*(2), 239–247.

Prochaska, J. O., Redding, C. A., Harlow, L. L., Rossi, J. S., & Velicer, W. F. (1994). The transtheoretical model of change and HIV prevention: A review. *Health Education Quarterly, 21*(4), 471–486.

Resnick, B. (2002). Geriatric rehabilitation: The influence of efficacy beliefs and motivation. *Rehabilitation Nursing, 27*(4), 152–159.

Thomas, R. J., Miller, N. H., Lamendola, C., Berra, K., Hedbäck, B., Durstine, J. L., et al. (1996). National survey on gender differences in cardiac rehabilitation programs. Patient characteristics and enrollment patterns. *Journal of Cardiopulmonary Rehabilitation, 16*(6), 402–412.

Vella, J. (1994). *Learning to listen, learning to teach: The power of dialogue in educating adults.* San Francisco: Jossey-Bass Publishers.

Whittemore, R. Q., Rankin, S. H., Callahan, C.D., Leder, M. C. & Carroll, D. L. (2000). I pointed out there is a tomorrow: The peer advisor experience providing special support. *Qualitative Health Research, 10*(2), 260–276.

Staff Development in Patient Education

LEARNING OBJECTIVES

After reading this chapter, the student should be able to:

1. Discuss three roles for staff development in planning organizational approaches to patient education.

2. Outline four JCAHO standards for patient and family education and corresponding teaching targets.

3. Describe continuing education interventions that prepare staff to provide quality patient and family education.

4. Identify four barriers perceived by health care providers in the provision of patient education, and interventions to overcome those barriers.

5. Provide examples of educational and institutional support to promote patient education expertise for nurses identified in Benner's four stages of skill acquisition.

6. Provide examples of age-specific approaches for teaching pediatric and geriatric patients.

INTRODUCTION

Patient Education Standards for Health Care Professionals

Licensed health care professionals are expected to provide patient and family education. Professional standards and job descriptions may vary in the details, but teaching always seems to be included. Box 5.1 provides specific examples of patient teaching in a variety of disciplines.

JCAHO Guidelines for Patient Education: Implications for Staff Development

To achieve accreditation by the Joint Commission on the Accreditation of Healthcare Organizations (JCAHO), health care organizations in the United States must show evidence that all patients receive teaching in which learning occurred. In addition to individualized teaching, JCAHO requires an organization-wide patient and family education focus and evidence of the impact of education on the patient and family. JCAHO standards require an interdisciplinary approach that includes the patient and family as a part of the health care team. Merged hospitals and hospital systems are surveyed as a single entity, requiring integration of patient education resources and programs (Joint Commission on Accreditation of Healthcare Organizations, 2001b).

JCAHO standards emphasize the need for all health care professionals to provide patient education as part of quality care. The responsibility to educate patients and families has broad implications for all who hold leadership and management positions in health care organizations (Box 5.2). Many education directors and staff development specialists have been challenged to develop their staff to be skilled teachers and to demonstrate patient learning outcomes. They

facilitate the coordination of patient education between members of the interdisciplinary health care team. They have been instrumental in helping merged organizations integrate education programs and coordinate patient education across the continuum of care.

This chapter reviews JCAHO Standards and Scoring Guidelines for Patient and Family Education and examines ways that staff development specialists can provide support and leadership in achieving successful JCAHO accreditation surveys. This information is also useful for those readers not in the United States because the principles of quality patient education are universal. This chapter also addresses key elements of individual and organization-wide teaching and the value of leadership in staff development to promote patient education within an organization. Along with this information, a plan for a patient education workshop is provided. The workshop addresses patient-centered approaches to patient education, including learning objectives, agenda, content outline, and teaching methodologies. The workshop plan illustrates how Chapters 7 through 11 of the text can be incorporated in a continuing education program.

The method by which nurses develop clinical expertise in patient teaching is also examined in this chapter, specifically by addressing the work of Benner and her colleagues (Benner, 2001). This discussion generalizes to all health care professionals. Finally, this chapter provides suggestions for motivating and developing staff competencies as patient teachers, and tailoring patient education with age-specific approaches.

Need for Innovation

Health care is now delivered across multiple settings, with only short hospital stays. There is no time to implement patient education programs designed to be delivered during the long hospitalizations of the past. Although the literature identifies considerable potential for nurses to take a lead role in patient

BOX 5.1 Examples of Professional Patient Education Expectations

Nurses
- Assist the patient to understand information related to a specific disease process
- Development, implementation, and evaluation of a patient teaching program for a group of individuals experiencing the same health condition
(McCloskey & Bulechek, 2000)

Pediatric Nurse Practitioners
- Identify realistic and achievable health goals for children and their families
- Evaluate individual readiness to learn
- Provide age-appropriate education based on growth and developmental factors, cultural and belief variables, and family systems
- Modify educational intervention as needed
- Provide families with guidance to learn skills that foster healthy behaviors
- Function as a resource person in health-related issues
- Evaluate the educational interventions provided and outcomes achieved
(The Association of Faculties of Pediatric Nurse Practitioner/Associate Programs & National Association of Pediatric Nurse Practitioners, 2000)

Nephrology Nurses
- Facilitate health promotion by providing education about, and assessment of, risk factors and early indicators of renal disease
(Canadian Association of Nephrology Nurses and Technologists. [2001, October 2001]. *Standards of Nursing Practice*. Retrieved 5/14, 2001, from http://www.cannt.ca/nursing_standards.htm)

Family Physicians
- Provide effective patient education by mastering a variety of practical skills. These include ascertaining patients' educational needs, identifying barriers to learning, counseling concisely, evaluating and utilizing written, audiovisual and computer-based patient education materials, and incorporating education into routine office visits.
(American Academy of Family Physicians, 2000)

Pharmacists
- Elicit the needs, values, desired level of care and desired outcomes of the patient
- Encourage and support the patient's right to make choices
- Provide appropriate information to facilitate the patient's understanding of his or her drug therapy and ability to comply with the therapy regimen
(National Association of Pharmacy Regulatory Authorities, 2003)

Physical Therapists
- Educate patients/clients, family, and caregivers, using relevant and effective teaching methods to assure optimal patient care outcomes
(Federation of State Boards of Physical Therapists, 2002)

Registered Dietitians
- Provide dietetics education in supervised practice settings
- Supervise counseling, education, and/or other interventions in health promotion/disease prevention for patients/clients needing medical nutrition therapy for uncomplicated instances of common conditions, eg, hypertension, obesity, diabetes, and diverticular disease
- Supervise education and training for target groups
- Develop and review educational materials for target populations
(Commission on Accreditation for Dietetics Education, & American Dietetic Association, 2002)

BOX 5.2 Management Responsibility for Patient Education

- Incorporate patient education in the mission and strategic priorities of the organization
- Assure an environment that regards patient education efforts and outcomes
- Provide an organizational infrastructure to oversee, deliver, and support patient education
- Incorporate patient and staff education into policies, procedures, and protocols
- Ensure that performance improvement efforts address patient education
- Provide critical resources (eg, staff, materials) for patient education

Source: Adapted with permission from *Educating Hospital Patients and Their Families* by Joint Commission on the Accreditation of Healthcare Organizations; 1996. Oakbrook Terrace, IL.

education, this is rarely achieved in practice (Nolan, Nolan, & Booth, 2001). For example, one study of nurses in a rehabilitation hospital found teaching was an ad hoc activity, with heavy reliance on giving information without evaluation of understanding, and documentation of teaching activities and outcomes was a low priority (Turner, Wellard, & Bethune, 1999). This may reflect actual practice in other settings.

Health care providers become frustrated when they try to teach too much material in too short a time. Many do not know how to streamline teaching, or how to coordinate teaching with other members of the health care team. They need continuing education and coaching to learn to collaborate, and to focus their teaching on survival skills and patient outcomes. Hospitals must refine patient education programs and devise teaching interventions that reach homes and outpatient clinics, so patients can learn, within the time available, how to manage their own care.

Patient education has a pressing need for innovation. Research can help us identify effective and efficient teaching methods. For example, in one study, clinical areas with a patient-centered philosophy of care and some degree of continuity of contact provided more developed medication teaching than clinical areas with brief and episodic contact between health care providers and patients. This study suggested the acuity and workload challenges to teaching could be offset by a patient-centered, partnership-focused philosophy of care (Rycroft-Malone et al., 2000).

BEYOND MEETING JCAHO STANDARDS: PRINCIPLES AND STRATEGIES FOR STAFF DEVELOPMENT

The Challenges for Staff Development

Staff development and training are comprehensive terms used to describe all the different ways in which people can be encouraged to increase, update, and adapt their knowledge, skills, personal abilities, and competencies in order to fulfill both current and possible future demands at work (Staff Development and Training, 2003). Within the health care professions, employers provide staff development to expand and improve competencies (see Box 5.3).

Organizations cannot afford for staff development to stand on the sidelines of patient education efforts. Staff development can help improve the competencies of health care professionals to provide patient teaching in a rapidly changing health care delivery system. Powerful staff development activities may include:

1. Providing leadership, oversight, or coordination of organization-wide approaches to patient education
2. Evaluating the skills of health care professionals in providing patient education, through competency measures, and

---

BOX 5.3 Staff Development Issues and Roles

Issues:

- Motivate health care professionals to teach
- Determine staff education and training needs
- Promote documentation of evaluation of understanding and outcomes of learning
- Streamline outdated teaching protocols
- Motivate health care professionals to collaborate their teaching, and communicate the status of teaching to other team members
- Use clinical nurse specialists and patient education specialists efficiently and effectively

Roles

- Formal, ongoing training related to work responsibilities (eg, JCAHO standards)
- Socialization into work setting to increase competence and excellence (eg, coaching, feedback, mentoring staff)
- Improving group performance to achieve quality and excellence (eg, making sure patient education programs are visible and valued)

---

enhancing skills as needed

3. Identifying barriers that health care providers perceive in the delivery of patient education, and designing strategies in partnership with management to create an environment that facilitates teaching
4. Providing ongoing training about standards for patient and family education
5. Teaching managers, supervisors, and health care providers how to meet standards and show evidence of patient learning

6. Helping the organization develop interdisciplinary patient education programs and interventions that are focused on patient survival skills, and realistic for the patient's length of stay
7. Raising awareness of the need for innovative approaches to patient education based on patient needs. Models for patient teaching must span both inpatient and outpatient settings and involve patients in prioritizing learning needs along a continuum of care. They focus on health promotion, risk factor reduction, and disease management.

In the context of JCAHO standards, this chapter outlines the developmental needs of an organization and its staff relative to patient education, and offers suggestions for staff development interventions. These principles apply to readers outside of the United States as well.

JCAHO Standards for Patient Education

The Joint Commission on the Accreditation of Healthcare Organizations supports the notion of patient-centered care with patient education as the centerpiece for involving patients as important members of the health care team. Health care providers can bring this concept to life by providing patients with information in the right place at the right time.

Table 5.1 outlines the JCAHO 2001 patient and family education goals. As members of the management team, staff development professionals must interpret an overall approach and ensure that quality patient education services are provided. Table 5.1 is useful for teaching managers and staff about JCAHO's expectations for outcomes. The organization must provide evidence that it assesses the need for focused programs and allocates resources to accomplish them. Health care providers who have the skills, interest, and time to teach patients are the organization's most important resource.

TABLE 5.1 Organizational Approach to Patient Education

Goal of the patient and family education:

To improve patient health outcomes by promoting healthy behavior and involving the patient in care and care decisions.

Education should:	Practical applications:
• promote interactive communication between patients and providers • enable and encourage patients to be involved in decisions about their own care • improve patients' understanding of their health status, options for treatment, and the anticipated risks and benefits of treatment • maximize patient self-care skills, which support recovery and a speedy return to function • increase the patient's ability to cope with his or her health status • increase the likelihood that patients will follow their therapeutic plans of care and participate in continuing care • promote healthy behaviors and lifestyles • inform patients about their financial responsibilities for treatment when known	• Assess organization-wide patient education programs and activities • Formulate patient education program goals • Allocate resources for patient education • Determine and prioritize specific patient educational needs • Provide education to meet identified patient needs

Source: Joint Commission on Accreditation of Healthcare Organizations (JCAHO). (2001b). *2001 Comprehensive Accreditation Manual for Hospitals Update 3: Joint Commission on Accreditation of Healthcare Organizations.*

The JCAHO standards recommend a systematic approach to patient education be demonstrated throughout the organization, with a philosophy that views the educational function as an interactive one in which both parties are learners. JCAHO does not describe specific structures or personnel titles. Organizations are encouraged to focus on their current processes and on how continuity of care is best accomplished (Box 5.4).

JCAHO standards address patient-focused care, including organizational approaches and individualized patient and family activities. Table 5.2 lists three standards that relate to specific educational needs of patients and families, with targets for patient-centered interventions, and evidence the standards have been met. To effectively assess and evaluate understanding to ensure these standards are met, the health care provider and learner must interact in two-way communication (Krozek & Scoggins, 2001).

Implementing an Organization-Wide Approach

The implementation process is key to successful patient education outcomes. The organization must assign responsibility for overseeing or directing the implementation of patient education, which may be assigned to a patient education coordinator or to the director of a department. This individual is referred to as the coordinator, although responsibility for patient education activities

---

BOX 5.4 Continuity of Care

• Interdisciplinary coordination
• Interunit and interservice coordination
• Interagency coordination
• Focus on discharge and patient safety

TABLE 5.2 2001 JCAHO Standards for Patient and Family Education

STANDARD	TARGETS	EVIDENCE
Standard PF.1 The hospital plans for and supports the provision and coordination of patient education activities.	• Learning environment • Staff competency to teach • Processes and procedures to identify and respond to learning needs • Collaborative/interdisciplinary educational resources and services • Performance improvement process	• Patient education activities and resources provided • Resources provided based on patient needs • Health care team involvement • Education is continuous, safe, timely, efficient, caring, and respectful
Standard PF.2 The patient education process is coordinated among appropriate staff or disciplines who are providing care or services.	• Continuing care needs and provider identified • Instructions provided to continuing care providers	• Any discharge instructions given to the patient/family are provided to the organization responsible for patient's continuing care.
Standard PF.3 The patient receives education and training specific to the patient's assessed needs, abilities, learning preferences, and readiness to learn as appropriate to the care and services provided by the hospital.	• Survival skills for safe discharge • Safe and effective use of medications • Modified diets, potential drug–food interactions, oral health • Safe and effective use of medical equipment and supplies • Pain management • Community resources • How to obtain further treatment, care, or services • Ongoing health care needs, rehabilitation, hygiene and grooming • Patient informed consent • Patient informed of responsibilities • Patient/family understanding of current health problem/reason for admission • Patient/family understanding of treatment plan and the role they will play in it • Priorities for individual learning needs, sequencing with patient readiness	• Policies, procedures, progress notes, flowsheets, referral and consultation notes, interviews with staff and patients, written information given to patients and families • Patient assessment considers physical and cognitive limitations, language barriers, cultural and religious practices, emotional barriers, motivation to learn, and financial implications of care choices. • Patient learning needs identified • Educational plan implemented with patient feedback • Priorities for education identified for each patient • Information understandable to patient • Teaching is culturally appropriate • Written discharge instructions, understandable to patient, include lifestyle changes • Discharge planning involves patient/family • Discharge instructions clear: who is to do what • Academic needs met, if appropriate

Source: Joint Commission on Accreditation of Healthcare Organizations (JCAHO). (2001a). *2001 Hospital Accreditation Standards*: Joint Commission on Accreditation of Healthcare Organizations.

is shared throughout an organization and across disciplines. Many staff development directors have been assigned responsibilities as coordinators of the organization-wide approach.

Although we have instituted individual patient education programs to meet the needs of particular patient groups, we do not recommend this single-shot approach to implementing patient education at the organization level. A single-shot approach tends to be hurried and crisis motivated; staff efforts are typically directed toward the most obvious needy group. Instead, we suggest conducting a systematic patient education needs assessment.

Conducting a Needs Assessment for the Organization

A needs assessment is the cornerstone for planning and implementing patient education. A needs assessment allows long-range planning and direction, so that continuity of program planning is ensured, regardless of leadership or personnel changes. Box 5.5 offers the types of questions to ask before designing a comprehensive patient education program. These questions can be modified for use in assessing educational needs in many settings across the continuum of care.

Appointing a Steering Committee

The role of the interdisciplinary Patient Education Committee is two-fold. In the short term, the group can determine if the organization is meeting Joint Commission standards, and if not, what needs to be changed to do so. The interdisciplinary Patient Education Committee can also act as a resource for reviewing teaching programs and tools, and provide a system for managing teaching resources.

An interdisciplinary Patient Education Committee should be appointed early in the implementation process. The committee acts in an advisory fashion, and should include representation from each discipline of health care providers (such as nurses, physicians, nutritionists, and pharmacists), administrators, and others who have an active interest in patient education. A patient education coordinator, hospital education director, or clinical specialist is usually responsible for initiating the committee and should judiciously gather recommendations for committee members. Appointment of physicians should be made by the medical staff, with a preference for physicians who are known proponents of patient education. Nurses at the decision-making level should be appointed to the steering committee with the input of the nursing service coordinator. Include other health professionals along the continuum of care, because their cooperation can enhance patient education programs.

After the assessment is complete, the patient coordinator will have a database to help the advisory committee organize and direct the organization's efforts. While the needs assessment is conducted and the advisory committee is appointed, the committee coordinator should review the literature to learn about what types of programs have worked, why they have been successful, and where they have been implemented. A great deal of information can be gathered from the successes and mistakes of others, and it is limiting to ignore the ever-increasing quantity of material about diverse patient education programs. The perspective of staff providing direct patient care is critical to the development of realistic, effective, and creative patient education resources. One method of evaluating patient education is offered in Box 5.6. Ask staff nurses for their assessment of patient education needs and challenges, and their suggestions for areas needing improvement. Interviews may provide different information from written questionnaires; both can be useful. Contacting people involved with patient education efforts in other community and inpatient settings maybe helpful. These individuals can share ideas about the needs of the community and help prevent duplication of efforts.

Establishing Goals and Priorities

Once the patient education needs assessment is complete, the goals and priorities for program development must be set. Two levels of patient education need to be supported: individualized teaching for each patient and family, and programs targeting specific patient populations.

BOX 5.5 Assessing the Status of Patient Education in the Organization

1. Hospital philosophy, goals, and policies
   - What is the philosophy of the hospital and what are the goals for patient care? Do these goals require the implementation of patient education?
   - Documents that can be obtained from administrators or the board of trustees can provide this information.
2. Organization of the hospital staff
   - What types of staff members are employed?
3. Patient care support staff
   - Who is responsible for orientation of all new hospital patient care staff?
   - Data pertaining to this question can be obtained by contacting department heads or by sending them a questionnaire.
4. Characteristics of the patient population
   - What are the most common diagnoses, diagnosis-related groups (DRGs), and surgical procedures for the various hospital units? What are the high-risk or high-volume diagnoses, patient groups, or product lines that are commonly identified by staff in various departments?
   - Answers to these questions can be obtained from the admitting office and its computerized data banks and from medical records. Interviews of various nursing and medical personnel also may be helpful.
5. Patient admission
   - What information is made available to patients before admission to inpatient services, short-stay surgery, or outpatient services?
   - Contact a variety of sources to answer this question. Interviews can be conducted or questionnaires can be sent to admitting and short-stay surgery and outpatient services. Also, contact the public relations department, admitting staff physicians, and community referral agencies.
6. Patient care process
   - How are patient care goals determined and revised? Do the medical, nursing, dietary, and other staff groups use a team planning method to assist in determining goals? Are patients included in the goal planning process?
   - Answers to these questions can be obtained by interviewing head nurses and other unit managers involved in patient care services. Consider mailing questionnaires to patients who have been recently discharged.
7. Staff perceptions of current and needed patient education programs
   - What patient education programs or activities are currently implemented? Are they conducted on each shift? What resources, in terms of audiovisual, printed, and other media, are being used in these efforts?
   - Interview or send questionnaires to head nurses, appropriate department heads, and supervisors who may be involved with patient teaching.
8. Adequacy of existing patient education programs for specific populations
   - Are there written goals and objectives for each patient education activity and are they evaluated after the patient completes the activity?
   - Answers to these questions should be obtained for all programs or for activities presently being conducted in the institution. Sources of information include extensive interviews with the staff responsible for the programs, review of written program materials, and participation in a program.

(continued)

BOX 5.5 Assessing the Status of Patient Education in the Organization *(Continued)*

9. Patient education resources within the hospital
   - What types of media are available within the hospital for patient teaching? What types of appropriations have been made for the purchase of audiovisual media, closed circuit television, and software? Where are patient education materials located, catalogued, and reviewed? Does staff use the materials? Are materials up-to-date?
   - For the answers, contact department managers, hospital administrators, and staff on the units.
10. Patient education resources in the community
   - Which community patient care agen-

cies provide follow-up care on discharge from the hospital? How do they interpret their role in patient education? Is there a feedback mechanism between the community agency and the hospital?
   - Answers to these questions can be obtained by contacting the community agencies that have been identified by staff as being involved in follow-up care. Also contact case managers, discharge planning nurses, or social workers.

Source: Adapted from: American Hospital Association. (1979). *Implementing Patient Education in the Hospital.* Chicago: American Hospital Association.

The advisory committee should wisely identify objectives. When attempting to forge new alliances in patient education programs that involve multiple disciplines and care settings, it may be helpful to focus the attention and resources on one or two major issues at a time.

Creating Task Forces for Specific Programs

After priorities and goals are determined, and a specific patient education program is identified for creation, a task force should be appointed. For example, if the committee decides to develop a new education program for patients with chronic obstructive pulmonary disease (COPD), then the multidisciplinary task force to do it should include health professionals in all departments that care for COPD patients. It is essential that a physician be on this task force, because approval must be gained from the medical staff to implement the teaching program.

However, including physicians on these task forces does not always guarantee wide medical staff approval. Also, when planning the program, providers who care for patients in the community should be invited, such as those in physician's offices and home health, in order to promote continuity of care.

Evaluating the Program

Evaluation of patient education programs presents some of the most difficult problems encountered in the entire patient teaching venture. (Chapter 11 discusses the many aspects and issues associated with the evaluation of patient learning.) Evaluation design is an integral part of program planning. Including a design for evaluation in any proposal for funding will make administrators more likely to approve the program. Evaluation frequently occurs after a patient education program has been well established. This type of evaluation procedure should augment a formative evaluation procedure

BOX 5.6 Staff Questionnaire Regarding Patient Education

This questionnaire asks for your assessment of patient education needs and challenges. It is part of an organization-wide effort to strengthen patient education programs and resources. The perspective of front-line staff is critical to the development of realistic, effective, and creative strategies for patient education.

   Please answer all of the questions from your own experiences in your department, service, or unit. If a question does not apply to you, please write N/A/. Feel free to add any thoughts, feelings, or opinions to your answers. Whenever possible, please offer suggestions for areas that need improvement.

1. Are you satisfied with the quality of education that your patients receive?
2. Do you think that patient education resources are adequate to prepare patients for discharge from your service?
3. For what **percentage of patients** on your service are interdisciplinary teaching plans (or critical paths) used for patient education?
4. Are current teaching plans realistic based on the average length of patient stay or the number of home visits?
5. Please list three most frequent patient diagnoses on your service.
6. Please identify three learning outcomes, or survival skills, that are essential for patients with the diagnoses listed in question 5.

7. What is one thing you have done during the past year to improve the patient education that is provided on your service? Feel free to list more than one, if you wish.
8. How would you rate interdisciplinary communication regarding patient education on your service?
   Excellent   Good   Fair   Poor
9. How would you rate the documentation of patient learning outcomes on your service?
   Excellent   Good   Fair   Poor
10. What opportunities are needed for staff to gain additional skills in patient education? Please list specific topics, issues, or needs.
11. Do you think that providing good patient education is valued and recognized by your supervisor?   Yes   No
12. What problem or challenge most frequently prevents patients and families from receiving needed education? Feel free to mention more than one.

   _____
   _____
   _____
   _____

Thank you for taking the time to complete this questionnaire. If you have any other ideas or concerns that are not addressed in the questions, you are encouraged to offer additional comments below and on the back of the page.

that aids refinement of the educational interventions during a pilot phase.

   Many different outcomes exist, and it is impossible, if not inappropriate, to evaluate all of them. Many nurses and physicians view the outcome of patient education in terms of desired patient compliance. Although compliance is desirable, many other positive outcomes of patient education exist. Therefore, a major issue in evaluation is deciding which

outcome should be evaluated and whether this outcome indicates that the program is beneficial.

   The desired outcome must be related to the type of intervention. For example, if you are educating a group of 13-year-olds on the relationship of cigarette smoking to cardiovascular disease and lung cancer, the desired outcome is prevention of smoking. If you are educating a group of the teenagers' smoking parents, however, the desired outcome is cessation of smoking. Outcomes must be measurable, and reflective of the goals of the program.

As more research is conducted on the relationship of knowledge acquisition to behavioral change, it becomes clear that acquisition of knowledge does not always guarantee the desired behavioral change. When we apply this concept to our group of cigarette-smoking patients, we may decide that a realistic short-term outcome is simply knowledge about the effects of smoking. Perhaps later a behavioral change, cessation of smoking, will occur; this may or may not be related to the knowledge acquisition.

Regardless, an argument can be made for improving and increasing the patient's knowledge and understanding of his or her health status, even if it does not lead to improved adherence to and cooperation with the medical regimen. Increasing the patient's understanding of his or her health can be interpreted as part of the patient's legal right to know. A patient deserves the information even if he or she chooses not to act on it.

JCAHO (2001b) defines the following outcomes as important:

- Patient participation in decision-making about health care options
- The increased potential to follow the health care plan
- The development of self-care skills
- Increased patient and family coping
- Enhanced participation in continuing care
- Healthy lifestyle

Evaluating the costs of patient education is imperative. Hospital administrators must calculate staff time, materials, and education equipment as part of the cost of care. In most cases, well-planned and executed patient education can be shown to decrease length of stay and costs of hospitalization. Documentation of this can be used to justify the professional staff time needed to teach. This information also can be used to determine the efficacy of specialized outpatient teaching programs versus inpatient teaching.

It is helpful to consider which outcomes to measure for whom, and what should be done with the findings.

Staffing for Patient Education

The types of staffing needed for patient education must be addressed. It requires more registered nurse (RN) hours to provide high-quality patient education. Nursing education provides the critical thinking skills needed to teach patients and families. Most licensed practical nurses (LPNs) have not been taught the fundamentals of patient teaching during their formal educational programs, and are not prepared to assume this role without additional training and supervision. An organization heavily staffed with LPNs and aides cannot deliver as much high-quality patient education as can a larger or more professionally staffed institution.

The registered nurse cannot delegate patient education to personnel who are not prepared to conduct a thorough assessment of learning needs. We have found that LPNs involved in prenatal education in an outpatient setting were willing and enthusiastic about attending classes but were unprepared and unable to lead patient discussions or to teach or lecture components of the class. LPNs can frequently reinforce patient education performed initially by RNs, but they should not be delegated the primary teaching responsibility.

The debate about the appropriateness of delegating patient teaching to multi-skilled workers or other unlicensed (less expensive) staff is often encountered by staff development professionals. Patient education is not a procedure, but an interactive process that involves knowledge about the topic being taught, assessment, critical thinking, negotiation, and evaluation of understanding. Health care professionals need time to provide patient education. The amount of staff time needed for patient education varies with the number of disease processes covered, and the sophistication and experience of the health care professionals. Patient teaching protocols or care maps and the amount of preparation the staff has in teaching and learning theory also influence the amount of staff time required to accomplish teaching. When health care professionals document the learner's response to education, they can also document the amount of time spent teaching. This information can help evaluate the overall effectiveness of the patient education program.

How well are nurses prepared to implement standardized teaching plans and individualize them based on patient needs and length of stay? Assess whether the staff who teach patients has received formal preparation in the use of standardized teaching plans, what teaching resources are provided in the organization, and where staff gets assistance with teaching for difficult patient situations.

Political and Financial Issues

Political and financial issues are often encountered in the planning of organizational approaches to patient education. For example, if those who control a budget are opposed to a patient education effort, implementing a program may be more difficult. Our experience is that if health care administrators and key physicians believe in the efficacy of patient education, then implementation is fairly straightforward. However, if these individuals think that patient education is not cost-beneficial, patient education programs may be extremely difficult to initiate, especially in light of budget shortfalls and competing demands for scarce resources.

Promoting patient education as a strategy to reduce the high cost of health care through prevention, as a purveyor of better patient services, and as a way of securing more consumer participation is helpful. In some communities with many medical facilities, patient education has been used as a marketing tool. Programs have sought the interest of the middle-class, well-educated learners with programs on cholesterol reduction, stress

abatement, parenting, and women's health issues. Efforts to address health education issues related to social problems (such as homelessness, teen pregnancy, AIDS, and substance abuse) have been largely ignored by both proprietary and nonprofit hospitals, because they address uninsured and underinsured populations.

With rising health care costs, decisions about the expenditure of increasingly tight funds must be made. The public, urged on in many cases by health professionals, is demanding greater technocracy and more lifesaving assistance devices, which cause the costs of health care to skyrocket. To health care professionals who have been committed to patient education and who have been actively promoting it in their organizations, the JCAHO standards and surveys provide important support and ammunition for the effort. The mandates and priorities of JCAHO have required attention to assessing the learning needs of patients and families and evidence of effective responses to these needs.

JCAHO Standards and Scoring Guidelines

Joint Commission surveyors look for adherence to the patient education standards. They look for evidence that health care providers identified priorities for teaching and provided individualized care for patients. They look for evidence of the patient and family's response to care. For example, does the medical record indicate how the patient responded to teaching, what he or she understood? It must be shown that teaching related to survival skills for safe discharge and strategies to enhance continuity of care was provided to all patients.

Patient education outcomes should be evident in 90% or more of patients' records. To score well in a survey, the organization strives to demonstrate that patient education is an integral part of care for every patient, not just patients who receive a specialized teaching protocol.

Hospitalization is a learning experience for every patient and family. Patient outcomes include evidence of the patient's response to teaching. (Chapters 8 through 12 offer examples of the range of needs, interventions, and outcomes that can be documented.) JCAHO surveyors look for evidence that information is understandable and usable to the patient, including considerations of non-English-speaking patients, patients with low literacy skills, and patients with sight, hearing, and processing difficulties. Educational needs and opportunities along the continuum of care should be viewed, and opportunities to incorporate health promotion for patients and families should be identified.

Evidence of individual patient and family learning include organizational policies and procedures, patient progress notes, flow sheets, referral and consultation notes, interviews with staff, written information provided to the patient and family, and interviews with staff and patients (Box 5.7).

Three standards comprise the directives for patient-focused teaching. Review the standards to appreciate the many examples of practical application. The following tips will help educators emphasize key points with staff.

JCAHO Standard PF.1

The hospital plans for and supports the provision and coordination of patient education activities.

BOX 5.7 JCAHO Focus

- Adherence to standards
- Evidence of priorities, individualized care
- Evidence of patient/family response
- Information understandable, usable to patient
- 91%–100% patients taught
- Continuity of care

TEACHING TARGETS

The organizational assessment described earlier in this chapter has resulted in the provision, coordination, and evaluation of quality learning interventions that are based on specific needs. They may include classes, community resources, videos, reading materials, presentations, and various other formats. The staff is provided with education to become skilled patient educators.

EVIDENCE

Documentation reports evaluation of effectiveness of individual teaching sessions, participation in classes, and the use of closed circuit television. (Chapter 12 provides examples of documentation.) Learning activities should be selected based on individual priority needs and length of stay. Nursing staff and other team members should acknowledge that they might not meet all the learning needs of the patient; instead, the focus is to assess the individual's learning needs, teach essentials, reinforce more, and communicate remaining teaching needs to continuing care providers. The organization-wide needs assessment should be documented and resulting programs should include standardized approaches, and educational resources used to promote learning. Well-prepared staff is the most critical resource for providing patient education.

Standard PF.2

The patient education process is coordinated among appropriate staff or disciplines that are providing care or services.

TEACHING TARGETS

Patient education is interdisciplinary, collaborative, and coordinated across the continuum of care. The process of patient education should not overwhelm the patient. Health care team involvement strengthens, streamlines, and individualizes care to address the patient's functional problems. Continuing care needs and instructions must be provided to continuing care providers.

EVIDENCE

Documentation reflects collaboration between interdisciplinary health care providers in educating the patient. All discharge instructions given to the patient and family are provided to the organization responsible for the patient's continuing care.

Standard PF.3

The patient receives education and training specific to the patient's assessed needs, abilities, learning preferences, and readiness to learn as appropriate to the care and services provided by the hospital.

TEACHING TARGETS

The patient and family should understand the current health problem or the reason for admission. This sounds obvious, but many patients do not know why they are hospitalized or cannot express it in their own words. Understanding the purpose of the hospitalization, and acknowledging the episode or symptoms that precipitated it, are important lessons in managing chronic illness.

To address health promotion goals, consider the following question: What brought this patient to this place at this time, and could the acute episode have been prevented? The answer to this question helps formulate an individualized teaching plan. The patient and family should be taught about the proposed treatment plan and the role they would play in it. Before a final drug, diet, or exercise regimen is prescribed, teaching should include the expectation the patient will participate actively in his or her recovery. Patients should receive an overview of the survival skills needed for discharge and explore their individual learning needs. Teaching priorities are based on survival and safety issues, and patient assessment is key. (Chapters 7 and 8 discuss the process of assessing critical learning needs.) The targets indicate priority areas that must be addressed if they apply to the patient, such as medications, medical equipment, food/drug interactions, diets, rehabilitation

skills, community resources, and ongoing health care needs. When appropriate, patients should receive written instructions that they can understand. (See Chapter 9 for information on preparing one-page discharge instructions that promote patient understanding.)

The patient and family receive individualized education specific to their assessed needs, abilities, readiness, and length of stay. Patient teaching is not dictated by medical diagnosis, but focuses on each patient's functional problems. Ask the question: How does this diagnosis affect this patient? The patient and family are also asked to contribute to this assessment, are actively involved in setting goals for their learning, and indicate preferences for the teaching methods to be used. The patient and family are educated to increase their knowledge of their diagnosis, treatment options, and skills needed to participate in their recovery and rehabilitation. The assessment considers cultural and religious practices, emotional barriers, physical and cognitive limitations, language barriers, growth and development of the patient, financial implications of care, and patient and family motivation.

Patients must be informed about how to obtain further treatment, including possible emergency treatment and follow-up appointments. Discharge planning clearly involves the patient and family, and instructions promote safe and continuing care.

EVIDENCE

All patients receive instruction. Documentation reflects assessment of patient's learning needs, evaluation of understanding, and readiness for self-care.

Patient assessment should include the patient's current understanding of the health problem; prior knowledge, beliefs, or values that influence care; statements in the patient's own words that reflect an understanding of the health problem; and willingness to participate. Documentation includes quotes from the patient and family about their needs and progress.

A copy of discharge instructions should be in the patient record and should also be forwarded to appropriate parties. Instructions should be readable, usable, and understandable. A JCAHO surveyor might ask a patient what kinds of written information have been provided, and to explain what other instructions he or she has been given about care.

Teaching priorities are based on the reason for admission, individual safety needs, and length of stay. The JCAHO surveyor may ask patients why they are in the hospital, what staff is doing to help them prepare for discharge, and what things the patients expect they will need to do to participate in their own care.

Preparing for Patient-Centered Care: Profile of a Teaching Program for Nurses and Other Staff

A formal teaching program may be effective in centralizing organizational values and approaches for patient education. The authors have found that full-day workshops best meet this need, with content and learning activities carefully planned to promote teamwork and critical thinking. Table 5.3 outlines an interdisciplinary workshop developed by Karen Stallings, one of the authors of this book.

TABLE 5.3 Workshop: Patient-Centered Approaches to Patient Education

OBJECTIVES	CONTENT	TIME	METHODOLOGY
I. List three goals of patient education.	I. JCAHO Standards and Scoring Guidelines	8:40–9:40 AM	Lecture, discussion, handout
II. Identify four levels of patient learning outcomes.	II. Four levels of evaluation	9:40–10:00 AM	Lecture
III. Describe how the Health Belief Model can be used to understand and influence patient behavior.	III. A. Cooperation vs. compliance B. Barriers to cooperation C. Patient motivation D. Application of model E. Patient decisions	10:15–11:00 AM	Lecture, group exercise, dyads, discussion, handouts
IV. List five concerns of hospitalized patients	IV. A. Pain B. Cure C. Scarring/deformity D. Burden on others E. Dying	11:00–11:30 AM	Discussion, handouts
V. List four questions a nurse can ask to determine priorities for patient teaching.	V. A. Safe discharge B. Complications/readmission C. Past experience D. Equipment used at home	12:45–2:00 PM	Lecture, case studies, discussion
VI. Discuss guidelines to improve the effectiveness and safety of videotapes and written discharge instructions.	VI. A. Content B. Format C. Organization D. Emergency plan E. Follow-up	2:15–3:30 PM	Lecture, discussion video preview/evaluation
Wrap-up/Evaluation	Review Objectives I–VI	3:30–4:00 PM	Q & A discussion

Goals of a Workshop

Workshop participants should include direct care providers of all disciplines, managers, and administrators. Participants are instructed that regardless of setting, three universal goals of patient education always exist:

- Developing survival skills
- Recognizing problems
- Making decisions

Focusing on three critical items in a workshop promotes learning retention. The workshop begins with a simple set of concepts, which are reinforced throughout the day. Participants may come to a workshop feeling overwhelmed at the prospect of teaching sick patients in limited time. The workshop is intended to give health care providers permission and skills to teach smarter instead of faster and harder. The three universal goals are applied to the JCAHO standards, demonstrating how the goals are a template for accreditation. Using small-group discussions and case study analysis, participants examine how the JCAHO might survey for outcomes and develop examples of learning outcomes that could be accomplished in various settings, from intensive to long-term care. Participants review key compliance challenges common to the JCAHO survey and how they are addressed in their practice area (Box 5.8).

Principles to Application

Workshop attendees discuss methods to streamline documentation and provide a snapshot of the patient's involvement in learning. How participants currently provide patient education is explored, often exposing issues over discipline turf battles and lack of coordination, which adversely affect patient-centered approaches. The focus of the workshop shifts to the process of patient education from a patient's perspective. The issue of compliance is highlighted as workshop participants are asked to answer a survey about their own health behaviors, including smok-

> **BOX 5.8** Hot Buttons: Key Compliance Challenges in JCAHO Surveys
>
> - Policy on how teaching is to be accomplished across the continuum of care
> - Teaching about potential food and/or drug interactions
> - Culturally relevant strategies and resources
> - Age-appropriate teaching (especially for older patients, children, adolescents)
> - Assessment of readiness to learn; emotional, physical, cognitive, and language barriers to learning
> - Teaching about medications patients will manage at home
> - Diet teaching for patients who are on a new or modified diet
> - Documented evidence learners understood teaching
> - Teaching about personal hygiene for patients who can no longer follow normal routine

ing, seat belt use, diet, exercise, and medication use. Participants, in analyzing why they often do not practice what they preach to patients, identify the challenges of motivating patients to change their behaviors. The wisdom of expecting three or four simultaneous lifelong behavior changes is questioned. The steps of the Health Belief Model are reviewed, with strategies for influencing patient decisions toward healthy lifestyles. Patient concerns are also discussed. Recommendations are offered to sequence patient education, based on the priority concerns of patients. Education about pain and pain management is discussed.

Critical needs for patient teaching are identified, based on the content of Chapters 7 through 11. Principles for streamlining teaching are introduced and applied to case studies. This part of a workshop often evokes lively discussion and differing opinions, based on the practice and education backgrounds of the participants. With the use of case studies, practice and feedback are provided to identify no more than three or four critical learning objectives for each patient, find ways to teach and observe performance as an integral part of care, and document based on what the patient accomplished or demonstrated.

Because of the importance placed on media for patient learning, the workshop concludes with a lecture and critique of patient education handouts and videos. These teaching tools must reflect the same targeted, streamlined approach based on length of stay, and the effectiveness of these tools must be evaluated. The information presented to participants is derived from Chapter 9 of this book. Examples of short, effective instructions are provided. The importance and challenges of creating a single, one-page, interdisciplinary set of discharge instructions is emphasized. As video and computer-assisted instruction become more sophisticated and affordable, they will allow practical application for patient education in both homes and hospitals. Continuing education offerings must prepare staff to use these technologies wisely and to evaluate their effectiveness. Throughout the workshop, participants are asked to describe barriers in their work setting that may prevent them from effectively providing patient education. As staff development practitioners know, learners often identify administrative and educational issues. Educators must carry the messages between staff and management to facilitate creation and maintenance of an environment that supports patient education.

Confronting Barriers to Patient Teaching

These workshops conducted by the authors identified four recurring themes as barriers that limit staff nurses' abilities to teach patients effectively: time restrictions, need for teaching skills, uncoordinated teaching efforts, and lack of notice or reward. When these barriers are addressed with ongoing training and management support, patient education and staff satisfaction can be significantly enhanced (London, 1999).

BARRIER 1: TIME RESTRICTIONS

Outdated protocols and teaching plans are impossible to implement in today's environment. Consequently, teaching is often reported as unrealistic, time consuming, and competitive with other facets of work. Health care providers often perceive patient education as a formal activity separate from routine care. Because of this perception, health care providers benefit from coaching to learn how to incorporate teaching into every patient encounter. They need to see role models demonstrate how to informally teach.

Staff development must assess the work setting and determine how to destroy barriers. For example, do teaching plans need to be streamlined? Are new teaching materials needed? Do the demands of paperwork, staffing, and supervision prevent staff from the patient contact required for teaching? Who are the patient education experts that can coach staff?

BARRIER 2: THE NEED FOR TEACHING SKILLS

Nurses state they lack the skills needed for teaching. Specifically, they ask for modeling and coaching from experienced teachers, such as clinical nurse specialists and patient educators. Many health care providers have stated that they have little confidence in their teaching and would like to observe expert teachers. This request goes beyond a class in which the expert shares tips for teaching. A preceptor model of observation, demonstration, and coaching can potentially create much greater productivity from the expert teachers as they develop a staff of confident teachers and become resources for difficult teaching situations. Abilities should be evaluated using competency measures that verify the health care professional has the technical, critical thinking, and interpersonal skills to assess learning needs, individualize teaching, and evaluate understanding (Wright, 1998). Health care providers who are skilled at individual and family teaching may lack skills for group teaching.

BARRIER 3: UNCOORDINATED TEACHING EFFORTS

Nurses often identify patient teaching efforts as haphazard, uncoordinated, and not directed to discharge priorities. Appropriate teaching materials are not readily available or are outdated; many teaching programs are also outdated. For example, one postpartum nursing unit had a flow sheet designed to streamline documentation of patient teaching with a check-off format. However, it contained more than 40 learning objectives that staff felt responsible for teaching. Because most patient stays were less than 72 hours, these teaching goals were not feasible, and the staff felt frustrated. Upon inspection, some items on the flow sheet were repetitive and some were best taught after discharge. The remaining items were divided into four topical areas with four key learning objectives related to (1) feeding, (2) hygiene and rest of mother, (3) managing the baby's schedule and the mother's needs, and (4) trouble signs that needed immediate attention. The staff felt confident focusing teaching and assessing patient outcomes on only four areas. To accompany the streamlined teaching plan, a new discharge instruction sheet was developed, following the old format.

When teaching plans are unrealistic, the creation of new documentation forms will take more work before the ongoing work of teaching is streamlined. Staff development personnel may need to advocate for revised teaching plans.

It should be asked: Do certain health care providers insist on keeping well-established programs that are no longer realistic, because of memories of past success, or political pressures? Successful interdisciplinary approaches to patient education depend on strong leadership, an honest appraisal of sacred cows, and a willingness to change to meet current conditions.

It is also important to assess the views of the staff, and bring them to a consensus on the purpose of patient education before introducing changes. Each health care provider's educational preparation and clinical experience may emphasize different priorities. For example, nurses who graduated in the 1970s were taught that informed consent is the primary aim of patient education, and teaching always begins with an anatomy and physiology lesson. In the 1980s, basic nursing education stressed discharge planning for high-risk patients, and offered less emphasis on individualized teaching for low-risk patients. Case managers and nurses educated in the 1990s have a heightened awareness of the need to focus on survival skills. Teaching also expanded beyond topics relating to acute illness, to include promotion and disease prevention.

In every practice setting, various approaches to patient education exist. This variety often causes disagreements among health care professionals on the priorities for patient teaching and which teaching interventions to provide. Many nurses attempt to follow patient education programs and standards based on long hospital stays. Some nurses entered the profession at a time when all patient teaching for specific health problems, such as diabetes, cardiac, and prenatal care, was delegated to a clinical nurse specialist. These nurses may have no formal teaching training, and may not accept that their role includes teaching. In addition, few health care professionals have been offered continuing education opportunities aimed at developing interdisciplinary approaches. Because all direct care providers teach patients and families, it is important that they learn to communicate with one another and coordinate teaching to optimize effectiveness and efficiency of their educational efforts. Continuing education provides an avenue for uniting practitioners with different perspectives and centralizing efforts to provide innovative new approaches to patient education.

BARRIER 4: PATIENT EDUCATION IS NEITHER NOTICED NOR REWARDED

Nurses state that patient education is neither noticed nor rewarded. They believe that more recognition should be given to involvement in patient education and it should be evaluated in the performance appraisal system. Patient education is creative work, requiring astute assessment and energetic involvement with the patient and family to make every moment count. If health care providers perceive that rewards and recognition are based on the number of patients cared for, the number of committees served on, or the ability to troubleshoot technical equipment, they are not likely to place priority on patient education activities.

Patient education is often invisible in management's eyes because it is frequently undocumented, unmonitored, and underappreciated for the skill and experience it demands. The positive impact of effective patient education on health outcomes and costs is not taken into account in day-to-day health care delivery.

Interdisciplinary patient education efforts should be described, evaluated, and marketed so health care providers receive credit for their work, and strive to improve their teaching. Staff development's role includes enhancing the visibility of teaching efforts, improving interdisciplinary communication of the status of teaching through documentation, promoting accountability of all staff through performance reviews, and sponsoring special events that recognize patient education efforts. An annual Patient Education Week that includes displays, guest speakers, and administration's recognition of outcomes and commitment to patient education can provide a needed boost for staff.

Promoting Skill Acquisition in Patient Education

Patient and family teaching must focus on survival skills. Patients and families should know the three or four critical behaviors they need to survive, how to recognize the prob-lems that may occur, and how to respond if these problems do occur.

Health care providers must be teachers and coaches. The practice of novice health care providers can be best supported with realistic teaching plans, critical paths, appropriate teaching tools, and interdisciplinary support. Overly ambitious teaching plans frustrate staff and overwhelm patients.

Anatomy and physiology lessons do not keep patients safe when they go home. They need psychomotor and problem-solving skills. Health care providers must help patients to integrate these behaviors in their daily lives so that, first, they will remember how to do them, and second, they will be skilled enough to exercise them properly.

Despite intensive educational efforts to teach, coach, and standardize approaches for patient education, staff development professionals recognize that nurses have different developmental needs in the process of becoming expert teachers. Patricia Benner (Benner, 2001) has convincingly explained that nurses live in different clinical worlds.

The clinical judgment and intuition needed to engage with patients and families, provide culturally sensitive care, and streamline teaching requires that nurses move from a theoretical, abstract base to a concrete world. Developing judgment and intuition occurs as the nurse learns through experience and reflection. Only by passing these developmental milestones can nurses eventually arrive at the expert stage of practice. The expert nurse can grasp the whole situation, set priorities, and confidently individualize patient care.

Staff development efforts can apply Benner's work by incorporating the strategies that most effectively promote development of expertise in patient education. Staff development can be targeted to different clinical worlds and can build a team approach to patient education (Figure 5.1).

Figure 5.1 is based on Benner's description of the process of skill acquisition. Although Benner applies this process to nursing, her work can be generalized to all

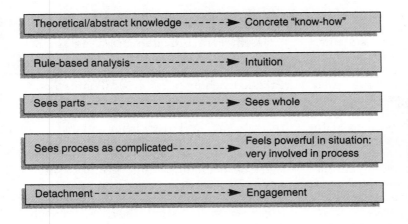

Theoretical/abstract knowledge	Concrete "know-how"
Rule-based analysis	Intuition
Sees parts	Sees whole
Sees process as complicated	Feels powerful in situation: very involved in process
Detachment	Engagement

FIGURE 5.1 Patient education science and art: a process of skill acquisition. The *arrows* refer to the process of skill acquisition as a nurse moves from beginner to expert. (Adapted with permission from Benner, P., Tanner, C., & Chelsa, C. [1992]. *From beginner to expert: Clinical knowledge in critical care nursing* [Video]. Athens, OH: Fuld Institute for Technology in Nursing Education (FITNE).

health care providers. One cornerstone of this process is the ability to translate theoretical knowledge into the practice and art of patient care, and to be guided by principles rather than explicit directions. The expert nurse can detect subtle cues, and becomes able to use intuition, recognizing what is salient in a specific situation. Clinical knowledge enables the nurse to attend to the patient's needs as a whole, with teaching the patient and family as an integral part of care. Rather than feeling overwhelmed, expert nurses feel confident and powerful in complex situations and adapt care based on individual patient priorities. Clinical judgment is embedded in practice. The question to answer is: What is required for a novice nurse to successfully progress to expert practice? Benner describes the developmental steps associated with each of four stages: advanced beginner, competent, proficient, and expert. When the nurse understands each stage, his or her capacity to accomplish patient education is better appreciated. This understanding also helps staff developers design effective coaching and preceptor interventions to support a health care provider's development of expertise in patient education. Benner's work helps educators carefully choose preceptors who best match the needs of their learners. Although many organizations tra-

ditionally assign preceptor responsibilities to their experts, Benner leads one to question this wisdom and to consider using the expertise of health care providers at all stages of development to support one another in practice.

Table 5.4 applies Benner's work to identify both the interests and educational needs of nurses at each stage of development.

ADVANCED BEGINNER STAGE

The advanced beginner must master technical skills and learn to organize patient care. Nurses are generally in this stage for the first two years of practice. Attuned to rules and procedures, the nurse is dependent on the availability of a preceptor to provide teaching and coaching in each situation. The nurse does not feel fully responsible and is often overwhelmed with the simultaneous demands of a clinical situation.

Staff development efforts for advanced beginners are often best fulfilled by unit-based preceptors. They focus on awareness of agency standards, resources, standardized teaching programs, and critical paths; ways to integrate patient and family teaching into all aspects of care; how-to aspects of teaching individual patients; developing explanations of diagnoses and procedures to share with families; and documenting the outcomes of learning.

TABLE 5.4 Promoting Skill Acquisition in Patient Education

BENNER'S STAGES	DEVELOPMENTAL FOCUS	EDUCATIONAL/INSTITUTIONAL SUPPORT FOR:
Advanced beginner	• Develops technical mastery and organization. • Needs other staff to delegate up. • Manages situations by rules, procedures. • Learns by situation. • Does not feel fully responsible.	• Awareness of agency standards, resources, programs for patient education • Skills for integrating patient and family in patient's care • How to teach skills
Competent	• Sees relationships among aspects of a situation: pattern analysis. • Desires to limit unexpected. • Deliberately plans and sets goals. • Notices patient/family in new ways: personalizes care. • Feels whole burden of health care team.	• Developing explanations to share with family • How-to of documentation • Family assessment • Group teaching skills • Home visits • Negotiating learning contracts • Case study analysis, exemplars
Proficient	• Recognizes patterns. • Sees changing relevance. • Increasingly senses what is salient. • Is attuned to situation: not detached.	• Leading/participating in health care team processes and critical path design • Documentation that supports individualized care
Expert	• Develops clinical grasp of whole situation. • Is at home in rapidly changing situations. • Attends to context and environment. • Makes decisions based on qualitative distinctions/what it means for this patient.	• Clinical career ladder based on exemplars that illustrate critical thinking • Permission to break the rules • Support for complex patient situations • Roles in case management • Teacher for competent-proficient • Facilitates patient care rounds • Designs product line models

Source: Adapted with permission from Benner, P., Tanner, C., Chesla, C. (1992). *From Beginner to Expert: Clinical Knowledge in Critical Care Nursing.* [video]. Athens, OH: Fuld Institute for Technology in Nursing Education.

COMPETENT STAGE

Nurses in the competent stage of practice begin to see patterns and recognize relationships among the various aspects of a situation. They have experienced similar situations, and have learned from them. The nurse no longer views the patient and family as adding to the demands of providing care, but begins to interact with them and personalize care. Desiring to limit the unexpected, the nurse in this stage engages in deliberate planning and goal setting, and feels responsible for all aspects of the patient's care.

Staff development efforts to support the competent nurse may include classes or workshops in family assessment, group teaching skills, learning contracts, and case study analysis. The nurse may be interested in and may benefit from making home visits, leading health care team conferences, and serving on committees to design new critical paths. Competent nurses should be engaged as preceptors for beginners, because they can remember how they learned and can still appreciate the needs of novice and advanced beginner nurses.

PROFICIENT STAGE

Nurses in the proficient stage recognize patterns. They can see differences in patients and the need to individualize teaching. They confidently streamline teaching, redefine priorities, and break the rules in ways that benefit the patient. Proficient nurses have an increased sense of what is salient in a situation, and can teach in ways that are culturally sensitive. They detect subtle cues (such as patient stress, pain, denial, depression, and family dynamics) and are attuned to the situation.

Staff development efforts for these nurses should focus on achieving documentation that reflects and supports individualized care. Clinical career ladders, based on exemplars that illustrate critical thinking, help proficient nurses demonstrate their significant contributions and development of clinical judgment. Although proficient nurses may still need support and resources for complex patient situations, they are skilled at coaching and precepting other nurses in most patient education situations, and should be involved as teachers and mentors. Proficient nurses should define patient education successes based on the patient's learning and right to choose, rather than on compliance. The failure to define patient education in this manner may result in disillusionment and detachment, rather than in engagement of nursing practice. Proficient health care providers must be encouraged to respect intuition. In truly listening to the patient and family, the proficient health care provider may decide to put aside the teaching checklist.

Expert Stage

Expert nurses demonstrate an excellent clinical grasp of the whole situation, including the patient, family, and environment, and are comfortable in rapidly changing situations. They attend to context and environment and can make the qualitative distinctions that are crucial in complex situations.

Experts are able to collaborate with other health care professionals to develop innovative patient education programs that achieve health outcomes. Expert nurses can provide valuable coaching for competent and proficient nurses; however, they are not the best choice to precept beginners because they are developmentally distant from the issues beginners experience. Beginners strive to learn and follow the rules, but experts have learned the conditions under which to safely bend or break rules to meet patient needs. Expert nurses are suited to roles such as case manager and clinical specialist, where they are asked to handle complex situations. They also are valuable resources for facilitating

patient care rounds and developing product lines for patient education that cross services.

Expert nurse practitioners perform many of the functions performed by primary care physicians, such as health maintenance examinations, management of common acute conditions and some chronic conditions. In addition, nurse practitioners are expert in patient teaching and counseling. For example, one study compared care between physicians and nurse practitioners, and found nurse practitioners had significant additional patient satisfaction, and better compliance with antibiotic therapy. This was attributed to the nurses' communication, counseling, and health education skills (Caine et al., 2002).

CLINICAL APPLICATIONS

Motivating Staff

How can we motivate staff to become more involved in patient education? Health care professionals frequently complain that they cannot improve their patient education skills because of heavy patient loads and difficulty scheduling time to attend continuing education programs. However, workshops are not the only effective means to impart teaching and learning principles to secure interest in patient education. Effective strategies for staff development include self-directed learning packages, computer-assisted instruction, computerized inventory of teaching materials and checklists, a newsletter with teaching tips, and opportunities for staff to team with experienced educators for peer review of their teaching. For example, one multimedia self-learning module available on compact disk is available from the University of Utah for a very small fee (Smith, 2003).

Continuing Education, Seminars, and Classes

One way to hone discharge-teaching skills is to give acute care staff the opportunity to make home visits with a seasoned home care nurse. Continuing education units should be offered with this activity, to enhance its attractiveness in states with mandatory continuing education requirements.

We have offered many successful brief seminars to nurses as a means of teaching cultural assessment, goal setting, and documentation strategies. We typically used case studies and role-play in these seminars to enhance the learning process. Sometimes we ask participants to apply the content learned in the seminar by developing their own teaching programs.

The actual disease process or health promotion content that must be conveyed to patients is another problematic aspect. Many health care providers say they do not know what to teach. Most know the pertinent information, because they apply it in their assessments and the care they provide. Their anxiety may be decreased by helping them identify, review, and organize the information the patients need. Teaching priorities should be identified by focusing on the goals of patient education:

- Developing survival skills
- Recognizing problems and knowing how to respond
- Making decisions

Frequently, staff members become so enthusiastic about teaching after attending these classes that they recognize other areas of need and develop teaching protocols with little assistance from the patient educator. Seminars and classes satisfy both intrinsic and extrinsic motivational factors for the staff. Negative intrinsic factors, such as anxiety about lack of knowledge, are modified; positive extrinsic factors, such as gaining continuing education units, are resolved.

Patient Education–Oriented Rounds

Nursing rounds and grand rounds oriented toward patient education can be an effective motivating force. In these cases, health care professionals should be asked to prepare information about a patient with whom they are familiar. This is especially useful if the learner posed a particular challenge. Content may be related to assessment of the patient's education needs, goal setting, the process of teaching, evaluation of understanding, or any patient education task. Rounds are an excellent means of learning from others and of expanding one's repertoire of patient education behaviors.

Integrating Patient Education Components in All Continuing Education Programs

Just as patient education is integrated into all patient care, patient education should be integrated into all continuing education activities. For example, when introducing new equipment to the staff, the information that the patients who will be using it need to know should also be pointed out. When updating staff on revised policies and procedures, the impact on patient education should be included. If a revised procedure is taught to patients for self-care, methods health care providers may use to evaluate the learner's understanding of the skill taught should be reviewed.

Reward and Incentive Programs

Reward and incentive programs for staff who provide and communicate patient education can be a strong motivator. The reward may be a better performance evaluation, the ability to move to a more desirable shift, or to advance up a clinical career ladder. Rewards and incentives show that the institution values patient education activities.

Peer and Colleague Support

Peer support is an important motivating factor for the staff. At change of shift reports, team meetings, and care conferences, health care providers should share assessments and evaluations of the status of patient education for each patient. Team members who discuss their problems and their successes in patient education, either formally or informally, can add an impetus to the promotion of patient education efforts.

The nursing profession suffers from a lack of internal validation. Too often we think we are alone on the battle lines, and we refuse to let ourselves ask for support when we need it. Greater team efforts and support within nursing would improve patient education and would motivate inexperienced nurses who look for guidance.

The benefits that accrue from increased collegiality between physicians and nurses motivate staff. Nurses who know that physicians approve of their patient education efforts will be motivated by the confirmation and validation. Because collegiality is a two-way proposition, nurses also must validate the patient education efforts of physicians. Collegiality as a motivator can, and should, extend to all members of the health care team. Another extrinsic motivator is a nurse's better sense of his or her own professional identity in these collegial relationships.

Teaching the Older Patient

Individualizing teaching to adapt to the needs of the learner makes patient education more efficient and effective. This is why JCAHO mandates age-specific approaches. As the population ages, the need for teaching older patients increases. Staff education needs to prepare health care providers to teach the older patient and his or her family.

Although most health care professionals modify their teaching when dealing with older patients, many mistakenly approach the older patient as if he or she is a child. A health care professional who takes this approach displays a lack of sensitivity and insults the patient.

As healthy people grow old, they show no decline in cognitive skills such as wisdom, judgment, creativity, common sense, or coordination of facts and ideas. However, they may show a slight and gradual decline in cognitive skills such as abstraction, calculation, word fluency, verbal comprehension, special

orientation, and inductive reasoning (Barry, 2000). Older people may have increasing difficulty understanding complex sentences, be less proficient in drawing inferences, and may process information more slowly.

Institutionalized older persons do even more poorly on tests of cognitive ability than do their counterparts living in the community. When teaching older patients, the following points should be remembered:

- Reduce environmental distracters.
- Speak in a low tone of voice; older persons hear low tones better than high-pitched sounds.
- Present information at a much slower rate than you would with younger learners.
- Help them connect the new material to information they already know. Build on past experiences and current knowledge.
- Allow enough time for the assimilation and integration of conceptual material. Evaluate understanding frequently.
- Focus on the concrete, not the abstract.
- Present one idea at a time.
- Teach in frequent, short sessions.
- Keep in mind that older learners are cautious and do not make changes easily.
- Remember the ability to learn may be modified by many physical, emotional, and social variables, such as cerebral changes, hypoxia, social isolation, fatigue, distracting financial concerns, misunderstanding, and changes in self-concept that result in loss of self-esteem.

Although people over 65 make up 13% of the U.S. population, they consume 35% of the prescription drugs. Because of multiple medical conditions, many take a number of prescription drugs each day, often incorrectly (Raehl et al., 2002). Patients may not understand how to take the medicine correctly, or they may adapt their treatment regimen based on how ill they feel and whether they can afford a refill (Ryan & Chambers, 2000).

Older adults are often strongly motivated to remain independent and in control of their medication. Take advantage of this motivation. Assess self-medication regimens carefully in the older adult, and individualize teaching to meet the needs of the learner. If the patient does not take his or her medicine independently, involve the caregiver in teaching (Ryan & Chambers, 2000).

In deference to the cautiousness and reluctance to make changes in some older people, health care professionals should minimize making changes in the medical regimen, whenever possible, to maintain a constant environment and schedule.

Many older learners prefer to learn alone. If this is the case, provide them with printed materials. However, be certain to return to discuss the contents, evaluate understanding, and help them problem solve (London, 1999).

Teaching Children

How is the teaching of children and adolescents different from the teaching of adults? What principles should we prepare staff to apply in teaching these patients and their families?

Children are not small adults. Teaching them demands ingenuity and a different approach. An adolescent's learning needs vary from those of children and from those of adults, and, therefore, are discussed separately.

Teaching and learning principles, when applied to children, should always consider the growth, development, and cognitive levels of the child. Table 5.5 is based on Piaget's well-known work regarding the development of perceptual and cognitive processes from infancy through adolescence (Piaget & Garcia, 1974). We purposely chose Piaget instead of Erikson because of the belief that understanding the cognitive processes is of equal importance to understanding the developmental processes for pediatric patient education. Table 5.5 outlines the cognitive and perceptual stages of development and suggests an approach to pediatric patient teaching.

Before teaching children, remember they have shorter attention spans, have greater need for support and nurturing, and learn more easily through active participation than do adults. Therefore, material must be presented in abbreviated format during a short time. Consistently and persistently show affection and offer praise to young patients during education sessions. By actively involving children in the learning process, we help them to more readily assimilate the information.

Children integrate new and unfamiliar information through play. The child's play is his work. Play, therefore, becomes a primary vehicle through which a child learns about his disease or acute problem, about what will happen, and about how to take care of himself to the best of his ability. Play therapy should also be used to help the child integrate and understand the painful or frightening experience he has undergone. Follow-up to surgery and procedures is just as important as preparation for these events, because most children have many unresolved feelings and questions that need expression.

The following case study illustrates the appropriate teaching for a 10-year-old boy with newly diagnosed idiopathic recurrent seizures.

CASE STUDY

A CHILD WITH NEWLY DIAGNOSED IDIOPATHIC SEIZURES

HISTORY
Eric experiences his first generalized, tonic-clonic (grand mal) seizure during recess at elementary school. He is hospitalized immediately for observation and a diagnostic workup.

PATIENT EDUCATION
Eric's primary nurse initiates patient education. Remembering that Eric's stage of cognitive development had been characterized by Piaget as concrete operational thought, she begins by teaching him the basic pathophysiol-

TABLE 5.5 Cognitive States and Approaches to Patient Education with Children

COGNITIVE STAGE	APPROACH TO TEACHING
Ages Birth to 2 yrs—Sensorimotor Development	
Begins as completely undifferentiated from environment. Eventually learns to repeat actions that have effect on objects. Has rudimentary ability to make associations.	Orient all teaching to parents. Make infants feel as secure as possible with familiar objects in home environment. Give older infants an opportunity to manipulate objects in their environments; especially if long hospitalization is expected.
Ages 2–7 yrs—Preoperational Development	
Has cognitive processes that are literal and concrete.	Be aware of explanations that the child may interpret literally (eg, "The doctor is going to make your heart like new" may be interpreted as "He is going to give me a new heart"); allow child to manipulate safe equipment, such as stethoscopes, tongue blades, reflex hammers; use simple drawings of external anatomy because children have limited knowledge of organs' functions.
Lacks ability to generalize.	Comparisons to other children are not helpful, nor is it meaningful to compare one diagnostic test or procedure to another.
Egocentrism predominates.	Belief that he causes events to happen may result in guilty thoughts that he caused his own pain, hospitalization, and so forth; reassure child that no one is to blame for his pain or other problems.
Has animistic thinking (thinks that all objects possess life or human characteristics of their own).	Anthropomorphize and name equipment that is especially frightening.
Ages 7–12 yrs—Concrete Operational Thought Development	
Has concrete, but more realistic, objective, cognitive processes.	Use drawings and models; children at this age have vague understandings of internal body processes; use needle play and dolls to explain surgical techniques and facilitate learning.
Is able to compare objects and experiences because of increased ability to classify along many dimensions.	Relate his care to other children's experiences so he can learn from them; compare procedures to one another to diminish anxiety.
Views world more objectively and is able to understand another's position.	Use films and group activities to add to repertoire of useful behaviors and to establish role models.
Has knowledge of cause and effect that has progressed to deductive logical reasoning.	Use child's interest in science to explain what has happened and what will happen to him; explain medications simply and straightforwardly (eg, "This medicine [insulin] unlocks the door to your body's cells just as a key unlocks the door to your house. By unlocking the door to the cell, the insulin can deliver the food and energy in your blood to the cell.")

Source: Adapted with permission from (1980). *Emotional care of hospitalized children* (pp 38–50). Petrillo, M., & Sanger, S. Philadelphia: J. B. Lippincott and Kolb. L. C. *Modern Clinical Psychiatry* (9th ed. pp 90–91). 1977. Philadelphia: W. B. Saunders.

ogy of seizure activity. Eric does not have abstract thought processes, but he understands the simple drawings the nurse provides of the brain and her explanation that the seizures were caused by too much electrical activity in the brain.

The nurse does not stress the term electrical activity; instead, she compares the problem in his brain to "an electric toy train that goes so fast that it runs off the track." She completes her analogy by saying that the medication he was going to take every day would act on his brain as if it were "slowing down the speed of the electric train." Eric's nurse remains aware that at this stage of development in the child's language skills, he may not always manage to indicate whether he has fully comprehended her explanation. Thus, she uses much repetition and asks Eric many questions.

Children from ages 7 years to 12 years generally can handle many of the aspects of their medical regimen. Eric is made responsible for administering his own medication at the prescribed times. He begins preparing and taking the medication himself while he is still hospitalized.

Children of Eric's age are more socially involved with their peers than are younger children, and it is important not to disrupt their attempts to join groups and participate in team sports. Eric is told that he can ride his bike as long as he wears his bike helmet and is accompanied by another child or an adult. He is also informed that he can continue swimming as long as someone is with him.

Finally, Eric is taught to begin to recognize the signs of his aura. The nurse defines an aura as the peculiar sensations Eric would grow to know as a warning sign of a seizure. After determining that Eric has previously experi-

enced nausea and vomiting with the flu, she tells him that an aura is the special warning that takes place before a convulsion, just as there was a certain warning that occurred before vomiting. Eric is told that when he began to recognize his aura, which might be a smell, sound, color, or sensation, he should try to lie down immediately.

The teaching includes both of Eric's parents, so they can reinforce the information imparted to Eric and offer support to him during the teaching sessions. The nurse presents the material to Eric during three half-hour sessions, so that he has an adequate amount of time to assimilate the information and to ask questions. She also spends time with Eric's parents alone, giving them more detailed information and answering their questions.

DISCHARGE

Eric is discharged from the hospital; he and his parents are encouraged to call the nurse, the pediatric nurse practitioner, or the pediatrician if they have questions or if they experience any problems. The hospital librarian also helped, by providing articles and Internet resources.

Teaching Adolescents

Adolescents have a different cognitive style from that of the school-age child. Piaget asserts that at the age of 12 years, children develop formal operational thought (Piaget & Garcia, 1974). Adolescents develop the ability to think abstractly, and reason deductively. Their cognitive processes are more like those of adults. Therefore, when teaching adolescents, be aware they can be taught in the same ways as adults.

However, adolescents are clearly different from adults in their social development, and the importance of peer groups. Knowledge of the adolescent's psychosocial task—identity versus role confusion, as defined by Erikson—is of primary importance to the health care provider (Erikson, 1993). The adolescent develops his identity in relation to his peers and in opposition to his parents, so it may be more effective to teach the parents separately from the adolescent.

Use of support groups for families with children with type 1 diabetes has been found to be an effective strategy in dealing with younger (11 years to 14 years of age) adolescents. One author, Rankin, facilitated a family support group for 3 years, in which parents and children attended each month. Although parents and children were frequently separated for different activities, many parents stated that the opportunity for their children to be in contact with other adolescents who have diabetes was a singular experience occurring only during the meetings.

On occasion, parents and children met when there were topics of interest to both. For example, representatives from local diabetes summer camps attended the meetings to orient parents and children to camp possibilities. The most popular joint speaker, however, was a young man with diabetes, who had not been well controlled metabolically during adolescence and who, at the age of 23 years, was experiencing complications related to retinopathy. This speaker served a two-fold purpose: First, he allowed children and adolescents an opportunity to see a young adult who had participated successfully in all types of sports and was determined to live as fully as possible, thus modeling a realistic role to adolescents. Second, the speaker's retinopathy that had resulted from a period of multiple hyperglycemic episodes allowed the parents to understand that parental control would probably be inadequate to protect their children from the excesses of adolescence.

Frequently, we assume that adolescents have more knowledge about their own anatomy and physiology than they do. This applies to functions of body organs and to sexuality. Illustrations are helpful with this age group, although they can be more sophisticated than those used with the school-age population. Understanding should be carefully evaluated.

It is crucial to be honest with adolescents. If a change in body image is expected as a result of surgery or during the course of a disease, the adolescent must be adequately prepared; body image is most important to this age group. Because of the desire to be part of the group and to look like everyone else, the adolescent who faces a change in appearance may want health care professionals to help camouflage the change.

Adolescents should be collaborated with to agree upon the goals of teaching and expected outcomes. Rationales should be provided to help give them a sense of control. When possible, offer them choices.

Adolescents may respond negatively when they feel their self-image or self-integrity is threatened. Confrontations should be avoided. Instead of acting like an authority figure, and contradicting their opinions and beliefs, acknowledge their feelings and offer alternatives (Bastable, 2003).

Don't miss the opportunity for health promotion teaching with adolescents. Six types of behavior are the biggest contributors to mortality and morbidity in adolescents in the United States:

- Alcohol and drug use
- Intentional and unintentional injury and violence, including suicide
- Poor nutrition
- Physical inactivity
- Sexual behaviors that contribute to unwanted pregnancy and sexually transmitted diseases
- Tobacco use

These behaviors usually are established during youth, persist into adulthood, are interrelated, and are preventable (National Center for Chronic Disease Prevention and Health Promotion, 2003). Assessments of these areas should be incorporated with each adolescent you care for, and teach, as needed.

SUMMARY

Many health care providers are frustrated by their patient education efforts, because their assumptions and approaches do not work. Consequently, learners do not learn what they need to know, health care providers feel unsatisfied, and outcomes suffer. There is a great need for staff development. If all the expert health care professionals who feel very powerful about their teaching could be paired up with colleagues in mentoring relationships, we would come a long way in improving the welfare of patients and the job satisfaction of health care providers.

Health care professionals can have the most impact on health outcomes by helping patients and families effectively take responsibility for their own health behaviors. This is accomplished through patient and family education. Staff development practitioners are positioned to make important contributions to patient teaching efforts by providing leadership to assess needs, developing educationally sound programs, and advocating for needed resources. The work of staff development includes interpreting JCAHO standards, promoting patient-centered approaches, streamlining or replacing outdated programs, and forging interdisciplinary and multi-setting alliances.

The role of staff development goes beyond helping the organization achieve a successful JCAHO survey. All continuing education programs must address implications for patient education. Workshops should be offered that expose staff to innovative approaches and skills for patient education, and propose realistic strategies for teaching and communicating with the team through documentation. Because patient education is interdisciplinary, all health care professionals, not just nurses, need to be included. As barriers encountered in the provision of patient teaching are identified, staff development professionals must address those issues honestly.

Perhaps our greatest resource for improving patient education outcomes is the strength of expert educators as coaches and teachers of others. Unit-based teaching and coaching should be provided to health care providers to build the acquisition of skills and expertise in patient education.

Staff development can help the organization to tailor its patient education programs to a growing population that is culturally diverse and aging.

Finally, staff development can increase the visibility of patient education efforts in the organization. This can be accomplished by sponsoring special events and recognition, bringing in national experts as guest speakers, and promoting patient education activities as integral to clinical ladders and performance review systems.

The next chapter moves from the organization that provides health care to the community. It explores the identification and assessment of community health education issues, and how to implement and evaluate community health education programs.

STRATEGIES FOR CRITICAL ANALYSIS AND APPLICATION

1. How can the respective strengths of nurses in each of Benner's four stages contribute to the development of a new patient education program for prenatal patients?
2. Describe two strategies that could be used by a staff development coordinator to increase administrative support for patient education efforts.
3. Describe an age-specific approach for teaching a newly diagnosed 8-year-old girl about how to manage diabetes.
4. Describe an age-specific approach for teaching a newly diagnosed 14-year-old girl about how to manage her diabetes.
5. The key to improving the quality of patient education efforts is to assess learning needs. Use the staff questionnaire in Box 5.6 to interview five health care professionals. Based on the interviews, what patient education and staff education needs should be addressed? Describe strategies for meeting these needs.

To find the latest information

Key search terms

staff development, age-specific competencies, needs assessment, Joint Commission on Accreditation of Healthcare Organizations, JCAHO

Websites

- National Nursing Staff Development Organization (NNSDO): http://nnsdo.org/Index.htm
- Joint Commission on Accreditation of Healthcare Organizations: http://www.jcaho.org/
- Patricia Benner, R.N., Ph.D., F.A.A.N, F.R.C.N.: http://www.bennerassociates.com

REFERENCES

American Academy of Family Physicians. (2000). Patient education: Recommended core educational guidelines for family practice residents. *American Family Physician, 62*(7), 1712–1714.

American Hospital Association. (1979). *Implementing patient education in the hospital.* Chicago: American Hospital Association.

Association of Faculties of Pediatric Nurse Practitioner/Associate Programs & National Association of Pediatric Nurse Practitioners. (2000). *Standards of practice for PNPs.* Retrieved May 12, 2003, from http://www.napnap.org/practice/pnpstandards/

Barry, C. B. (2000). Teaching the older patient in the home assessment and adaptation. *Home Healthcare Nurse, 18*(6), 374–387.

Bastable, S. (2003). *Nurse as educator: Principles of teaching and learning for nursing practice* (2nd ed.). Sudbury, MA: Jones and Bartlett Publishers.

Benner, P. (2001). *From novice to expert: Excellence and power in clinical nursing practice* (commemorative edition). Upper Saddle River, NJ: Prentice Hall Health.

Benner, P., Tanner, C., & Chelsa, C. (1992). *From beginner to expert: Clinical knowledge in critical care nursing* [video]. Athens, OH: Fuld Institute for Technology in Nursing Education (FITNE).

Caine, N., Sharples, L. D., Hollingworth, W., French, J., Keogan, M., Exley, A., et al. (2002). A randomised controlled crossover trial of nurse practitioner versus doctor-led outpatient care in a bronchiectasis clinic. *Health Technology Assessment, 6*(27).

Canadian Association of Nephrology Nurses and Technologists. (October 2001). *Standards of nursing practice.* Retrieved May 14, 2001, from http://www.cannt.ca/nursing_standards.htm

Commission on Accreditation for Dietetics Education, & American Dietetic Association. (April 2002). *Foundation knowledge and skills and competency requirements for entry-level dietitians.* Retrieved May 14, 2003, from http://www.eatright.org/cade/

Erikson, E. (1993). *Childhood and society.* New York: W. W. Norton.

Federation of State Boards of Physical Therapists. (2002). *Standards of competence.* Retrieved May 10, 2003, from www.fsbpt.org/standards.htm

Joint Commission on the Accreditation of Healthcare Organizations. (1996). *Educating hospital patients and their families: Examples of compliance.* Oakbrook Terrace, IL: Author.

Joint Commission on Accreditation of Healthcare Organizations (JCAHO). (2001a). *2001 hospital accreditation standards.* Oakbrook, IL: Author.

Joint Commission on Accreditation of Healthcare Organizations (JCAHO). (2001b). *2001 Comprehensive Accreditation Manual for Hospitals Update 3.* Oakbrook, IL: Author.

Krozek, C., & Scoggins, A. (2001). *Patient and family education . . . amended to comply with 2001 JCAHO standards.* Retrieved August 11, 2002, from gateway2.ovid.com/ovidweb.cgi

London, F. (1999). *No time to teach.* Philadelphia: Lippincott Williams & Wilkins.

McCloskey, J. C., & Bulechek, G. M. (2000). *Nursing interventions classification (NIC)* (3rd ed.). St Louis, MO: Mosby.

National Association of Pharmacy Regulatory Authorities. (2003, 3/20/2003). *Model standards of practice for Canadian pharmacists.* Retrieved May 12, 2003, from http://www.napra.org/docs/0/95/123//124.asp

National Center for Chronic Disease Prevention and Health Promotion. (2003). *Adolescent & school health.* Retrieved May 26, 2003, from http://www.cdc.gov/nccdphp/dash/health-topics/index.htm

Nolan, J., Nolan, M., & Booth, A. (2001). Developing the nurse's role in patient education: rehabilitation as a case example. *International Journal of Nursing Studies, 38*(2), 163–173.

Piaget, J., & Garcia, M. (1974). *Understanding causality* (D. Miles & M. Miles, Trans.). New York: W. W. Norton.

Raehl, C. L., Bond, C. A., Woods, T., Patry, R. A., & Sleeper, R. B. (2002). Individualized drug use assessment in the elderly. *Pharmacotherapy, 22*(10), 1239–1248.

Ryan, A. A., & Chambers, M. (2000). Medication management and older patients: An individualized and systematic approach. *Journal of Clinical Nursing, 9*(5), 732–741.

Rycroft-Malone, J., Latter, S., Yerrell, P., & Shaw, D. (2000). Nursing and medication education. *Nursing Standard, 14*(50), 35–39.

Smith, J. A. (2003). Patient education workshop. Salt Lake City: University of Utah. Contact: jackie.smith@nurs.utah.edu.

Staff development and training. (2003). Retrieved May 18, 2003, from http://www.ucl.ac.uk/epd/sdtu/mission.htm

Turner, D., Wellard, S., & Bethune, E. (1999). Registered nurses' perceptions of teaching: constraints to the teaching moment. *International Journal of Nursing Practice, 5*(1), 14–20.

Wright, D. (1998). *The ultimate guide to competency assessment in healthcare* (2nd ed.). Minneapolis, MN: Creative Healthcare Management.

Community Health Promotion: Assessment and Intervention

Ronna E. Krozy

LEARNING OBJECTIVES

After reading this chapter, the student should be able to:

1. Describe the interrelationship between community assessment and identification of community health education issues.

2. Develop a needs assessment using several approaches of data collection.

3. Apply marketing techniques to improve the success of a health education program.

4. Incorporate empowerment strategies in health promotion programs.

5. Implement health promotion strategies that facilitate behavioral change in families, aggregate populations, or community groups.

PLANNING, ASSESSMENT, OUTCOMES, & EVALUATION RESOURCES

This chapter contains a number of tools, models, and organizations that support project planning, goal-setting, and outcomes measurement in community health.

INTRODUCTION

Patient health promotion represents an integral part of the health professional's role. Health promotion addresses activities that decrease the impact of risk factors and facilitate well-being and self-actualization. Healthy People 2010 is a major national initiative to improve the health of the United States. Initiated by the United States Department of Health and Human Services, it established priorities for health promotion, health protection, and preventive services. Issues addressed included smoking, violence, physical fitness, mental health, occupational safety, environmental health, human immunodeficiency virus (HIV) and other sexually transmitted diseases (STDs), cancer, and immunizations (U.S. Department of Health and Human Services, 2000). The overall goal was to help change behaviors that were unhealthy or a risk to health, to eliminate unequal access to comprehensive health services, and to eradicate many chronic, costly conditions that are essentially preventable. Ultimately, prevention of disability and suffering also improves quality of life.

Healthy People 2010 intends to strengthen the scientific basis for health promotion and disease prevention programs, improve methods for collecting comprehensive health statistics, and increase the government's commitment and provision of services to provide quality care for all citizens. To raise the standard of care for the consumer, increased consumer participation also will be needed.

Health education is an important aspect of health promotion. Community health education differs from patient or family education in that its focus may extend to global, nation-al, state, or local needs. The clients of community health strategies include groups and aggregates that cross all age, socioeconomic, and cultural strata. These clients are in homes, schools, occupational settings, shelters, prisons, or on the street. Health promotion initiatives may be aimed at an entire country or a small village; the learners may be comprised of people who are homogeneous or extremely dissimilar. Health educators must develop proficiency in group or aggregate teaching; many participants must be reached efficiently, and groups serve as more potential sources of support and sharing.

This chapter discusses factors that must be considered in promoting health in aggregate populations. Two health education projects in which the author was involved are described. In each of these two projects, the demographic factors and health promotion focus are different; therefore, the approaches to needs assessment and intervention also vary. In the first example, Gordon's 11 functional health patterns (Gordon, 1994, 1997) are used as the framework to assess the health education needs of a culturally diverse population in a poor Ecuadorian community. The second example demonstrates the use of force field analysis and behavioral change strategies with staff attending a university health promotion program.

COMMUNITY HEALTH PROMOTION AND EDUCATION

Definitions

Health education is a helping process using learning theories and teaching techniques that promote the client's knowledge, attitudes, and skill to voluntarily engage in a wellness lifestyle. Part of this process requires mobilizing resources and developing supportive relationships with clients. Another aspect is assuming the role of client advocate or political activist for the disenfranchised, in whom health education may be a resource for self-empowerment. The health educator must use tested learning theories and teaching techniques that are based on the population's specific needs, and are incorporated into the overall plan.

Health education outcomes include the client's learning factual information, developing self-confidence, re-examining or changing values, decreasing fear, developing competence to make informed decisions, and performing desired behaviors autonomously. Another important goal is to help clients develop resilience—the ability to withstand internal and external stress without adverse effects (Lindenberg et al., 1998). The overall goals are aimed at enhancing, maintaining, or restoring health and preventing disease.

Challenges to the Health of a Community

Poor Habits, Chronic Illness, and Disability

Poor health habits, chronic illness, and disability are costly to communities in terms of lost work and school days, financing of health care and service agencies, and unnecessary suffering. Therefore, primary prevention is the best way to preserve the health of any community. Primary prevention is defined as the activities that prevent an illness or negative condition. Approaches to community health education often focus on the role of individual responsibility, recognizing that many health problems result from diverse personal habits, such as smoking, unprotected sexual activity, or overexposure to sun. These habits represent complex behaviors arising from internal and external stimuli; they are not easily amenable to medical intervention or the advice of a health professional. Despite potential or real disease, many people have difficulty changing their behavior.

For example, many young people begin or continue smoking despite multifocused anti-smoking strategies. According to a national study of students in grades 6 to 12 (National Center for Chronic Disease Prevention and Health Promotion, 2000), almost 9 in 10 students saw anti-smoking media messages in the previous 30 days, but in that same time frame almost 9 in 10 students saw pro-cigarette ads. Of the students surveyed, 23% currently use some form of tobacco, 18% currently smoke cigarettes, and 15% currently use some other form of tobacco. Nine in ten students think smoke from others is harmful to them. Over half of smokers want to stop smoking, and 58.2% tried to stop smoking during the previous year. Smoking is clearly a complex behavior that many people have difficulty changing.

Resistance and Barriers

Both resistance (internal) and barriers (external) can pose challenges. Resistance occurs when a specific population believes a health behavior change interferes with perceived quality of life, when the population views the change as unimportant, or when the resources needed for change are not available.

The health care system sometimes creates barriers. Health professionals are expected to establish trusting relationships with clients and act as role models. However, some health care professionals express attitudes or behaviors that prevent clients from following advice. Health professionals may hold beliefs that certain people (especially those from different socioeconomic classes) do not value health, do not want to get well, enjoy their sick role, are too unintelligent to learn new behaviors, and are taking up valuable time. Incongruent or ineffective messages also may be transmitted when a health professional engages in the unhealthy behaviors being discouraged, such as one who smokes, is overweight, or who drives without a seat belt.

IMPROVING THE SUCCESS OF COMMUNITY HEALTH PROGRAMS

Chapter 4 describes specific teaching and learning principles that can be applied to health promotion programs. To optimize the success of any health education campaign, several basic issues need to be addressed.

Identifying the Need

After defining the community you want to impact, consider this question: Have needs been assessed to determine the community's perception of the problem? Specific issues can be identified using public forums, focus groups, surveys, and interviews with professionals and community leaders. Data can be collected from health departments, hospital admission and exit records, census data, Centers for Disease Control, and other resources (Community Tool Box Team, 2002).

Acceptance by the Majority

Are the health promotion goals and objectives clear? Will most people in the target community accept the idea or method? Can they implement the program? Is it congruent with their lifestyle, needs, and resources? What are the barriers and facilitators of behavior change? Are the behavior changes practical and realistic? Does the health innovation integrate local resources, customs, and environment? Are the positive healthy habits of people capitalized upon?

Involvement in Planning

Has the plan been developed collaboratively with the community, or representatives of subgroups? Can you partner with groups that are doing similar work? Discussion and compromise at the planning stage can help devise a plan that can work. Opposing views should be identified early in the process, and the plan adjusted to accommodate them.

Cost-Benefit and Cost-Effectiveness

Is the expenditure of time, energy, money, or other resources required to carry out the action worth the effort, yield, rewards, or inconveniences? Have competing demands that influence learning or behaviors been considered?

Community Enhancement

Will the process enhance the community with job opportunities, environmental protection, or by equalizing wealth? Is there enough consumer orientation reflecting the target audience's specific concerns? Consider the resistance that arises from tobacco farmers whose livelihood is the product that causes cancer and heart disease.

Self-Help

Are the ultimate goals self-help or self-determination? Who is included: those in greatest need, or just those who can take advantage because of sophistication, education, money, and maturity? Is there a plan for those who cannot act because of physical, emotional, or social impairments?

Use of Theory

What theories are used to guide the design, implementation, and evaluation of the health promotion effort? Some examples described in previous chapters include the Health Belief Model, Health Promotion Model, and Self-Efficacy Theory.

Media Effectiveness

What are the outcome-linked, measurable objectives of your communication strategy? Did the messages emerge from the target audience, recognizing message competition? Have the appropriate channels been selected, carefully considering visual and/or sound elements, and the overall design of the message? Is the message linked to themes and values familiar to the target audience? Has every message been pretested? Does your audience understand your message as you meant it? (Community Tool Box Team, 2002).

POLITICAL AND LEGAL INFLUENCES ON HEALTH PROMOTION

Political and legal influences refer to formal and informal sources of decision-making and control. Policymakers or special interest groups can influence the withholding of health promotion programs from segments of society. For example, as a result of selection bias, researchers have underrepresented older people, the poor, and ethnic minorities from study protocols. Consequently, they do not gather information on how these populations respond to the interventions they test. Legislators in tobacco-growing states have supported subsidies to tobacco growers and have opposed smoking restriction regulations, despite the evidence showing the association of tobacco smoking with cancer. In context of the AIDS epidemic, needle exchange programs have been barred, and parents and religious leaders have influenced school committees to vote down comprehensive sex education curricula. Drug companies and manufacturers have withheld information on adverse outcomes to gain a profit.

Sometimes decision-makers place higher value on profits, religious beliefs, or getting re-elected than on health promotion in their communities. They may be unconcerned about certain health problems, or opposed to specific interventions. They may fear offending others and losing status; they may also be uninformed. The influence of decision-makers can be assessed by asking:

- Is health promotion a value?
- Who is permitted to learn how to promote health?
- Who controls what is taught?
- Who is permitted to teach health promotion?
- Are sufficient resources allocated?

A needs assessment can answer these questions and determine whether the allocated budget, human resources, time, space, and materials are sufficient to address the health problem. Health professionals can influence policy by clearly defining goals, focusing on effective activities, conducting research, gathering support, identifying and communicating with policy-makers, staying updated, and following up (Center for Health Improvement, 2003).

COMMUNITY EMPOWERMENT

General Considerations

Community empowerment, also called community self-determination or community self-help, is an effective process of decision-making and problem solving. Please see the Community Empowerment Case Study below.

CASE STUDY 6.1

COMMUNITY EMPOWERMENT

FROM BLIGHT TO BLOSSOM PARK: A CASE STUDY OF COMMUNITY EMPOWERMENT

Alice Samuels, a public health nurse, walked along *Blossom Street,* past the boarded-up dilapidated house sitting back from the street in a yard filled with refuse. Despite the *Do Not Enter* sign posted on the rusting barrier fence, she noted several teenagers sitting on the rotting front stairs smoking and laughing. She had heard that small groups of teenagers entered the house at night through a broken window, using candles for heat and light. Just recently, one had fallen down the stairs in the dark, requiring emergency room treatment for a fractured leg.

Two houses away lived Ms. Jordan, an elderly client. Ms. Jordan had remarked on several occasions how unsightly and dangerous this property was. In addition, the teenagers became rowdy and made people feel uncomfortable. She mused, "What we need there is a little park for children to play in or for us old folk to sit in." The nurse replied, "Let's see if we can do this."

EMPOWERMENT COMPONENT	APPLICATION TO THE COMMUNITY
Sufficient knowledge to make rational informed decisions	The nurse identifies key community persons and groups who will "own" the project, which is called Friends of Blossom Park. Multiple community assessment strategies are used to identify awareness of health hazards; impact on neighborhood—eg, sense of identity, safety, property values; and community goals, resources, and needs. All data are shared with the planning group. A Blossom Park Media Campaign is initiated; posted and written notices are placed in churches, schools, supermarkets, health centers, and local news and TV. Participants in a school poster contest, "Paint the Park," will receive free ice cream, and the posters will be displayed at the Park's opening.
Sufficient control and resources to implement decisions	Government support from legal, building, and health departments is required to approve demolition of abandoned property. Voluntary assistance is solicited from Scouts and the local high school; local trash removal company/municipality, landscaping, and construction companies; and personal and business donors, for cleanup, blueprints, plantings, equipment, and funds. A Blossom Park Bash fundraiser is established with a community dance, supper, and raffle. All decisions result from collaboration among community membership.
Sufficient experience to evaluate the effectiveness of the decision	After the park is created, Friends of Blossom Park decide to create other beautification projects and will collaborate with City Park and Recreation Department. Nurse remains as resource.

Community empowerment strengthens the community and improves its ability to accomplish its goals, rather than encouraging it to remain dependent upon outside resources. This is accomplished through many steps, including awareness raising, organizing unity, training community leaders and workers, identifying priority problems, developing an action plan, implementing the plan, and monitoring and reporting progress until completion (Bartle, 2003).

Examples of Community Participation in Health Promotion Programs

Consortium for the Immunization of Norfolk's Children (CINCH)

In recent years, many successful health promotion programs have resulted from broad community participation of diverse citizens and institutions. In Norfolk, Virginia, the urban coalition CINCH involved the community in assessment, planning, and intervention, improving preschool immunization rates and prenatal care received in the first trimester (Consortium for Infant and Child Health, 2000).

The Falmouth Safe Skin Project

A multidimensional skin cancer prevention program for parents and children through age 13 was launched in an ocean community of Cape Cod, Massachusetts. Goals of the Falmouth Safe Skin Project included educating parents about sun protection for their children and themselves and the dangers of early childhood sunburn. The project used community activism, specific learning activities, and a broad educational initiative that included providing information at maternity hospitals, day care programs, schools, beaches, recreation programs, and through the media. A follow-up survey 3 years after the initiation of the project showed an improvement in community knowledge, attitudes, and behaviors and a reduction in reported childhood sunburns (Miller et al., 1999).

THE INFLUENCE OF MARKETING

General Considerations

The objective of marketing is to influence action. Actions are taken when the target audience believes the benefits they receive will outweigh the costs. Marketing is most effective when it is based on an understanding of the audience's perceptions, the competition, and the changing marketplace (Novartis Foundation for Sustainable Development, 2003).

As indicated earlier in this chapter, marketing of unhealthy behaviors such as smoking can be counteracted with positive messages. Health care professionals can promote health by applying technology and mass communications to their media strategies. Media can be used to raise awareness, influence opinion, provide information and advice, change attitudes, introduce skills, offer triggers, encourage maintenance of behavior change, and reward action by broadcasting achievements (Whitehead, 2000).

Social Marketing

When applied to health, the term social marketing is often used. Commercial marketing tries to steer existing patterns of thought and behaviors to prefer a specific product, such as the superiority of a specific toothpaste. Social marketing aims to influence ideas and behavior, such as the importance of brushing teeth regularly, so it is sometimes less effective than its commercial counterpart (Novartis Foundation for Sustainable Development, 2003).

Marketing Example: The Massachusetts Tobacco Control Program

Examples of marketing strategy may be seen in Massachusetts, a state that funds tobacco control programs with taxes from tobacco products. In November 1992, Massachusetts voters passed a ballot referendum to raise the tax on tobacco products, establishing the Massachusetts Tobacco Control Program with a portion of the funds raised through this referendum. The Massachusetts Tobacco Control Program (MTCP) is a comprehensive statewide initiative that incorporates advertising and community relations, statewide smoking cessation and education programs, and grants to local boards of health, schools, community agencies, and health advocacy organizations. Its services to the communities of Massachusetts included smoking cessation counseling, school-based education programs, paid media, and tobacco product regulations. When tobacco opponents won the referendum, the tobacco industry used a massive paid media advertising campaign to publicize its message. Despite a heavily funded counterattack by the tobacco industry, supporters have received an additional $66 million revenue to the state from increased cigarette tax ($1.51) in 2002. The 2003 budget was cut to $5.5 million or $0.95 per citizen.

This investment showed excellent results. Since the Massachusetts Tobacco Control Program was introduced:

- Adult cigarette consumption decreased 41% since 1992.
- The prevalence of current adult smokers (18.3.0%) in 2001 decreased from 20.0% in 2000, and remained below the base rate of 22.6% in 1993.
- The average number of cigarettes smoked per day fell from 19.7 in 1993 to 16.7 in 2001.
- Youth smoking decreased from 35.7% in 1995 to 26.0% in 2001.
- The number of women who smoked during pregnancy declined 58% from 1990 (25.3%) to 1999 (10.8%) (Massachusetts Tobacco Control Program, 2003).

Community health promotion aims to foster behavior that maximizes wellness and minimizes the development of disease. Health promotion at the community level requires an understanding of the needs and desires of the target population. It is important to consider the behavioral lifestyles and values of the various groups that make up the community and to maximize community involvement. Socioeconomic status, educational level, culture and language, formal and informal power structures, occupation, and marketing forces are some of the important factors that must be accounted for if a health promotion initiative is to be successful. The influence of these factors is demonstrated in the health promotion programs presented in the following section.

GLOBAL HEALTH PROMOTION

Despite growing international concern toward health promotion and disease prevention, there are many barriers to promoting global health. These barriers include over-population, social injustice, social disorganization, increasing poverty, and population shifts from rural areas to overcrowded shanty towns in which children are born into unsanitary, polluted environments. Consequently, health professionals must be prepared to practice in settings where environmental factors adversely affect health. They need to be able to make decisions at social, economic and political levels, and direct energies toward altering environments to prevent risks to populations.

The Por Cristo–BCSON Health Project

A collaborative venture between the Boston College School of Nursing (BCSON) and Por Cristo, a medical missionary group, was initiated by the author of this chapter in 1991. From a self-supported voluntary health education mission, the Por Cristo–BCSON Health Project has evolved into a credit-granting undergraduate clinical experience in community health nursing. This project takes place in Isla Verde, an impoverished South American community. Nursing students work with Father Fred, a British missionary priest, who also is a registered nurse, and with the chapter author, a professor of community health nursing at Boston College.

Students assess and care for families in the home, conduct community assessments, and present community health education programs. Students set up temporary clinics, diagnose illnesses, prescribe interventions, counsel, and refer. A simple dispensary now exists, and students work with a lay community health worker and part-time physician. This project also has established relationships with two local university schools of nursing. Both Boston College and Ecuadorian nursing students present seminars to one another and a small group of Ecuadorian students accompany the BCSON students to work in the Isla. The goals of this project are the following:

1. To provide basic health education and services to an underserved population

2. To develop creative teaching approaches
3. To be immersed in a linguistically and culturally diverse community
4. To develop sensitivity and awareness of cultural diversity and universality
5. To recognize the dignity of a person, regardless of his or her socioeconomic status
6. To help empower the community through enhancing its self-help capabilities
7. To observe firsthand the effects of poverty
8. To demonstrate the role of the community health nurse and family nurse practitioner

Assessing the Community

An official community assessment and census have not been done in Isla Verde. Although the demographic characteristics appear the same as those in neighboring squatter communities, we realize that an individualized assessment uncovers specific needs, interests, resources, and community capabilities (Association for Community Health Improvement, 2002). These data form the basis for community diagnoses and educational interventions. A descriptive approach to community assessment was planned with the approval of Fr. Fred and community leaders.

Choosing an Assessment Tool

For many years, the students of this program have used an assessment tool based on Gordon's Eleven Functional Health Patterns (1994, 1997) applied to the community (McCarthy, 2002) (Box 6.1). To account for language and lifestyle differences, the assessment tool required adaptation, and a Spanish version was developed (Krozy & McCarthy, 1999). A number of people helped to develop and test the tools, including a bilingual health professional and students (several of whom were bilingual), families, groups, and faculty and students in the host country. Translating the material back into English and audience testing assured that both nurse and patient would exchange exact meanings in their communication.

These tests help ensure the material conveys the information you want to convey, is understandable to those you are trying to reach, and is culturally accessible to your audience (Rudin, 2003).

Conducting the Assessment

Students conduct a walking assessment, speak with community residents and leaders, and tour the institutions in the surrounding city. This approach lets the students observe and record many aspects of community life. The data collected provide the background and basis for interventions.

Isla Verde is a poor coastal community of squatters who live on government-owned property. The community began in 1985 and is divided into cooperatives, each run by a council and president. The community has continually expanded and it is estimated that 400,000 people live in the Isla. The community lacks running water, electricity, sanitation services, and fire or police protection. Illness is rampant, and there is little employment and great educational disadvantage. Many children are malnourished, have multiple frequent parasitic diseases, and frequently die.

The birth rate in the Isla and surrounding areas is high. Some deliveries occur at home, and other births take place at a local maternity hospital. This hospital is considered the second or third largest maternity hospital in South America (approximately 120 births daily and more than 500 prenatal visits daily for problem pregnancies only). One student with a special interest in maternal-child nursing was permitted to return to this hospital for a portion of a day. She observed 16 births within 2 hours, with many differences noted in maternity nursing practices. One example was very limited use of pain medication.

Many children do not or cannot afford to go to school. These children play in the streets; swim or play in polluted waters; urinate and defecate on the ground without handwashing; and run barefoot. Children as young as 5 years of age are left in charge of

BOX 6.1 Community Assessment Guide

I. Health Perception–Health Management Pattern

1. History (community representatives)
   a. In general, what is the health/wellness level of the population on a scale of 1–5, with 5 being the highest level of health/wellness? Any major health problems?
   b. Any strong cultural patterns that influence health practices?
   c. Do people think they have access to health services?
   d. Is there a demand for particular health services or prevention programs?
   e. Do people think fire, police, safety programs are sufficient?
2. Objective data (community records)
   a. Morbidity, mortality, disability rates (by age group, if appropriate)
   b. Accident rates (by district, if appropriate)
   c. Current operating health facilities (types)
   d. Ongoing health promotion/prevention programs; utilization rates
   e. Ratio of health professionals to population
   f. Laws regarding drinking age
   g. Arrest statistics for drugs, drunk driving by age groups

II. Nutritional–Metabolic Pattern

1. History (community representatives)
   a. In general, do most people seem well nourished? Children? Older people?
   b. Are there food supplement programs? Food stamps: rate of use?
   c. Are foods reasonably priced in this area relative to income?
   d. Are stores accessible for most? Meals on Wheels available?
2. Objective data
   a. What is the general appearance of the population (nutritional appearance; teeth; clothing appropriate to climate)? Children? Adults? Older people?
   b. What food do people purchase (observations of food store checkout counters)?
   c. Are "junk" food machines in schools, fast food restaurants, etc.?

III. Elimination Pattern

1. History (community representatives)
   a. What are the major kinds of wastes (industrial, sewage, etc)? Are there disposal systems? Recycling programs? Any problems perceived by community?
   b. Is there pest control? Food service inspection (restaurants, street vendors, etc.)?
   c. How is water supplied and what is the quality? Are there testing services? What does water usage cost? Are there drought restrictions?
   d. Is there concern that community growth will exceed good water supply?
   e. Are heating/cooling costs manageable for most? Do help programs exist?
2. Objective data
   a. Communicable disease statistics
   b. Air pollution statistics

IV. Activity–Exercise Pattern

1. History (community representatives)
   a. How do people find the transportation here? To work? To recreation? To health care?
   b. Do people have/use community centers (seniors, others)? Are there recreation facilities for children? Adults? Seniors?
   c. Is housing adequate (availability, cost, size)? Is there public housing?

BOX 6.1 Community Assessment Guide *(Continued)*

2. Objective data
   a. Recreation/cultural programs
   b. Aids for the disabled
   c. Residential centers, nursing homes, rehabilitation facilities relative to population needs
   d. External maintenance of homes, yards, apartment houses
   e. General activity level

V. Sleep–Rest Pattern
1. History (community representatives)
   a. Is it generally quiet at night in most neighborhoods? If not, why?
   b. What are usual business hours? Are there industries operating around-the-clock?
2. Objective data
   a. What are the activity–noise levels in business districts? In residential districts?

VI. Cognitive–Perceptual Pattern
1. History (community representatives)
   a. Do most groups speak English? Are they bilingual? Other dominant languages?
   b. What is the educational level of population?
   c. Are schools seen as good/needing improving? Is adult education available/desired? Is vocational training available/desired?
   d. What types of problems require community decisions? How are decisions made? What is the best way to get things done/changed here?
2. Objective data
   a. Describe the school facilities. What is the dropout rate?
   b. How is the community government structured? Describe the decision-making lines.

VII. Self-Perception–Self-Concept Pattern
1. History (community representatives)
   a. Do people think this is a good community to live in? Is it going up in status, down, about the same?
   b. Is this an old community? Fairly new?
   c. Does an age group predominate?
   d. What are people's moods in general? Do people appear to be enjoying life, stressed, feeling "down"?
   e. Do people generally have the kind of abilities needed in this community?
   f. Are there community/neighborhood functions?
2. Objective data
   a. Racial, ethnic mix (if appropriate)
   b. Socioeconomic level
   c. General observations of mood

VIII. Role Relationship Pattern
1. History (community representatives)
   a. Do people seem to get along well together here? Are there places where people go to socialize?
   b. Do people think they are heard by government? Is participation in meetings high or low?
   c. Are there enough jobs for everyone? Are wages good/fair? Do people like the kind of work available? Do they seem happy in their jobs or appear to have job stress?
   d. Are there problems in the neighborhood with riots? Violence? Family violence? Child, spouse, or elder abuse?
   e. Does this community get along with adjacent communities? Do they collaborate on any projects?
   f. Do neighbors seem to support each other?
   g. Are there community get-togethers?

BOX 6.1 Community Assessment Guide *(Continued)*

2. Objective data
   a. Observation of interactions (generally or at specific meetings)
   b. Statistics on interpersonal violence
   c. Statistics on employment, income/poverty
   d. Divorce rate

IX. Sexuality–Reproductive Pattern

1. History (community representatives)
   a. What is the average family size?
   b. Do people think there are any problems with pornography, prostitution? Other?
   c. Do people want/support sex education in schools or in the community?
2. Objective data
   a. Family size and types of households
   b. Male-female ratio
   c. Statistics on average maternal age, maternal mortality rate, and infant mortality rate
   d. Teen pregnancy rate
   e. Abortion rate
   f. Sexual violence statistics
   g. Laws/regulations regarding information on birth control

X. Coping–Stress Pattern

1. History (community representatives)
   a. Are there any groups that seem to be under stress?

   b. What is the need/availability of telephone help lines or support groups (health-related, other)?
2. Objective data
   a. Statistics on delinquency, drug abuse, alcoholism, suicide, psychiatric illness
   b. Unemployment rate by race/ethnicity/sex

XI. Value–Belief Pattern

1. History (community representatives)
   a. Community values: What are the top four issues that people living here see as important in their lives (note health-related values, priorities)?
   b. Do people tend to get involved in causes/local fund-raising campaigns?
   c. What religious groups live in the community? What religious institutions are available?
   d. To what extent do people tolerate differences or socially deviant behavior?
2. Objective data
   a. Zoning laws
   b. Scan of public health department reports (goals, priorities)
   c. Health budget relative to total budget

Source: Adapted with permission from McCarthy, N. C. (1994). The 11 functional health patterns assessment guidelines for communities. Health promotion and the community. In Edelman, C. L., & Mandle, C. L. (Eds.), *Health promotion throughout the lifespan* (3rd ed.), pp. 209–210. St. Louis, Mosby-Year Book.

other much younger children while a parent works. A 1-year-old child was observed left in a house alone, unfed and dirty; other small children may be locked in from the outside. Many children and adults have lice, fungus, and other skin infections.

Living quarters are frequently one-room shacks built on sand or on stilts over the river's edge, reached by a network of rickety, narrow, broken catwalks. Accidental injuries and drownings have resulted from falls into the water. The shacks are constructed of new or salvaged materials, such as bamboo, wood, cement block, or cardboard. These shacks frequently do not prevent water or insects from entering. In heavy flooding, the shacks may collapse into the river. As many as 15 children and adults may live in one room, sleeping on rags on the floor or six in one bed. Chickens live in some homes.

Injuries and deaths from burns are considered a major hazard. They occur frequently because people cook on open flames situated next to bamboo walls; small children pull over pans of hot grease; rubbish is burned in the street, often injuring children who play nearby; and adults get electrical burns and shocks while pirating electricity from main lines.

Without a sanitation system, the people who live on the water have used the tidewaters in place of latrines to carry away human and material waste. The government has begun to permit people to live in this area and has filled in parts of the area with tons of sand, permitting housing to be built on a landfill base. The government contends that the sand is the foundation for water pipes to be laid in the future. However, the sand has prevented the natural clearing of waste by tidewater. Groundwater levels have increased particularly after tropical rains and ground waste is accumulating around the homes of families without latrines, increasing the medium for disease transmission.

There is currently no piped-in water system and water is delivered by truck and stored in a barrel outside, which may not be covered. Water is used for drinking, cooking, bathing, and cleaning. To be potable, water must be boiled for 20 minutes. If a lack of funds precludes buying fuel, water is often boiled for less than the recommended time or ingested from the barrel. Dysentery, cholera, and typhoid result from ingesting water contaminated with human and animal feces and often cause fatal diarrhea and dehydration. Some families cannot afford to purchase water.

Extreme poverty makes food purchase and safe storage equally difficult. Food is often eaten with soiled hands or left out uncovered, where flies contaminate it. Many houses have no food. One mother admitted to only eating a handful of peanuts the day before. Children are given cola drinks instead of the more costly milk; maternal nutritional deprivation often leads to ineffective breast-feeding; babies may be given coffee or diluted formula to drink. There is a large outdoor market in the city where vendors sell domestic goods, items in bulk, fresh fruits and vegetables, and meat. Students observed chickens being freshly killed and then left out without refrigeration. Unfortunately, the market is inaccessible to Isla residents, who must find and pay for public transportation to get there. This forces residents to buy goods at small stores in the community, where prices and quality of products are problematic.

Health care for the Isla is highly inadequate, although it has improved since the small dispensary was constructed in 1994. Many people cannot afford to pay the equivalent of 50 cents for a visit or for prescriptions. Home remedies, some of which are dangerous, may be used for a sick person. Even hospitalized patients may not receive medication, plasma, or bandages until the family prepays.

There are few avenues for rest and recreation in the community. Adults admit they are too poor or tired to do much that can be considered fun. Children have few toys. A day care center was established to assist working parents and provide socialization for some children. However, 35 children and infants are tended by 3 adults. Stress levels are admittedly high and many people, particularly men, use alcohol as a relaxant. Many families attend Sunday religious services or other activities held at the church. The church plays a prominent role in many of the residents' lives. They hold Fr. Fred in great esteem and frequently turn to him for spiritual, emotional, and economic assistance. Fr. Fred has also developed training programs to try to create job skills for interested residents.

Establishing Community Diagnoses

A community assessment by each student group demonstrates the numerous health hazards in the Isla Verde community, many of which are related to poor hygiene practices and risk-taking behavior. Students choose a functional health pattern, identify associated community diagnoses, and prioritize them according to community strengths and deficits. The students then establish health promotion projects. Box 6.2 is a selective list of community diagnoses identified by students.

Establishing a Community Health Promotion Intervention

It is challenging to develop successful health promotion programs for culturally and ethnically diverse populations. Language differences, poverty, prejudice, low literacy levels, traditional teaching and learning styles, alternative treatment modes and practices, and beliefs about illness are some of the many factors that must be considered if a program is to be effective. The students in the Por Cristo–BCSON project try to incorporate the community's needs, interests, values, beliefs, and resources into the health promotion programs while recognizing their own time limitations.

Preparing the Health Promotion Projects

Before arriving in the host country, students arrange themselves in teaching groups and begin planning their health promotion projects based on Fr. Fred's feedback and the priority community diagnoses identified by former students. They also incorporate many of the helpful suggestions found in *Where There Is No Doctor* (Werner, Thuman, & Maxwell, 2002) and *Helping Health Workers Learn* (Werner & Bower, 1995) into their teaching activities and materials. They also use the Spanish versions of these books.

Teaching groups are organized around various health issues, including infant and child care, nutrition, immunization, diarrhea and dehydration, breast-feeding, hygiene, and accident prevention. Adolescence and women's health issues addressed include education about and prevention of STDs and HIV/AIDS and sex education to prevent adolescent pregnancy. General health and safety issues, such as burn prevention and treatment, first aid for choking, when to seek medical attention, and principles of nutrition adapted to the customs, income, and available products of the region are also addressed.

Developing Relationships and Gaining Acceptance

Fr. Fred has helped the students gain acceptance by securing support of community leaders and residents. Students are warmly welcomed because of their willingness to roll up their sleeves and dig in. Students have paid for and helped construct latrines, cleaned a poor mother's backyard of broken glass where young children were running around barefoot, and even built a table out of new and used wood for a family who ate on the floor. Students have brought medical supplies, school books, and other items to distribute to the neediest. The Isla Verde community looks forward to the arrival of students and many people attend the community charlas, or chats, run by the students.

Implementing the Health Promotion Projects

Once the students are in the Isla Verde community, focus groups are formed to promote community participation, to self-select topics, and to provide insight on the dimensions of problems. This approach works well with the Latino population, and attendees welcome the opportunity to offer suggestions, admitting that few people ever ask for their input. Through the community suggestions, students of the Por Cristo–BCSON project conduct daily charlas (afternoon talks), which are publicized by word of mouth and posted notices. Classes take place in either the dis-

BOX 6.2 Community Diagnoses in Isla Verde

Health Perception–Health Management Pattern

Health Seeking Behaviors related to (r/t) faithful attendance at classes, active questioning, attentiveness

Injury: Actual and Potential r/t multiple sources of burns, abuse, drowning, broken glass and syringes on road, bare feet, broken boards in houses on stilts, getting hit by cars, violence (rock throwing, guns, etc.)

Altered Protection r/t wife abuse, child abuse, sexual abuse, lack of police or social protection

Impaired Home Maintenance r/t sense of hopelessness, lack of structural integrity, and inability to purchase repair materials

Infection: Actual and Potential r/t not cleaning wounds, bug bites, using inappropriate remedies for burns (i.e., toothpaste, mud, sputum), multiple sex partners and prostitution, and lack of condom use

Pain r/t lack of medicine, conservative use of analgesics

Nutritional–Metabolic Pattern

Altered Growth and Development r/t altered nutrition and sensory deprivation

Altered Nutrition: Nutritional Deficit r/t inability to purchase food, inability to obtain quality food, knowledge deficit in best use and preparation of local foods, diarrhea

Fatigue r/t nutritional deficit, overworking, etc.

Fluid Volume Deficit r/t diarrhea and knowledge deficit

Elimination Pattern

Alteration in Elimination: Diarrhea r/t environmental pollution, poor hygiene practices, barriers to implementing prevention strategies

Activity–Exercise Pattern

Diversional Activity Deficit r/t small overcrowded living situations and neighborhoods, deficit of play space or equipment

Ineffective Breathing Pattern r/t environmental dust, untreated asthma

Sleep–Rest Pattern

Sleep Disturbance r/t overcrowding, lack of adequate space, noise

Cognitive–Perceptual Pattern

Knowledge Deficit r/t AIDS transmission, basic hygiene

Cognitive Impairment: Potential r/t malnourishment before and after birth, child neglect, lack of stimulation

Self-Concept–Self-Perception Pattern

Fear r/t robbery, rape, abandonment, inability to support family units

Powerlessness: Severe r/t lack of education, social control, abuse of women and children

Role Relationship Pattern

Impaired Social Interaction r/t lack of community cohesiveness, inability to request help despite need

Altered Parenting r/t young pregnancies, no resources, unemployment, abuse cycles, single female-headed families of many closely spaced children

Violence: Potential for r/t dispiritedness, lack of protection against abuse and injustice, reports of weapons in community

Sexuality–Reproductive Pattern

Altered Sexuality Patterns r/t lack of sex education, frequent unplanned pregnancies, rape, prostitution, unprotected sex

Coping–Stress Tolerance Pattern

Family Coping: Potential for Growth r/t observation and report of families supporting and caring for one another and unselfishly sharing all their goods

Anxiety r/t deaths and debilitating diseases

Defensive Coping r/t deplorable living conditions

Value–Brief Pattern

Spiritual Distress r/t lack of basic human needs, human rights abuse, expressions of hopelessness

pensary or adjoining church and are well attended. Most attendees are women, many with children, and it is not unusual to see a standing-room-only crowd.

Teaching Strategies

The students use various approaches in their teaching projects. A large toothbrush and a set of teeth have been used to demonstrate oral hygiene to children. Each child receives a toothbrush for return demonstration and a sample of toothpaste. A doll is used to demonstrate infant care and breast-feeding positions. A realistic breast model worn over the chest permits the attendees to learn about appropriate positions for breast self-exam. Verbal instructions, posters, and handouts are used to teach how to prevent diarrhea in children and how to prepare and administer oral rehydration therapy. Donated microscopes help the students to teach about sources of bacterial contamination; children and adults are fascinated to see teeming microbes living in samples taken from an ordinary water barrel. By visualizing the organisms that make people sick, the community understands the basis for teaching them to cover food and to boil water.

Discussion groups have been organized by students and include coeducational adolescent support groups to discuss sexual development and prevention of unplanned pregnancy and rape; a parents' support group, with men attending, discusses community issues, such as stress reduction and domestic abuse.

Burn Prevention and Treatment Program

The burn prevention and treatment program is a crucial community-wide project for the Isla Verde. Nursing students present this program to children, adults, health providers and teachers, using the clinic, school, church, and day-care center for settings. The objectives of this program are for participants to identify sources of burn injuries and deaths, practice preventive strategies, and treat burns appropriately. Small groups of children are gathered and the nursing students appear in brightly colored clothing. Their orange gloves, red shirts, and yellow tights simulate fire colors. Participation is encouraged by a question-and-answer period before and after the program. The children are asked if they know anyone who has been burned. What happened to that person? What caused the burn? What could have been done to prevent it?

The children usually know a burn victim and mention pain and scarring. The causes of burns range from playing with matches to being scalded with hot liquid. Their knowledge of preventive methods is often limited. They are asked what they should do if their clothing catches on fire. Some of the students know the correct answer and are complimented. The student teachers role play with props, actually rolling on the ground or floor, while others recite the Spanish version of "Stop, drop, and roll." Volunteers from the audience are then selected.

Posters emphasizing burn prevention strategies depict storing matches away from children, turning pot handles inward, observing children when a trash or other type of fire is burning, and securing a metal shield behind a cooking fire.

Proper burn treatment includes understanding how to treat pain, keeping the wound clean, assessing severity, and knowing when to seek medical treatment. Posters depict first-, second-, and third-degree burns. Students emphasize protecting the burn from dirt, excreta, and insects; they also emphasize using clean cool water on first-degree burns and warm salt water as compresses for second-degree burns (Werner, Thuman, & Maxwell, 2002). They explain why grease, mud, oil, coffee, feces, urine, or toothpaste should never be used and that severe burns, signs of infection, or extended burns on small children should be treated at the clinic.

An oral quiz is given at the end of each session, and questions from the audience are answered. Children are instructed to share what they have learned with their siblings and parents. Teachers are also given materials for reinforcing the lessons.

Water Purification

Lack of potable water is a major public health problem in many poor countries that causes many deaths, especially to young children because of diarrheal disease and dehydration. Therefore, students now teach a water purification process, using an empty plastic soda bottle with half of its surface painted black from top to bottom. A bottle is filled with water that is filtered first if it comes directly from a river. It is then left under direct sun for 5 hours, painted side down. All microbes are killed and the water becomes safe to drink. The procedure has been shared with community residents, staff, and nursing students.

Outcomes

Evaluation of the various health promotion activities must be ongoing, and there are no statistics to demonstrate the outcomes. However, each year the Por Cristo–BCSON project has tried to reach as many children and families as possible. They continue to teach burn prevention and treatment and collaborate with a community pediatrician who has begun to collect data on burns; in a system in which people frequently self-treat except in major crises, data collection is a challenge. Teacher and learner satisfaction have been rated as high, and the community has consistently demonstrated the desire to learn and to promote self-help.

The author believes that the Por Cristo–BCSON Health Project has helped create a vehicle for health promotion by sharing all of our teaching projects with the staff of the dispensary and the students and faculty with whom we affiliate. In this way, we promote continuity in health teaching and nursing intervention from within the population. In 1999, the chapter author facilitated the first nursing diagnosis conference to take place in an Andean country. Dr. Marjory Gordon, the featured speaker, addressed the need for a thorough assessment to guide diagnosis and intervention at all levels. Particular emphasis was placed on the nurse's health teaching role. This conference and other workshops with nurses in practice aimed to increase the commitment of professional nurses to include health promotion and primary prevention in their patient care.

Most of the U.S. population will soon be comprised of people originating from Africa, Latin America, and Asia. An overseas immersion experience provides a milieu for health professionals to develop and incorporate cultural competence and language fluency into clinical practice. Successful health promotion strategies must be congruent with the health beliefs and practices of the target population, based on the population's fundamental concerns and needs, and aimed at results that are desirable and ultimately achievable. Nurses, irrespective of their clinical specialty, must accept health promotion and counseling as an integral part of their nursing practice. These principles will continue to guide our missions to Isla Verde.

Health Promotion Programs in the Workplace: Boston College "The Challenge"

General Considerations

Promoting healthy lifestyles is both a humanistic and an economic concern to employers and those who provide occupational health promotion programs. Although not mandated by federal regulation, many companies take a proactive approach to health promotion and offer employees various services that promote wellness.

Successful workplace programs employ preventive strategies to keep workers healthy and productive. They teach skills that encourage workers to take responsibility for their own health. These workplace programs also provide emergency care, follow-up, and referrals for job-related injuries and illnesses, counsel workers about work-related illness and injuries, substance abuse, and emotional and family problems (American Association of Occupational Health Nurses, 2003).

Description of "The Challenge"

The Challenge is an ongoing health promotion program for university faculty and staff at Boston College. It takes place during the spring semester and includes weekly discussions on health, diet, and exercise; organized exercise activities; and establishment of support groups. The model is based on a team approach, and points are awarded to those teams who lose weight within a predetermined range, engage in specific exercises, and attend weekly 55-minute presentations on a relevant topic. Each team consists of at least five members, headed by a team captain who tallies individual weight and exercise points weekly. Programs include a nominal registration fee and various prizes and rewards, such as a t-shirt with the program logo.

The School of Nursing faculty and students of the participating university provide consultation on various aspects of the overall program, conduct height and weight measurement and blood pressure screening at the first and last sessions, and present some of the seminars. Topics include principles of behavior modification, choosing the right exercises, understanding one's relationship to food, principles of nutrition, stress management, and maintaining one's health promotion program. Additional nutritional and health counseling and referrals are made available.

Force Field Analysis

As a member of Boston College's health promotion team, the author of this chapter incorporated Lewin's force field analysis and various health promotion strategies to teach participants how to plan and maintain wellness behaviors. Lewin's force field analysis has two main components. First, compliance increases when people identify both the stumbling blocks to their own behavioral change and the strategies for change they would find most acceptable. Second, knowledge of the forces that promote positive behavioral change and the strategies that are more likely to effect change help the health professional improve the target population's health outcomes.

Force field analysis, although developed in the 1940s by Lewin and associates, is still considered an important approach to planned change. It offers a way to look at variables to determine whether organizational change will occur. The forces are the perceptions that people in the organization have toward a variable and its influence. Driving forces are attempting to push it in a particular direction. These forces tend to initiate change or keep it going. Restraining forces act to restrain or decrease the driving forces. When the sum of the driving forces equals the sum of the restraining forces, a state of equilibrium is reached (Enock, 2002).

Lewin proposed three phases to change:

1. **Unfreezing**—developing an awareness of the need to change, increasing readiness or willingness to change
2. **Experiencing the change or moving**—exploring the alternatives, defining goals and objectives, planning how to accomplish the goals, and implementing the plan for change
3. **Refreezing**—integrating the change into one's own work or life, internalizing the change (Habel, 2000)

Force field analysis is best applied to the unfreezing stage. It addresses those driving forces that will assist the change and those restraining forces that will impede change. There are three ways to facilitate change:

1. add forces that promote change
2. reduce forces that impede change, or
3. redirect forces that support change.

Driving and restraining forces are rarely equal. For example, resistance to change may be weakened when the behavior is deemed as culturally appropriate, pleasurable, or easy to maintain. When the suggested action is deemed as a loss, painful, culturally incorrect, expensive, beyond the resources of the target population, or without value, resistance will be stronger.

Health Promotion Strategies

The literature suggests a variety of health promotion techniques for the community. No single technique has been found superior; therefore, successful interventions often incorporate several approaches. A combination of strategies that provide factual information, stimulate motivation, help change attitudes and behavior, and promote competence may better address the multifaceted nature of health behavior (Behavioral Change Strategies, Table 6.1).

Identifying Personal Barriers, Enhancers, and Strategies for Change

The Challenge program was introduced with the notion of how challenging it is to advise people to change lifelong habits. In considering stress reduction, health professionals often suggest changing one's lifestyle without assessing the availability of options or resources for making these lifestyle changes. However, the interest in improving health and fitness shown by Challenge participants was a positive sign of motivation. The attitudinal framework for Challenge sessions would therefore be positive thinking and positive reinforcement rather than negative thinking and reinforcement.

It was explained in multiple Challenge sessions that what people do is a result of what people believe or value and the meaning attached to the behavior. The more value attached to the behavior, the more difficult it is to change the behavior. Value may be measured by pleasure, reward, satisfaction, or relief of emotional or physical pain. This connection between behavior and value leads to habits, both good and bad, for example, buckling your seat belt every time you get into a car, or reaching for snacks every time you sit in front of a television. Therefore, changing attitudes and customary behaviors requires knowledge, motivation, resources, and skill.

The purpose of these sessions was to help participants identify their particular strengths and weaknesses, uncover their values, examine the bases for their actions, and identify some of the strategies they could use in reaching and maintaining their individual goals. Force field analysis was explained as a method that helps people identify the forces that promote or prevent their own behavior change. Many of these forces are common to all of us. Participants began to identify barriers to change, such as fear of failure and sense of loss.

For the Challenge, forces that promote or impede change were combined into three categories: biologic-physiologic, emotional-cognitive, and social-cultural-economic. Examples of biologic-physiologic factors included genetic makeup (such as body type or metabolism), gender, existing disease processes, and age. Emotional-cognitive factors address coping styles, mental status, long- and short-term health goals, and knowledge deficits. Social-cultural-economic factors included cultural food patterns, job-related activity patterns (such as sedentary work or frequent restaurant dining), and access to health services.

As the beginning step in self-knowledge, participants in the Challenge were instructed to identify a realistic goal and note on an assessment form the positive and negative factors particularly relevant to them (Figure 6.1). Participants were then instructed to assign a level of importance to each factor in accordance with how easy or difficult it would be to accomplish. These steps were based on the research reports that suggest the belief one is capable of carrying out the action (self-efficacy) is one of the strongest determinants of successful behavior change. (Bandura, 1997). Finally, each participant received a worksheet to list the factors perceived as barriers and the behavioral strategies he or she thought would help.

Because of the group's diverse makeup, many different health-related issues, diets, and types of exercise were identified. Participants viewed the university's commitment to health promotion, the availability of excellent resources, and supportive fellow staff as external motivators. Written evalua-

TABLE 6.1 Behavioral Change Strategies

Informing

Direct learning	Commonly uses a group setting such as the classroom and allows material to be shared and discussed by several individuals.
Audiovisual material	Include written instructions, videos, tapes, structural models, computerized instruction, or even cartoons where the concepts being taught can be demonstrated.

Motivating

Self-instruction	A popular method but difficult to evaluate. An example of self-instruction is the use of "how to" books.
Bibliotherapy	A promising area of research using a combination of self-instruction and directed reading, evaluation, and group discussion. May involve inspirational story where crisis situation is resolved; reading about health risk information with follow-up counseling.
Mass media	Uses persuasion and power of the written word in newspapers, radio, or TV. Influential in changing some behavior but readers who experience cognitive dissonance may ignore the message or refute it. Mass media may also have a negative effect because of sensationalist themes of sex and violence and high-powered advertising.

Skill Building

Demonstration/return demonstration	Experiential method commonly used for teaching procedures, such as how to prepare foods or engage in low-impact aerobics.
Simulation	A representation of a real-life situation to teach new behavioral responses. Practice sessions on responding to emergencies or conducting one's activities of daily living while blindfolded are examples.
Role play	A form of simulation whereby each participant assumes the characteristics of a player in a situation. Through role play, individuals can be taught in a nonthreatening atmosphere how to respond in an effective way.
Inoculation	Also known as refusal skills training and assertiveness training are methods that prepare people for setbacks and challenges. Individuals role play potential stressful situations or exposure to real-life stress, and rehearse protective responses that will prevent backsliding. Assertiveness promotes the ability to say "no" in a comfortable and gracious way (such as upholding the decision to abstain from alcohol or refusing a high-calorie food) while respecting others' rights.
Activism participation	Requires participation in activities such as letter writing or lobbying that create an unfavorable environment for the activity such as smoking. Also stimulates participants to resist or terminate the behavior.

Modifying Attitudes and Behavior

Imagery	Creates a mental picture of a habit-free self by focusing on the competing behavior and visualizing the self without the habit. For example, individuals giving up smoking must imagine themselves as nonsmokers; seeing themselves with a cigarette in their hand or mouth must be incongruent with their picture of wholesomeness.
Cueing	A stimulus–response-based approach using human or computer-generated telephone calls, wall-charts, or other types of messages to remind an individual to continue an activity. This intervention has been used to enhance medication compliance, immunizations, or appointments.
Tailoring	Uses compromise as an interim step to change. Valuable when a suggested change is viewed as extremely difficult or impossible (such as a stringent dietary restriction of salt or sugar).
Contracting	A verbal or written agreement toward one or more specific actions. Requires feedback to be effective.
Contingency contracting	An "if-then" approach that states a behavioral goal as well as the rewards for its achievement. Each step of change and reward are shared with a health care provider.

(continued)

TABLE 6.1 Behavioral Change Strategies *(Continued)*

Graduated regimens	Implements the desired behavior changes in intermediate steps and goals. Acknowledges each level of success.
Self-monitoring	A method of self-tracking (such as one's daily intake or weight) using a journal or diary. Frequently short-lived.
Self-confrontation	Consciously interrupts negative thinking. Person says "stop," claps hands. Works in conjunction with self-reinforcement.
Self-reinforcement	Acknowledges positive behavior and verbalizes it frequently out loud.
External reinforcement	Uses social support or continuity of care system to help maintain behavior change.
Self-generated aversive behavioral control	A method of urge control using a negative stimulus such as snapping an elastic band on the wrist or stimulating an acupressure point. Permits time to intervene between urge and acting. Is enhanced by urge replacement/response substitution with another behavioral strategy, such as taking a walk in lieu of smoking.

Other

Hypnosis	A method of behavior modification that requires the individual to be put into a receptive mental state where suggestion influences the behavior.
Acupuncture	Behavioral response believed to be a neurochemical reaction to endorphin production released by stimulating various superficial nerve endings.
Pharmacotherapy	Prescribed therapies often used with drug addictions, eg, nicotine patches or gum for tobacco addiction, Antabuse for alcoholism, and Methadone for heroin addiction.

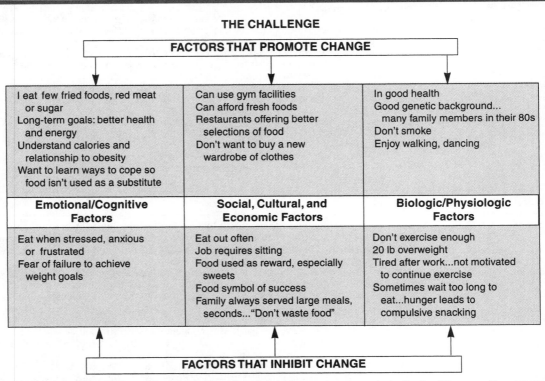

FIGURE 6.1 Behavior change self-assessment, using weight loss as an example in the health promotion program *The Challenge*.

tions indicated that self-assessment of behavioral barriers and motivators provided insight into behavior patterns that had not been considered.

Given the success of this approach with the Challenge, this method has been taught to nursing students for use with individuals or community groups. It remains important that follow-up be done to identify stumbling blocks that may arise and to ascertain that the intervention(s) selected are appropriate, realistic, accessible, and used.

SUMMARY

Health professionals are often responsible for helping patients learn new ways to improve their health and to achieve a higher level of wellness. This chapter presents two health promotion projects that demonstrate how to assess areas in which health education is needed, how to teach people to identify their own behavioral barriers and enhancers to change, and how to promote health through techniques of behavior change. Health promotion occurs in many different settings with diverse population groups. The health educator must therefore develop cultural competence and the ability to act as advocate to help the community acquire necessary resources to successfully achieve health promotion goals. Although personal responsibility for health is recognized, consideration is given to external factors that arise from the political climate, the social environment, the economy, and the resources that may or may not be available from the health system.

The next section of this book provides the details of how to apply these principles in practice. Chapter 7 details how to assess learning needs.

STRATEGIES FOR CRITICAL ANALYSIS AND APPLICATION

1. Compare the differences in planning a health promotion program for a person, a family, or an entire community. What are the advantages and disadvantages of each approach?
2. You work in a community comprised of many low-income families and older people. How would these demographic variables be used to develop a health promotion campaign? What other information would you obtain to prioritize the community's needs?
3. What are the goals of health promotion programs in accordance with the developmental stage?
4. Discuss how culture and language influence health education programs in a community.
5. Identify the persuasive methods that advertisers use to convince consumers to buy such products as tobacco or alcoholic beverages. How could these same methods be used to foster health-promoting behaviors, such as the use of seat belts?
6. What strategies are necessary to achieve a smoke-free society by the year 2020?

To find the latest information

Key search terms
community health, health promotion, community self-determination, community self-help

Websites
- Association for Community Health Improvement: http://www.hospitalconnect.com/communityhlth/resources/planning.html
- Planned Approach to Community Health (PATCH): http://www.cdc.gov/nccdphp/patch/. An effective model for planning, conducting, and evaluating community health promotion and disease prevention programs, the PATCH Guide is designed to be used by the local coordinator and contains "how to" information on the process, things to consider when adapting the process to your community, and sample overheads and handout materials
- Making Health Communication Programs Work: A Planner's Guide: http://cancer.gov/pinkbook

REFERENCES

American Association of Occupational Health Nurses. (2003). *Occupational and environmental health nursing profession fact sheet*. Retrieved June 10, 2003, from http://www.aaohn.org/press_room/fact_sheets/profession.cfm

Association for Community Health Improvement. (2002). *Planning, assessment, & evaluation resources*. Retrieved May 26, 2003, from http://www.hospitalconnect.com/communityhlth/resources/planning.html

Bandura, A. (1997). *Self-efficacy: The exercise of control*. New York: W. H. Freeman.

Bartle, P. (2003). *Community self-management, empowerment, & development*. Retrieved June 8, 2003, from http://www.scn.org/cmp/site.htm

Center for Health Improvement. *Bringing policy change to your community*. Retrieved June 8, 2003, from http://www.healthpolicycoach.org/

Community Tool Box Team. (2002). *Community Toolbox: Bringing solutions to light*. Retrieved July 12, 2004, from http://ctb.ku.edu

Consortium for Infant and Child Health (CINCH). (2000). *2000 report on the health of children in Hampton Roads*. Retrieved June 8, 2003, from http://www.chkd.org/about_us/cpr_report.asp

Enock, K. (2002). *Force field analysis*. Retrieved June 10, 2003, from http://www.healthknowledge.org.uk/knowledgebase/Part1/Organisation9_change_management.htm#Lewin

Gordon, M. (1994). *Nursing diagnosis: Process and application* (3rd ed.). St. Louis: Mosby–Year Book.

Gordon, M. (1997). *Manual of nursing diagnosis: 1997–1998*. St. Louis: Mosby–Year Book.

Habel, M. (2000). *Developing your leadership potential*. Retrieved June 10, 2003, from http://www.cyberchalk.com/nurse/syllabus.cfm?CourseKey=1106

Krozy, R. E., & McCarthy, N. C. (1999). Developing bilingual tools to assess functional health patterns. *Nursing Diagnosis: The Journal of Nursing Language and Classification, 10*(1), 21– 29, 34.

Lindenberg, C. S., Solorzano, R. M., Krantz, M. S., Galvis, C., Baroni, G., & Strickland, O. (1998). Risk and resilience: Building protective factors. *MCN: American Journal of Maternal Child Nursing, 23*(2), 99–104.

Massachusetts Tobacco Control Program. (2003). *Massachusetts tobacco control program accomplishments*. Retrieved June 9, 2003, from http://www.state.ma.us/dph/mtcp/home.htm

McCarthy, N. C. (2002). The 11 functional health assessment guidelines for communities. In C. L. Edelman & C. L. Mandle (Eds.), *Health promotion throughout the lifespan* (5th ed.). St. Louis: Mosby–Year Book.

Miller, D. R., Geller, A. C., Wood, M. C., Lew, R. A., & Koh, H. K. (1999). Falmouth Safe Skin Project: Evaluation of a community program to promote sun protection in youth. *Health Education and Behavior, 26*(3), 369–384.

National Center for Chronic Disease Prevention and Health Promotion. (2000). *United States national youth tobacco survey (NYT) fact sheet*. Retrieved June 4, 2003, from http://www.cdc.gov/tobacco/global/GYTS/factsheets/2000/US_factsheet.htm

Novartis Foundation for Sustainable Development (NFSD). (2003). *The social marketing concept*. Retrieved February 10, 2003, from foundation.novartis.com/leprosy/social_marketing_print.htm

Rudin, D. (2003) *Translating materials for non-English speaking audiences*. Retrieved June 10, 2003, from http://www.medicareed.org/Resources.cfm?RT=CMEPub&Detail=61

U.S. Department of Health and Human Services. (2000). *Healthy People 2010: Understanding and improving health*. Retrieved July 10, 2004, from http://www.health.gov/healthypeople; http://www.healthypeople.gov/

Werner, D., & Bower, B. (1995). *Helping health workers learn: A book of methods, aids, and ideas for instructors at the village level*. Berkeley, CA: The Hesperian Foundation.

Werner, D., Thuman, C., & Maxwell, J. (2002). *Where there is no doctor: A village health care handbook*. Berkeley, CA: The Hesperian Foundation.

Whitehead, D. (2000). Using mass media within health-promoting practice: a nursing perspective. *Journal of Advanced Nursing, 32*(4), 807.

Application of the Principles in Nursing Practice

Assessment for Patient Education

LEARNING OBJECTIVES

After reading this chapter, the student should be able to:

1. List red flags used to identify patients with complex discharge planning needs as part of the assessment process.

2. Identify the four steps of the assessment process and describe how they relate to patient education.

3. List four questions that obtain vital assessment data.

4. State two benefits of using a Patient and Family Assessment Guide.

5. Discuss how patient education relates to all nursing diagnoses and the limited circumstances in which you might select the following nursing diagnoses: knowledge deficit, noncompliance.

6. Describe benefits of home visits for patient assessment.

INTRODUCTION

Patient Education Process

Patient education plans are part of the total plan for patient care. The patient education process has the same steps as the nursing process: assessment, planning, intervention, and evaluation. Patient education activities are an integral part of each of the four phases of patient care. Figure 7.1 illustrates how a nurse might apply the patient education process.

The medical diagnosis initiates early screening on admission. It is used to determine what is likely to cause trouble for the patient after discharge. The focus should be shifted from medical diagnosis to functional problems and the question asked: How the medical diagnosis affects *this* patient?

The anticipated length of stay should be looked at realistically and it should be determined how much and when you might teach each patient. The patient education process encourages the application of protocols and standards that will direct, rather than dictate, patient care. The components of the patient education process offer a framework for modifying care so health care providers and patients grow in a cooperative relationship. When this cooperative relationship exists, patients are cared for as individuals

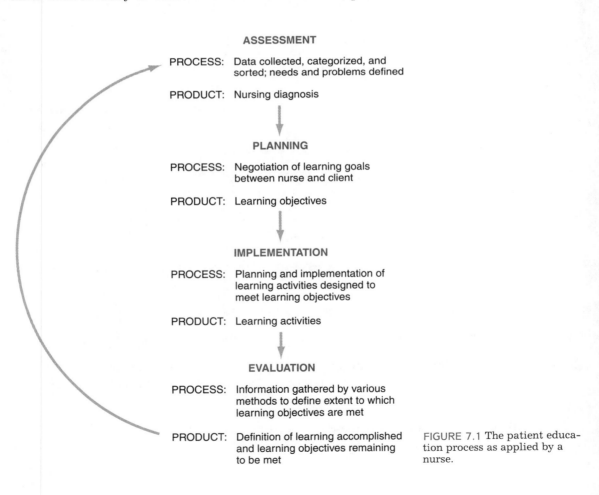

ASSESSMENT

PROCESS: Data collected, categorized, and sorted; needs and problems defined

PRODUCT: Nursing diagnosis

PLANNING

PROCESS: Negotiation of learning goals between nurse and client

PRODUCT: Learning objectives

IMPLEMENTATION

PROCESS: Planning and implementation of learning activities designed to meet learning objectives

PRODUCT: Learning activities

EVALUATION

PROCESS: Information gathered by various methods to define extent to which learning objectives are met

PRODUCT: Definition of learning accomplished and learning objectives remaining to be met

FIGURE 7.1 The patient education process as applied by a nurse.

and can learn to participate in their own care in a meaningful and satisfying manner.

This section illustrates the use of the patient education process, highlighting the important skills of assessment, planning, implementation, and evaluation. Although the principles may appear simple, application of the patient education process involves a broad understanding of the patient and family, and considerable clinical expertise to provide individualized care. Individualized care fulfills the following criteria:

- It includes a care plan that is specific to the individual patient.
- It requires critical thinking to meet the patient's unique needs.
- It cannot be accomplished in a cookbook approach.

The case studies offered in this chapter illustrate principles of patient education, but are not intended to be used as a cookbook. As health care providers continue training in their specialty areas and continue learning more about patient problems they encounter, they can use this text to complement their education of patient and family and to develop individualized teaching plans.

Discharge Planning

Discharge planning occurs not just in inpatient acute care settings, but also in emergency rooms, home health care, surgical centers, and long-term care. Discharge planning is an important evaluation of actual or potential problems that must be dealt with before a safe discharge is made. All members of the health care team have a responsibility to contribute to the discharge assessment process. Usually discharge planning and patient education are intertwined. The patient and family will be taught survival skills and will assume functions of health care management.

As soon as patients are admitted to the hospital, assessment of the potential for discharge begins. For some patients, post-discharge needs are complex. Early detection of special assistance and resources and making

timely arrangements for continuing care are essential, especially in light of decreased lengths of stay.

One method of ensuring coordinated care is to ask questions upon admission to screen for discharge concerns. These concerns are referred to as *red flags*. Interdisciplinary case conferences can also be used to identify red flags. Nursing rounds have become increasingly popular to continue the screening, and to coordinate discharge planning and patient teaching efforts. Interdisciplinary discharge planning, a part of routine patient care, also helps patients and their families develop and implement a feasible post-hospital plan of care.

Interdisciplinary health care team meetings may be regularly scheduled to review patient cases. If not, any health care provider who identifies the need to better coordinate care may organize a meeting of interdisciplinary team members. Depending on the identified patient needs, disciplines that may be represented include nursing, physicians, nutrition, social work, pharmacy, physical therapy, occupational therapy, recreational therapy, and home health. Sometimes patients and family members are included.

In these meetings, both learning needs identified by the health care team and those identified by the learners should be considered. It might be helpful to ask the patient and family to complete the Patient Learning Needs Scale (Galloway et al., 2003) before the meeting. This scale does not delineate specific content to be taught, but helps identify areas of discharge information that the learner wants to know more about, such as medications, diet, activity, and follow-up resources. Responses on this scale can help focus group discussion on perceived needs. The responses should be shared with the health care team members before the meeting, so they can come prepared.

The health care team members identify learning needs through assessment, with high priority to red flags. Box 7.1 provides examples of patients who are high risk and need intensive discharge planning. Patients with red flags may be identified before or during admission, during routine patient care, or through the expressed concerns of significant others. The plan of care for these patients usually requires social services and a highly individualized approach.

Every patient, including those without red flags, needs to be assessed for vital information (Box 7.2). Teaching how to perform physical care at home is critical to successful discharge planning.

Throughout hospitalization patients and families must be prepared to evaluate their

---

BOX 7.1 "Red Flag" Patients

Older patients (older than 70; may include younger patients with disabilities)
Older patients suspected of being abused or neglected
Patients living alone
Children abused, neglected, or with birth anomalies
Patients transferred from other institutions
Recent admissions
Multiple readmissions
Patients who depend heavily on community resources
Patients with financial problems
Patients with terminal illnesses
Patients who live out of state or out of the country
Patients with care-intensive disease, catastrophic illness, or chronic illness
Patients with multiple chronic illnesses
Patients with newly diagnosed disease
Patients who receive few or no visitors
Substance abusers
Patients suspected of being abused, including domestic violence
Patients with family problems
Patients with psychiatric disorders
Patients with poor living conditions
Patients who speak little or no English
Patients with recent disabilities

BOX 7.2 Assessment: Vital Information

- What information does the patient need?
- What attitudes should be explored?
- What skills does the patient need to perform health care behaviors?
- What factors in the patient's environment may pose barriers to the performance of desired behaviors?
  - Is the patient likely to return home?
  - Can the family or significant others handle the care that will be needed?
  - Is the home situation (or environment) adequate or appropriate for the type of care needed?
  - What kinds of assistance (eg, financial resources, medical equipment, manpower, community support) will be needed?

---

family resources, understand their illness and treatment, help them make behavioral changes, and manage their continuing care.

At-Risk Patients

In complex situations, strategies should be developed to follow-up with the patient, family, and community services to determine the outcomes of discharge planning. High-risk situations, such as domestic violence or other forms of abuse, require skilled observation and appropriate questioning (Taliaferro, 2003; Yeager & Seid, 2002).

During the assessment process, the patient often hides the signs of abuse or makes excuses for injuries, which may be life-threatening. Domestic violence, a pattern of assault and coercion, includes physical, sexual, and psychological attacks. The patient may attribute recurrent episodes of injury to being "accident-prone." There may be substantial delay between onset of injury and presentation for treatment. Suicidal thoughts and depression are also common. Patient groups at special risk for abuse are children, pregnant women, and older people.

The patient should be assessed alone in a safe and private environment. The following questions, asked in a nonjudgmental way, can help patients break the silence about abuse, while acknowledging that violence is not the victim's fault (Taliaferro, 2003; Yeager & Seid, 2002).

"At any time, has a partner or parent kicked, hit, or otherwise hurt or frightened you?"

"Have you ever been emotionally or physically abused by your partner or by someone important to you?"

"I noticed your bruise. How did your injury occur? Did someone hurt you?"

"Often patients with these types of symptoms have a history of having been hurt by another person. Has that ever happened to you?"

It is important to document the findings of suspected domestic violence with objective data. Use the patient's own words regarding the injury and abuse and include the name of the assailant and his or her relationship to the patient. Legibly document all injuries using a body map and take photographs of the injuries. Notify the patient's physician immediately. In states with a reporting law, any person who suspects abuse or neglect of a child is required by law to report this suspicion to the county Department of Social Services. This includes instances of physical abuse causing physical harm; neglect causing failure to provide for the child's basic physical, medical, educational, and emotional needs; sexual abuse, such as fondling, intercourse, incest, rape, sodomy, and exhibition; and emotional maltreatment, such as bizarre punishment, belittling, or psychological rejection. Be certain to assess a patient's safety in returning home. Ask if weapons are kept in the house and determine if children are in danger.

THE ASSESSMENT PROCESS

The first step of the patient education process is *assessment:* the collection of data to identify actual or potential health problems. All members of the health care team gather data, and share it through conversation and documentation. A strong assessment process ensures the patient's inclusion in the health care team. The patient is the primary source of information. Families play an important role, especially when the patient is sedated, in pain, or unable to provide crucial information. Families can inform the health care team about the patient's typical behavior and responses, daily patterns, and sources of comfort. A spouse may describe a particular fear the patient is unwilling to disclose, thereby helping health care providers address it and promote the patient's readiness to learn. The needs of family members are included in the assessment, to optimize their ability to best support the patient. When the patient is a parent, the caregiver in the family may be a child or adolescent. When this is the case, the assessment needs to include the child's perspectives and needs.

The assessment process involves continuously collecting information from different sources, validating these data, and sorting, categorizing, and summarizing or interpreting the information. We make assessments every day in our personal and professional lives, often without realizing it. While driving to work, we quickly note the fuel gauge is almost empty, and drive to a gas station. We take inventory in the pantry and make a list before grocery shopping. We walk into a patient's room, notice shortness of breath, and elevate the head of the bed. All of these actions are based on assessment.

Nurses often lead the team in coordinating patient education efforts. The practice of nursing is founded on the ability of nurses to carry out nursing interventions based on the assessment of individual situations. Nurses respond to patients and their families who cannot meet their own needs. The goals of nursing care are to reinforce the patient's strengths, assist the patient in meeting basic human needs, and help the patient regain the ability to meet these needs to the greatest degree possible. Appropriate nursing care requires an accurate assessment of strengths and needs, and clearly defined patient problems.

It is vitally important to make an accurate assessment of strengths and problems, so teaching may be tailored to the learner. In patient education, the nurse's goal is to ensure that patients' rights to information are upheld, and that they are taught the skills that will help them meet basic human needs. Therefore, thorough assessment is essential to accomplish these goals. The three steps of the assessment process are:

1. Gathering data
2. Sorting and categorizing data
3. Writing a summary statement (nursing diagnosis or diagnoses)

We now look at each step in the assessment process as it is applied to patient education.

Gathering Data

It is important to collect data in an organized and efficient manner because data collection can be time consuming. It is imperative to collect only useful information in the assessment process. Data should be gathered while keeping in mind how the information is to be used.

Assessment defines learning needs. The assessment for patient education does not have to be separate from other patient assessment activities. Information about the learning needs of the patient and family is gathered with other data about the patient's condition. To collect information vital to an assessment of learning needs, the nurse must consider the questions listed in Box 7.2.

Assessment Guides

Data should be gathered using criteria that direct the health care provider to the areas to be assessed. Many guides are helpful in assessing the learning needs of patients and families. Some are directed toward a particular patient population, such as patients with diabetes, stroke, or ostomy. Some nurses construct their own assessment tools, which may better meet individual situations. Good assessment tools guide the health care provider to view the patient holistically, within the contexts of the family and environment. The tool should help the health care provider focus on the total person and direct data collection into specific areas related to what the patient must learn.

The health assessment instrument often begins with physiologic data: chief complaint, history of the present illness or problem, and a review of systems. It is also important to note who is the informant, if other than the patient. Assessment often uses many informants, including other health professionals, and, of course, the patient and family. During or after physical appraisal, the health care provider also gathers psychosocial data that affect the educational process. The skill of taking a patient's history improves with practice and experience. Over time, health care providers learn to fine-tune the reporting of problems and to look for significant negatives, ruling out possible problems. For example, a nurse told us about her experience assessing an older patient in a long-term care setting. The patient's daughter reported: "My mother can't walk." When the nurse had the patient attempt to walk, she found the patient could balance herself but was short of breath and dizzy. The problems were dehydration and shortness of breath rather than a musculoskeletal weakness. Other problems to be ruled out include depression, social isolation, pain, and functional dependence.

The assessment instrument may be a checklist with space included for responses, or it may be in guide form with an accompanying flow sheet for summary in the patient's chart. Hand-held or bedside computers may be used to document assessment data. The health care provider should use the tool that seems most helpful and most appropriate to the care setting.

Depending on the setting and the amount of time the health care provider spends with the patient, the assessment is completed in several phases. Data are gathered at different times and are used to update the plan of care. At the first encounter, a nurse screens for the most obvious and acute needs. This is a starting point for beginning care. As time permits, a more comprehensive assessment can be made, and some data gathering may be delegated to other health care providers working with the patient. During assessment is a good opportunity to look for potential problems that can be anticipated in the plan of care. Particularly in the hospital setting, registered nurses often ask how nursing assistants and licensed practical nurses can participate in this process. Both can contribute observations; however, the registered nurse should help them know what to look for and should validate their data, rather than use them as the only source of information.

We constructed our own guide for assessment in patient and family teaching and demonstrate its application in this chapter. This guide applies to various situations and prompts a thorough consideration of factors that will either promote learning or pose barriers to behavioral change.

Patient and Family Education Assessment Guide

Various guides have been drawn up for assessment of individual learners' needs, and family assessment guides are abundant in the literature as well. Box 7.3 is an assessment guide developed by the authors—*Patient and Family Education Assessment Guide*. This guide is based on material contained in educational, nursing, psychological, and sociologic writings. The guide considers the patient and family as a system in a potential learning environment. It also illustrates the importance of evaluating the family as a system, while considering the impacts of the community, the health care industry, and sociocultural influences as suprasystems. It is not necessary, or possible, to obtain answers

to every question for every patient. However, it is important to assess every major category (such as physiologic data, family profile, resources) to ensure the whole context is considered. When a potential problem is discovered, questions are provided to help assess the topic in greater depth.

A model of patient and family education was constructed to help the reader visualize the related components that influence learning. Figure 7.2 illustrates the components of assessment found in the assessment guide. This model represents a healthy educational situation, in which the family has reasonable resources and family functioning demonstrates strengths.

We have observed in our clinical experience that patients who have the support of family members in the learning process cooperate better with the medical regimen. Many studies confirm that support, whether from families, peers, or health care professionals, improves outcomes (Haynes, McDonald, & Garg, 2002; Krumholz et al. 2002; Rankin & Fukuoka, 2003).

Most health professionals now include families in the process of patient education. A systems approach to patient education mandates the inclusion of family members. Teaching one isolated subsystem without dealing with the important family system can, in some instances, negate all teaching efforts. We believe that educating the patient without including the family frequently results in poor rehabilitation and poor cooperation with self-care measures, whether the patient is acutely ill or faces life with a long-term chronic illness. Patient education should be conducted with the family present, whether in the hospital, ambulatory care setting, or at home.

We developed the assessment guide to set the stage for such a teaching environment. It was first used for an adult patient and his family who were dealing with a chronic illness. With some minor changes, the guide in Box 7.3 can be adapted to a family dealing with a patient who has just suffered an acute illness or to a family trying to establish every-

BOX 7.3 Patient and Family Education Assessment Guide

I. Physiologic data
   A. Chief complaint
   B. History of present illness or problem
   C. Review of systems
   D. Functional, cognitive, and sensory abilities (anxiety, ability to concentrate)

II. Family profile: a word picture of the family
   A. Household composition
   B. Gender and age of members
   C. Occupations of family members
   D. Health status of family members; physical limitations
   E. Genogram: a diagram showing family relationships

III. Resources available to the family
   A. Ability to provide for physical needs
      1. Home: space, comfort, safety?
      2. Income: sufficient for basic needs and important extras?
      3. Overall ability to perform self-care
      4. Health insurance: available to the family?
   B. Neighborhood/community resources: friends, neighbors, church, and community organizations helpful and involved?
      1. What kinds of support are provided?

IV. Family education, lifestyle, and beliefs
   A. Educational backgrounds and attitudes toward education
      1. Do all adult family members have basic reading and writing abilities? Check ability to read aloud from patient education material.
      2. To what extent is education, formal or informal, valued? How much education does each family member have?
      3. Are there language barriers to verbal communication among the patient, family members, community, and medical personnel?

   B. Lifestyle and cultural background
      1. Does the family subscribe to folk medicine beliefs?
      2. Is there a conflict between cultural and lifestyle approach and the health professional's teaching?
      3. What are the normal diet patterns of the family?
      4. What are the family's sleep habits?
      5. What are the activities, exercises, occupations, and hobbies of family members?
   C. Learning abilities of family members
      1. Do they assimilate information easily?
      2. Are they able to apply what is taught?
   D. The family's self-concept
      1. Are family members lacking in self-esteem?
      2. Do they have feelings of powerlessness as a result of either life situation or patient's sick role?

V. Adequacy of family functioning
   A. Ability to be sensitive to the needs of the family members
      1. How is the identified patient perceived?
      2. What are the relationships of other family members to the identified patient and to each other?
   B. Ability to communicate effectively with each other
   C. Ability to provide support, security, and encouragement, especially pertaining to the learning environment
   D. Ability for self-help and acceptance of help from others when needed
      1. How open is the family to the health professional's teaching?
      2. How likely are family members to request help in the future, if needed?

(continued)

BOX 7.3 Patient and Family Education Assessment Guide *(Continued)*

E. Ability to perform roles flexibly
F. Ability to make effective decisions
G. Ability of the family to readjust ideas about family status, goals, and relationships
H. Ability to the family to handle crisis situations
  1. Has the family been confronted with chronic illness in the past?
  2. How have family members reacted to situations such as accidental injury or death? Who helped them through it?
VI. **Family understanding of the present event**
  A. Current understanding of the problem:
    1. What do you think has caused your problem?
    2. Why do you think it happened when it did?
    3. What do you think your illness does to you? How does it work?
    4. How severe is your illness? Will it have a short course?
    5. What kind of treatment do you think you should receive?
    6. What are the most important results you hope to receive from this treatment?
    7. What are the chief problems your illness has caused for you?
    8. What do you fear most about your illness?
  B. Point in the life cycle of the family at which the problem occurred

C. Type of onset of the illness or problem: gradual or sudden?
D. Prognosis for survival or prognosis for restorative training
E. Nature and degree of limitations imposed on the patient's functioning
F. Level of the family's confidence in the health system with which it affiliates
VII. **The identified patient, health problem, and educational needs**
  A. The patient's educational and cultural background, especially if different from the family's
  B. The patient's self-concept and reaction to stress
  C. Physical limitations that are barriers to learning or self-care
  D. Information base of the patient
    1. Does he or she understand the health team management and the health team's advice?
    2. Does he or she know others with the same problem and have knowledge of their treatment?
    3. What is his or her position and role in the family?
    4. Has he or she had past illnesses?
    5. What kind of physiologic feedback does he or she use?
  E. Are the patient and family members willing to negotiate goals with the health care team?
  F. Are the patient's perceptions and expectations congruent with those of family members?

day health maintenance, such as one with a newborn.

Systems Theory Applied to Patient Education

Using a systems perspective, this guide moves from the family system, its structure, func-

tion, and processes, and how the family relates to education, to the patient as a subsystem of the family, and to some of his or her educational needs. Integrated in the guide are factors that commonly affect the teaching of older patients (Best, 2001).

Systems theory has gained prominence among family therapists as a method of

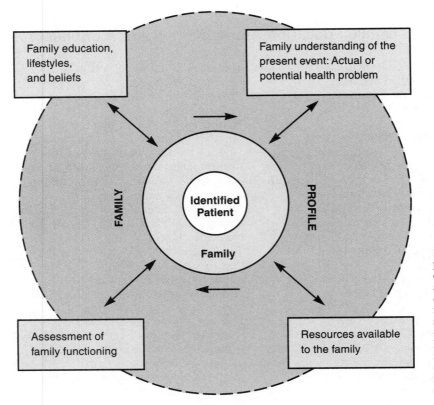

FIGURE 7.2 A model of patient and family education. The two-way arrows between each component and the family system demonstrate their dual effects on each other. The broken line indicates the interactions among all of the components; the family encircles the entire model.

understanding the effects of family members on one another during their ongoing interactions. The interactions of the individual members, or *subsystems,* produce the beliefs, goals, roles, and norms that form the *family system.* Systems theory states the system is more than the sum of its parts. This means the patient educator must assess the family system and include the family in the intervention if the patient (subsystem) is to learn to adapt. For example, if the spouse and children of a patient with hypertension are unwilling to prepare and eat low-sodium, low-fat meals, the patient will have difficulty complying with the medical regimen.

Another aspect of systems theory that is important to the patient educator is the concept of the suprasystem. When we consider the family as a system, the suprasystem is the community to which the family relates, such as the school, church, economic, legal, and health institutions. Assessment of the suprasystem is important because it provides the patient educator with information about support systems that may be implemented to aid in rehabilitation and financial assistance.

Family Structure and Function

Families, like other social systems, have structures and functions. The effectiveness of a family's organization can affect the extent to which new health behavior is assumed. Problems with family organization and role definition often pose obstacles to learning. Differentiation and specialization of roles are important in assessment. For example, the patient's roles may have to change with the onset of a chronic illness, and the provider must recognize this to help the family adapt.

Family functions are closely related to family structure. The structure and function of a family changes over time, as the family moves through the phases of marriage, raising children, launching children, and entering later life. Sometimes the stress associated with daily living, or coping with an acute or chronic medical condition, will disrupt the normal cycle (Rowett, 2001). Family strengths relate closely to family functions and are covered in Part V of Box 7.3. If the desired family strengths are absent, the wisdom of including the family in patient education must be reconsidered or planned in a careful way, because the family may be more destructive than beneficial, posing barriers to the patient's learning process.

The family processes of adaptation, integration, and decision-making are important to patient and family education. A family faced with the illness of one of its members must adapt and change in a healthy fashion. When anxiety is high, it could interfere with the family's ability to receive and comprehend information, maintain patterns of adequate family functioning, use effective coping skills, and provide support for each other and the patient. To positively influence patient outcomes, the family is the most important social context to consider (Leske, 2002).

Boundary maintenance, or the ability to meet needs by obtaining, containing, retaining, and disposing of resources, reflects important data about the ability to adapt. Assessment questions about obtaining and containing resources are found throughout the assessment guide. Dealing with neighborhood and community resources is of special importance. Human resources outside the family are necessary during illness or stress, and they also are indicative of the family's ability to form trusting, caring relationships with others outside of the family.

The family process of integration is covered mainly in parts IV and VI of Box 7.3, and chiefly refers to the family norms and beliefs that help to form the bonds in well-integrated families. A high degree of family integration, built through cultural beliefs and lifestyles, may complicate the teaching process if the beliefs and values differ widely from those of the health care provider. When these beliefs and values are identified and defined, they can be addressed through individualization of teaching (London, 2002).

Culture and Beliefs

The cultural assessment in section IV B of Box 7.3 brings to light the diversity of backgrounds among patients. Values and beliefs influence health and the patient's care. When nurses encounter patients with beliefs and values different from their own, the cultural assessment section must be expanded to include the following significant variables:

1. **Time.** In some cultures, there is a "right time" to do things, and the Western concept of time and clocks is disregarded. Patients may not arrive for appointments at the scheduled time, but when the time seems right to do so.
2. **Religious beliefs.** Some religious beliefs may prevent the patient from seeking health care or accepting treatments and must be considered.
3. **Cultural remedies and healers.** It is important to know about any remedies or healers the patient currently uses or consults and their meaning to the patient. Diet and dietary remedies should be fully explored.
4. **Language and communication.** Note what language is spoken and what nonverbal signals are used.

Cultural differences make each patient unique. When ignored, health care providers treat all patients in a similar way, often resulting in a failure of patient education. Those who hone assessment skills and become sensitive to the patient populations they serve can plan care creatively, and are more likely to achieve successes in patient and family education. This can be accomplished by:

1. Clarifying awareness of the cultures of the health care provider and professional health care.
2. Learning the patient's understanding of the situation, interpretations of illness and symptoms, symbolic meanings, and expectations about treatment (section VI A of Box 7.3).
3. Mutually exchanging information, openly comparing the patient's perspectives with those of the health care provider, and collaborating and negotiating to develop a plan to achieve the patient's goals (Bastable, 2003).

To ensure implementation of a consistent plan of care, information gathered and negotiations agreed upon in these exchanges need to be communicated to the rest of the health care team through conversation and documentation. Chapter 3 addresses challenges and approaches to working with patients whose cultural and belief systems differ from those of the nurse. In addition, we recommend that health care providers seek continuing education to enhance skills to care for patients from other cultures.

Decision-making in the family during events of stress or illness can affect the family's future. If decision-making is not organized adequately, the family may be unable to make important choices related to health care plans or be unable to assume responsibility in health care practices. When patient education is involved, it is frequently necessary for the family to decide, whether by consensus, accommodation, or de facto decision-making, who will learn the required skills (such as how to irrigate a colostomy or give an insulin injection). The importance of assessing the patient as a subsystem of the family is covered in part VI of Box 7.3.

The patient's perception of his relationship to the family, whether realistic or unrealistic, can alter the educational process and should be determined before the teaching plan is begun.

Data should be gathered as objectively as possible. Collecting these data, using fact or measurement, rather than feelings or judg-ments, will guide the health care provider to define needs or problems accurately. Words such as *seems, appears, acts,* and *looks* should be avoided. More useful data would note direct observations or actual behaviors. Whenever possible, the health care provider should document what the patient said in his or her own words. What is heard, smelled, seen, and felt should be described, and the source of the information noted. Observations should be shared with the patient to validate what is observed.

Several effective methods of gathering data exist:

- Observation
- Interviews with patient, family, and significant others
- Review of patient records and literature; continuing education
- Collaboration with the health care team

Observation

Much information can be collected through the senses. Assessments can be made of the patient's affect, and abilities to perform self-care activities and maintain physical appearance. Observation will also provide information about the patient's literacy level, leisure activities, and the role assumed within the family. The home health nurse can gather valuable information by observing the comfort and safety afforded by the patient's dwelling, the facilities available to meet basic needs, and the interactions of family members.

Although the most common method of observation is through sight, nurses also rely on information from things they hear, feel, and smell. Verbal and nonverbal cues gathered by observation provide us with valuable information about what the patient thinks, feels, and believes. Questionnaires and tests may be used to assess a patient's knowledge of facts and to explore attitudes.

Interview

The most reliable methods of obtaining data are taking a patient history or interviewing a patient and family. When patients cannot supply information about their physical or emotional condition, family members should be asked to supply as much information as possible. Whether one is interviewing the patient or family members, several skills and activities apply: establishing trust, asking open-ended questions, reviewing records, reviewing the literature, and collaborating with the health care team.

Establishing a Trusting Environment

Patients must feel secure to confide information. They must feel their concerns are taken seriously and their needs are important and respected. The health care provider communicates trust and respect to patients by concentrating attention on them, maintaining eye contact, and actively listening.

The health care provider should speak in language comparable to the language the patient uses. Trying to impress the patient with medical expertise is not an effective relationship-building strategy. Abbreviations or medical terminology should not be used, except to explain the meanings of terms the patient may hear. When speaking to a child, the nurse should tailor the explanations to the child's level of understanding.

The nurse should speak slowly and clearly, taking time to think about the questions. If the patient wanders off-track, questions may be gently repeated. The purpose of the interview should be explained to the patient, including that the nurse wants to get to know him or her better to provide care in the best manner possible.

The necessity of establishing a trusting relationship is illustrated by the situation that develops when dealing with a patient with a sexually transmitted disease (STD). The health care provider must convince the patient that all information will be held in strict confidence. After assuring the patient of confidentiality, he or she must then explain the importance of notifying the patient's sexual contacts so they can be treated. Such situations are delicate, and if the patient does not trust the health care provider, it will be impossible to provide assistance.

The best settings for effective interviews are private and free of distractions. Obstacles to effective interviewing arise when the patient is too tired or ill to share his thoughts comfortably, or when the interviewer is distracted. Extremely lengthy interviews are difficult for both the patient and interviewer. The interview should be planned so that critical information is obtained first. It may be necessary to have several short sessions. For example, counseling related to STDs must be accomplished discreetly and without family members or anyone else present. The patient should be alone with the health care provider in a private room where there will be no interruptions.

Family members can be included in assessment when they visit the patient, or if this is not practical, by telephone. The health care provider might say, "Staff members are planning care for your mother, and we would like to know what you think. Can you answer a few questions to help us?"

The patient's perceived needs and problems should be explored by the health care provider. Objectivity should be maintained about what the patient says. Pain and perceived needs are subjective; the patient's statements are always correct and accurate from his or her point of view. Opinions or judgments should not be imposed into this conversation.

For example, the adult patient with chronic obstructive pulmonary disease (COPD) and asthma should be allowed to explain his or her perception of the problem. The patient may believe the recent onset of severe symptoms is related to a specific activity, such as walking or sexual intercourse, when, in fact, the blood level for the medication is not in the therapeutic range. Once we learn what the patient believes, we may correct significant misconceptions.

Notes from the interview make documentation more accurate; however, writing too many notes during the interview should be avoided, because this may disturb the patient. Before beginning to record data during an interview, the nurse should say, "I am going to write down a few things you say so I don't forget anything important." Taking notes during an interview frequently makes patients uncomfortable; an explanation can alleviate such discomfort and prevent misunderstandings. Facts, symptoms, times, names, and short quotes from the patient may be recorded quickly and can be used when the nurse is ready to document the results of the interview. When using a computer at the patient's bedside, eye contact should be maintained with the patient. The focus is the patient, not the computer.

Open-Ended Questioning Skills

Open-ended questioning skills help the health care provider to learn the patient's thoughts, which are needed to be understood to best individualize teaching. Open-ended questions elicit the patient's description, in his or her own words, of symptoms, concerns, or needs. When done well, the phrasing of the question does not bias the response.

Both nonfocused and focused questioning have a place in assessment. Nonfocused questioning skills include silence, nonverbal encouragement, and neutral utterances or continuers, such as "uh-huh." Nonfocused questioning skills encourage the patient to choose the topic to discuss. Skills that focus the patient on a specific topic while minimally influencing the content include reflection, echoing, open-ended requests, summarizing, and paraphrasing (Smith, 2002). Open-ended requests can help determine what is most important or most troubling to the patient. For example, the nurse may ask, "If you could change one thing, what would it be?" or "Please tell me what is troubling you the most."

A closed-ended question, which could be answered yes or no, might not get to the most valuable information. If we continue with our example of the patient with an STD, an appropriate open-ended request would be, "Can you tell me what you know about STDs?" In contrast, the closed-ended question, "You know how you got this, don't you?" would probably elicit the response, "Yes," because the patient is embarrassed, does not want to admit ignorance, and feels uncomfortable. To most effectively educate patients, the health care provider should behave in ways that do not reveal disapproval of or disagreement with the patient's choices.

Review of Patient Records

The patient's medical records are often the first source of information. Although information can be gathered quickly from the patient's chart, it should be supplemented by information from other sources. Medical records supply data about the patient's health history, previous hospitalizations, past experience with the health care system, and observations others have made. They can provide clues to finding additional sources of information, such as a public health nurse or community agencies that have worked with the patient. Observation and the patient interview should validate information gathered from the patient record.

Review of the Literature: Continuing Education

Reading texts and journals to update knowledge and skills is a professional responsibility. Education is a foundation for practice, but the ability to anticipate and intervene in areas of need depends on willingness to increase the knowledge base through continuing education.

To intervene responsibly with patients and their families, the health care provider must be prepared with an understanding of the disease or health problem, its medical management, and its impact on lifestyles. Textbooks are valuable resources. Many journal articles describe new approaches to teaching patients and their families, or increase our awareness of self-help groups and other resources that assist in preventing, resolving, or coping with health problems. Workshops and other continuing education programs offer good opportunities for learning from experienced colleagues about patients' problems and the causes and management of these problems. The Internet has the potential to provide much valuable information and resources. (See Chapter 10.)

Collaboration with the Health Care Team

Data gathered by nurses, physicians, dietitians, pharmacists, physical therapists, and other health care professionals can combine many points of view to provide a multifaceted understanding of the patient and family. Insights can be shared and validated, and misperceptions corrected. Whenever possible, team members should collaborate to plan the care of the patient and family. Communication through conversation or documentation helps health care providers share assessments, and build on one another's teaching progress. Coordination of efforts is especially important when time to teach is limited. Collaboration is facilitated by clear verbal and written communication, team conferences, updated care plans, and effective use of rounds to discuss the patient teaching plan.

For example, a patient with multiple chronic illnesses may have prescriptions from several physicians. The hospital social worker who interviews the family may obtain the long list of medications. The social worker then gives this list of medications and prescribing physicians to the nurse, who is responsible for sharing the list with the patient's admitting physician. "Think big. Who else can you involve in the patient and family education process? Go beyond traditional organizations and boundaries. Who can you invite to join the health care team?" (London, 1999, p. 68.)

Sorting and Categorizing Data

Data gathered from various sources must be carefully considered, validated, and grouped into problem areas. In optimal circumstances, the health care team agrees on assessment of patient problems, learning needs, and factors affecting behavioral change for health promotion.

Patients are often overwhelmed by the barrage of information they receive upon discharge from the hospital, particularly if they suffer from an illness that requires permanent lifestyle modification, such as cardiovascular disease. They are expected to make many changes at once, which is difficult for most people. A dietitian, physical therapist, lipid specialist, and nurse might all advise a patient. A good assessment can help identify the one or two most important modifications a patient can make to reduce risk factors. Helping patients prioritize and focus on short-term goals can make the recovery plan seem more manageable.

Writing the Nursing Diagnoses

The summary statements that describe problem areas in which the nurse can intervene are called *nursing diagnoses*. A nursing diagnosis is different from a medical diagnosis because it focuses on a patient's response to a health problem that can be prevented or altered by nursing intervention. A medical diagnosis, by contrast, describes the illness, focuses on its pathology, and guides medical orders or protocols (Carpenito, 2002).

Nursing diagnoses, statements of actual or potential health problems, are derived from the data collected in assessment. These diagnoses are validated with the patient and family who, while doing so, prepare to negotiate goals.

The North American Nursing Diagnosis Association (NANDA) provides a standardized list of nursing diagnoses. This taxonomy has been developed by nurses in all specialties, working together since 1973. Each diagnostic category contains descriptions of etiology, contributing factors, and definitive characteristics that help the nurse select the correct nursing diagnosis. Many health care organizations have established policies and procedures supporting the use of nursing diagnoses and incorporating them in documentation systems.

Nursing Diagnoses

The nursing diagnosis *knowledge deficit* identifies the primary problem as the lack of knowledge, which is rarely the case. *Knowledge deficit* most appropriately applies when the only focus of attention is the promotion of knowledge, such as in prenatal education or parenting skills classes. In these cases, the desired outcome is an increase in knowledge.

In contrast, all nursing diagnoses have implications for patient and family education. When the problem is identified as something other than knowledge deficit, such as "alteration in mobility," interventions often include the provision of information and the coaching of behavioral changes. By framing problems with these nursing diagnoses, the outcomes measured are not the acquisition of knowledge, but more meaningful measures, such as the patient's adaptation to the alteration in mobility. Consequently, patient education is integrated into the total plan of care, and is not separated out as an extra problem and task.

The diagnosis *noncompliance* should be used carefully and specifically after a thorough assessment to describe the patient who wishes to follow a recommended plan but cannot do so because of physiologic or situational reasons. This diagnosis should not be used if the patient has made an informed decision not to comply (Carpenito, 2002).

When patients' readmissions are related to medication noncompliance, the health care team must identify the source of the problem. If a patient has not taken medications correctly or does not maintain a therapeutic drug level, the health care provider must help the patient and family determine what went wrong. Did the patient take the medicine as prescribed? Ask the patient to recall, in the last day or week, when and how much of the medication was taken. Was financial assistance needed to obtain the medication? Were there unanticipated side effects, causing the patient to stop taking the medicine? Instead of only teaching the patient about the medicine, the appropriate educational intervention might be to work with the prescribing physician. Without a good assessment, the teaching may be misdirected (O'Hara, 2002).

Management of the Assessment Process

Prioritizing Needs and Problems

When an individual is faced with problems in several areas, it is often difficult to set priorities. A consideration of a hierarchy of human needs helps rank the priority of problem areas, and offers guidance in how and where to begin patient teaching.

All people have common needs that must be satisfied. The ability of patients and their families to survive depends on their effectiveness in meeting these basic human needs. When they cannot meet basic needs, problems arise that they often cannot resolve alone. At that point, health professionals are called on to intervene. The goal of the health care team, especially nurses, is to help patients regain the ability to meet their own needs and to foster their maximum development, both as individuals and in their relationships with others.

Maslow suggests that needs exist in various levels, and that these groups of needs can be visualized as a hierarchy in which lower-level needs must be at least partially met before a person can meet higher-level needs (Maslow, 1987). One study (Acton & Malathum, 2000) suggests that persons who are more fulfilled and content, have physical need satisfaction, and have positive connections with others may be able to make better decisions regarding positive health-promoting self-care behaviors. Considering these needs helps to prioritize care and patient teaching. Many of us have discovered that learning is hampered when the family faces problems with housing, finances, or threatened self-esteem. Patients who are in pain or are fearful of pain place high priority on managing it; they will learn little else until this need is met. In the assessment process we identify the learner's needs, then prioritize our interventions. We often find the learner's identified needs are consistent with Maslow's hierarchy of needs. Figure 7.3 illustrates examples of nursing assessment for individuals, families, and communities based on Maslow's work.

Learning During the Assessment Process

When the patient and family have an active role in defining their problems, learning occurs. Self-care activities depend on the ability of the patient and family to solve problems by gathering information and categorizing signs and symptoms into problem areas. Health care providers can help them build skills by verbally sharing thoughts during the assessment process. The health care provider should let the patient and the family witness and contribute to a systematic collection of data and definition of problems. They should be informed about the rationales for collecting certain kinds of data and the best ways for discovering and documenting them. The promotion of learning during assessment builds problem-solving skills, encourages validation of data with the patient and family, and serves as a motivator for future learning.

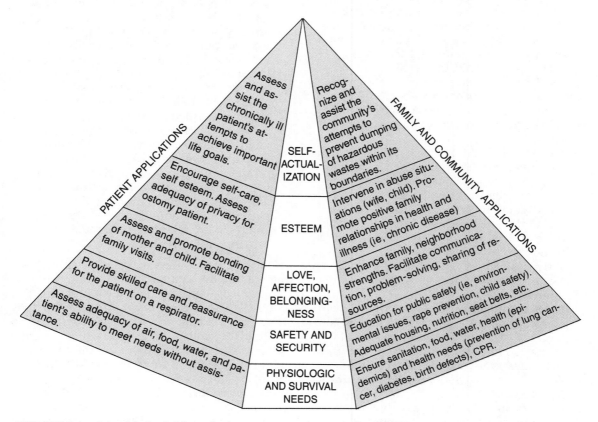

FIGURE 7.3 Applying Maslow's hierarchy in assessment of patient, family and community.

When adults can identify their own needs and contribute toward planning a program tailored to their circumstances, they are more motivated to learn. The questions asked by the nurse provide families with a sense of what is important and what they need to do to prepare for discharge.

Time Management

Health care providers often identify lack of time as an impediment to the assessment process. They find it difficult to justify dedicating an hour to collecting information in an interview or to making a detailed assessment. Here are some insights to counter that point of view:

- **A good assessment is a time-saver.** Although assessment requires spending time in astute observation and active listening, time will be lost if the care plan is constructed without input from the patient and family. In these cases, interventions are often ineffective, and additional time is spent going back to the assessment process to discover barriers to change that were preventing progress all along.
- **The patient and family must have time to tell their story.** They must be given time to offer their perceptions of their own problems. This information is necessary to tailor teaching to meet the patient's needs and abilities. Time should be taken to help them understand what is expected of them if they are to take charge of self-care activities. This is critical in the management of chronic illnesses that affect children, such as asthma.
- **Assessment can be made any time a health care provider interacts with a patient and family.** Gathering information should not be restricted to the formal interview. Bath time, meal time, rounds, visiting hours, and medication times are all opportunities for assessment.
- **Patients are sensitive to the time pressures of health professionals.** Patients often do not know what is expected of them, whether (or for how long) they will have your attention, or how to contribute important information. Health care providers can teach patients to help with time constraints by offering statements such as the following: "Mrs. Wise, I have set aside 15 minutes this morning at about 10:00. I will ask you and your husband to answer some specific questions for me about your health problems so I can better plan your care with Dr. Mason and the nursing staff." This gives the patient an idea of what is expected and informs her she will be asked specific questions instead of being put in the position of not knowing what information is important. In some instances, a questionnaire can be given ahead of time to collect initial data, which will be discussed during the interview. Whatever can be done to minimize interruptions and distractions during the interview will help to maximize productivity. Fifteen minutes of well-planned, well-used time accomplishes more toward assessment than does an hour with interruptions and lack of direction.
- **Assessment varies based on the setting and the patient.** Even in the most brief encounter, the nurse can ask "What brought you here at this time?" and gain the wealth of information outlined in the assessment guide. In outpatient clinics, patients and families may be asked to complete brief written or computerized assessment instruments.

Health care providers in pediatric clinics recognize the best time for patient education is during well-child visits. Education is focused on safety and prevention. During the first visit, they assess the home environment as part of the initial history. Teaching at each immunization visit is based on the age of the child and key information from the assessment, such as whether guns, lead paint, or poisonous houseplants are found in the home. The physician or nurse practitioner continues further assessment and teaching during the examination of the child. For instance, she might ask about pets in the home, stressing that pet dander is a cause of child allergies.

CASE STUDIES

How can the wealth of information offered by patients and families be used during short inpatient experiences in the hospital? The assessment guide in Box 7.3 is a comprehensive tool for identifying clues for individualizing the teaching plan. Even with this tool, it is difficult to gather all pertinent information at one time, and the health care team often cannot cover every aspect. The more information the team can access, the better able they will be to understand and influence patient behaviors. The guide offers direction for discovering such information during the initial assessment and throughout ongoing assessment as part of the relationships among the provider, the patient, and family.

Nurses who work on hospital inpatient units typically do not have the time and opportunity for extensive patient and family education assessments. Patients are often so ill and families so stressed in an acute episode that assessment must be conducted in bits throughout the hospitalization. This information is helpful, not just in planning, but during the inpatient phase. With good documentation, the information benefits other providers along the continuum of care, such as home health nurses, who can build on the assessment data during home visits. The following case study is an example.

CASE STUDY 7.1

THE SMITH FAMILY

PHYSIOLOGIC DATA
The Smith family was in the Newborn Intensive Care Unit. The wife recently gave birth to 34-week premature twins, Joshua and Sarah. Both babies do well and are soon discharged after 2 weeks of birth.

At the initial encounter with the nurse, Mrs. Smith says she wakes up every 3 hours to breast-feed Joshua and console him. Sarah is still learning to suck and swallow, and is working on feeding with the nurse so the mother can concentrate on Joshua. They both receive initial respiratory assistance.

Joshua goes home first and Sarah soon follows, but she still cannot breast-feed. Mrs. Smith appears determined to learn the skills required in caring for these two infants. After the twins' discharge, the nurse follows up with them for 6 months to assess their needs and coping abilities.

PERTINENT HISTORY
Joshua and Sarah: Normal pregnancy until 8 months, when Mrs. Smith's membranes ruptured prematurely and the babies were delivered the same day, 2 hours apart. Joshua is intubated initially and Sarah is put on continuous positive airway pressure (CPAP). Overall, Joshua's recovery is quicker and smoother. Sarah is sicker and requires oxygenation for a longer time, delaying her ability to latch and suck at the breast. The mother has two lactation consultations since Sarah's discharge. She believes they "didn't tell me anything new, they just said I was doing everything right."

At the nurse's first home visit, however, the mother plans to bathe with Sarah that evening to "recreate the womb," because of a suggestion given to her from the lactation consultant.

The Smiths have been married for 12 years, with 6 moves during that time. Both families of origin live on the East Coast. The Smiths moved to the West Coast 2 years ago and are happy in their location.

FAMILY PROFILE

FAMILY STRUCTURE (FIGURE 7.4)

The family is composed of the husband, Lad, 52, a successful businessman; wife, Karen, 38, a full-time mother; and children, Max, 3, and Joshua and Sarah, 3 weeks. Health status for all is well with the exception of a lack of sleep for both parents, lack of patience for Max, and occasional colds acquired by Max at school. Both newborns are healthy and growing, but Sarah continues to have difficulty breast-feeding and both twins are on different sleep/feed schedules.

RESOURCES AVAILABLE TO THE FAMILY

The family can meet its physical needs. They live in a modest home in the suburbs that has enough space for three children and two adults. It is child-safe and appears comfortable, although the mother complains about the disorganization and clutter around the house. Lad's income is sufficient for basic needs, but the family can also access some community resources for additional needs. These resources include twin and breast-feeding support groups, friends and neighbors who bring over meals in the evenings, Max's school friends, and Jewish community center contacts. These support networks help the Smiths with babysitting and house cleaning.

Karen expresses concern about the extent of their family's needs and her support network's ability to maintain this intensive amount of help. Health insurance is available to all family members and has paid for the few lactation consultant visits at the home and several at the hospital. The Smiths' overall ability to perform self-care is limited because Lad is gone all day and Karen cannot meet all the children's needs alone. Max attends preschool 8 hours a day, 5 days a week, which reduces Karen's workload. Still, she needs help with the twins during the day and at night, because neither she nor Lad sleeps longer than 2 to 3 hours at a time during the night. Karen has presently organized a schedule for help she receives 3 days a week from a college-aged neighbor in the afternoons when Max gets home from preschool, but still feels overburdened and overwhelmed.

FAMILY EDUCATION, LIFESTYLE, AND BELIEFS

Both parents have college degrees, and Lad has a graduate degree. Education appears to be important in this family. The parents have no language barriers between them, but they are still teaching Max how to communicate his needs and are learning how to understand the twins' communication of their needs. Karen emphasizes her needs with any-

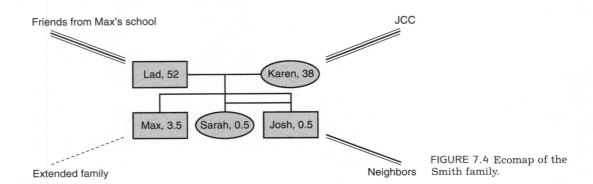

FIGURE 7.4 Ecomap of the Smith family.

one: friends, medical personnel, or family. Lad is more reserved than Karen, but does communicate when asked. This family subscribes to Western medical ideals, and their cultural and lifestyle approach agrees with their health professional's recommendations, although Karen did express frustration with Sarah's inability to breast-feed and the health profession's lack of help in this area. Normal diets include food from the four basic food groups, eaten generally three times a day with snacks throughout the day. Karen often drinks large amounts of fluids to help her with breast-feeding.

The family's sleep patterns are a concern. Lad has been sleeping on the first-floor couch to get some sleep, although Karen is up every 2 hours breast-feeding Joshua and Sarah. Lad is in charge of Max in the evenings and nighttime; recently, Max has been waking up during the night. Consequently, no one in the house is getting enough sleep. Lad has continued to maintain his exercise routine, but now must wake at 5:00 A.M. to get his workout in. He then helps get Max ready for school, and then takes the ferry to work. He works in the city, approximately 45 minutes from home.

Karen is too exhausted to exercise, and is concerned whether she is eating enough because of her current stress level. She worked in retail for years before having children and always believed she would return, but never did, once she had Max. She enjoys being a mother, has Max involved in many community programs (such as art classes), and encourages him to be creative. The family is active in the Jewish temple and enjoys many friendships from this association.

Both Karen and Lad are bright, assimilate information easily, and apply what they learn. For instance, Karen took the information a lactation consultant gave her and attempted to breast-feed in the bath with Sarah, which was successful. Both parents and Max present with strong self-esteem. Karen feels overwhelmed with her situation at times, but she always tries to learn new ways to make things work and is receptive to new ideas. She stated, "I know this is temporary, so I am trying to enjoy this time because I know it will fly by quickly."

ADEQUACY OF FAMILY FUNCTIONING
Because of the lack of sleep, no one is particularly sensitive to the needs of the other family members at present. Karen and Lad often take things out on each other and sometimes even on Max. Max has been biting children at school. In addition, he was home for a week with a bad cold, and felt sick and neglected. Both Karen and Lad are aware of their lack of patience with each other and they are also aware of Max's need for attention. Max has never acted angrily toward either twin, but will do anything to get Karen's attention when she is breast-feeding. One solution she discovered was to breast-feed wherever Max was playing, so they could talk to each other without her having to choose between Max or one of the twins. She also left the twins once a week with a babysitter for an hour and spent that time with Max. Since Karen and Max began having one-on-one time together, Max has stopped acting out and is more independent of his mother. Karen believes this is because he feels more secure in his relationship with her. During the weekends, Lad spends most of his time with Max.

Lad and Karen's relationship has suffered the most since the twins came home. They have not slept in the same bed since that time. Karen considers Lad's job a vacation compared with being at home; Lad disagrees. They are both sleep-deprived, impatient with each other, and severely in need of time alone. Karen copes well, but with all her overwhelming responsibilities, she is presently in survival mode. She told me the only people who could visit were those that would help. This was one of the reasons her family had not been to visit, because she believed they would not be helpful to her and she could not handle it. Karen is adept at asking for help and would be likely to ask for future help if someone could provide assistance. Lad is less likely to ask for help and at times doesn't understand why Karen is so needy.

Karen and Lad have had numerous discussions about seeking help from a community-based program called Mother's Help, which sends someone to the house night or day to assist with infant care. Lad has offered to stay at home 2 days a week, but Karen says she would rather have him at work, because he would be bored and unhappy. She also says she would rather have someone else, such as a nursing assistant or a trained babysitter, helping her rather than him. Lad has tried to be flexible in his role as a father, but is less so in his role as manager of the family budget. Karen would rather spend money on extra help and have him go to work to make up the difference. She thought they both would be happier if they had outside help. Both parents can make effective decisions, but it became apparent they had different values that caused difficulty in making this decision.

The Smiths had a great ability to readjust ideas about family status, goals, and relationships. Both parents realize Lad won't sleep on the couch forever, that Sarah and Joshua will one day sleep through the night, and that

Max will soon enjoy a relationship with his siblings without feeling threatened about his current relationship with his parents. Overall, the Smiths exhibited a good response while handling this crisis situation. Karen's positive outlook extends to all of the family members.

When the nurse commented that it was surprising in only a year and a half of living in the neighborhood that this family has built such a strong support system and awareness of community resources, Lad smiled and said, "You wouldn't be surprised if you knew Karen. This is how she handles everything."

FAMILY UNDERSTANDING OF THE PRESENT EVENT
All family members are aware of how dramatically their lives changed when Joshua and Sarah were brought home from the Newborn Intensive Care Unit 2 weeks after their delivery. Their present challenge is to figure out what will work out for them emotionally, physically, and financially as far as getting more help during the day or night, getting more sleep, and meeting each other's needs during this temporary crisis. Considering how well the Smiths have handled the situation thus far, their survival prognosis is excellent. One aspect of this event that is different than in other health care settings is that the changes are happy changes and the family is happy and enthusiastic about working out the problems, despite the stress. In addition, these choices were made consciously, so they could prepare for the changes. The level of the Smiths' confidence in their affiliate health system is high, and they receive frequent pediatric and obstetric visits.

HEALTH PROBLEMS AND
EDUCATIONAL NEEDS
Nursing Diagnoses:
- Knowledge deficit related to care of premature newborn twins

- Ineffective breast-feeding related to unsatisfactory breast-feeding process, secondary to inability to attach
- Altered family process related to gain of new family members, secondary to need to meet physical needs of all family members and seek help appropriately
- Fatigue related to interrupted sleep patterns secondary to feeding and care needs of newborns
- Altered nutrition (less than body requirements) related to increased maternal needs during breast-feeding

Both babies must be placed on a consistent schedule. Sarah must continue practicing breast-feeding until she no longer needs supplementing, if Karen continues to have the patience and desire to do so. The twins' are progressing appropriately and growing with each pediatric visit. The nurse addressed concern to the family about Karen not taking care of herself (such as lack of sleep, nutrition, and stimulation). By educating both parents about Karen's physical needs for breast-feeding alone, the nurse could discuss Karen's desire for outside help and weigh this possibility against the challenge of meeting financial obligations. The nurse discusses with Lad and Karen the possibility of getting away together for just 1 night or 1 day and letting someone else care for the children. The nurse encouraged them to let family members help with the children, if possible, and stay for extended periods.

CONCLUSION

By the end of 6 months, Karen had help during the nights and several days during the week. Both she and Lad were sleeping better and feeling better emotionally and physically, although they were still sleeping in separate rooms. They did allow their family to visit and were surprised at how helpful they were. With this extra support, Lad and Karen left for 2 nights together while the grandmother watched the children. Sarah learned how to breast-feed, and both babies were well established with breast-feeding and gained an enormous amount of weight, which helped them sleep through most nights. Max established relationships with both siblings, and couldn't wait for them to play with him and be more mobile. Karen was feeling better, and was meeting her physical and emotional needs as well.

How can nursing students gain practice in assessing patients and families for the purposes of patient education? We recommend home visits as a helpful way to learn assessment skills. The authors worked with students who identified a patient in the family medicine clinic and then conducted a follow-up visit at home. A pair of students made each visit, and then wrote a summary based on the assessment guide.

CASE STUDY 7.2

THE DAWE FAMILY

HISTORY

Mrs. Dawe comes to an outpatient clinic for her regular appointment. She tells the nurse she has "to keep check on my sugar and have my blood pressure checked." She states she has diabetes and needs help with her "weight problem." The physician shares with the nurse some of his frustration in caring for Mrs. Dawe. He refers to her as a "delightful lady" who is just "not compliant," despite numerous patient education efforts.

The nurse suggests a home visit as a means of identifying factors that might influence Mrs. Dawe's cooperation with her self-care management in the areas of diet, exercise, medication, and blood glucose monitoring. The physician agrees this is a good idea and together the physician and nurse suggest it to the patient. The following information is collected using *the assessment guide.*

FAMILY PROFILE

FAMILY STRUCTURE

Mrs. Dawe is a 73-year-old, Caucasian, obese woman. At 157.5 cm (5 ft 3 in), she weighs 77 kg (169 lb), 30% more than her ideal weight of 52.3 kg (115 lb). Her manner in the outpatient clinic is matter of fact. Mrs. Dawe is a retired RN. She makes certain that the nurse immediately recognizes her status and competence.

An appointment for the first home visit is made during the visit to the outpatient clinic. The following information is obtained during the home visit.

Mrs. Dawe meets the nurse at the door in a house dress with sandals and no stockings, her white hair neatly combed. Mr. Dawe is dressed in denim overalls. He is smaller than his wife and considerably outweighed by her. He is slightly deaf, but makes every effort to keep up with the conversation, although he is neither as verbal nor as articulate as his wife. Mr. and Mrs. Dawe were both born in the South and lived there all their lives.

Mr. and Mrs. Dawe are both retired. Their last jobs were at a medical center, where Mrs. Dawe worked as an RN floater and where Mr. Dawe was a maintenance worker. Mr. Dawe's occupational history included various skilled and semiskilled jobs; he had worked for railroads, textile mills, and during World War II, for the Army at a military camp.

The household once included the Dawes' four children. The oldest child (and only daughter) is presently employed at a local government agency. She was educated at a local private university, and was married and widowed within 4 years. A daughter from this marriage, now 20 years old, is presently a freshman at a local state university. The Dawes' daughter remarried, and the second marriage was unhappy, involving physical abuse and separations. The Dawes' second child is married with three children, and lives and works in the same county as his parents. He is employed in the electronics industry. The third child seems to be the "fair-haired boy." He graduated from a local state university and then went to work for a large insurance company, which had steadily promoted him and transferred him around the country. This son, his wife, and three of their four children are living in Arizona, and are greatly missed by Mrs. Dawe. The Dawes' youngest child is living nearby with his wife and son. He works as a painter, and recently painted the exterior of his parents' house.

The health status of the Dawes is important to consider in assessment because it influences other areas in the analysis. Both Mr. and Mrs. Dawe were in robust good health well into their 50s. After that, however, Mrs. Dawe's genetic heritage and the effects of Mr. Dawe's physically demanding work caught up with them.

At age 56, Mr. Dawe had a power-tool accident that resulted in permanent loss of function of his left hand. Ten years after surgery, Mr. Dawe suffered a myocardial infarction, from which he fully recovered. Two years later, emphysema developed and persisted, limiting

Mr. Dawe's ability to engage in yard work or gardening. Mr. Dawe had smoked approximately a pack and a half of cigarettes per day, but quit. Glaucoma had been a problem, but was arrested by medications. Mr. Dawe is amazingly spry considering his ailments.

Mrs. Dawe's health history is not as long and complicated, but its implications for the future are probably more negative. Mrs. Dawe's diabetes was first diagnosed at age 56, and she was placed on insulin (premixed 70% intermediate and 30% long acting) at the time of diagnosis. Her insulin requirements have steadily increased, and she has been on a long-term regimen of 44 units/day. She takes 29 units in the morning and 15 units each evening. Her weight has steadily increased from 65.9 kg (145 lb) to 74 kg (163 lb), and her attempts at weight reduction using an American Diabetes Association (ADA) diet have been fruitless. Retinopathies and a cataract requiring removal had developed since the onset of diabetes. Mrs. Dawe's written records of home blood-glucose monitoring show few periods of diabetic control. Hypertension was diagnosed about 8 years earlier. She currently takes Prinivil (30 mg/day) and enteric-coated aspirin daily. She has exercised progressively less during the years, and the combination of obesity, diabetes, and coronary artery disease has left her in poor physical health. The slightest amount of exertion makes her short of breath, and she states she cannot participate in any guided exercise program.

RESOURCES AVAILABLE TO THE FAMILY
The Dawes' seven-room home, which they own outright, is situated in a small, rural community and has aged comfortably during its 30 years. The interior is well kept, with additions such as carpeting and a new furnace added since they first built the house themselves "piece by piece." The furniture is comfortable and in good repair, and provides a homey feeling, accentuated by a pleasant clutter of family photographs, trophies, and knick-knacks. Prominently displayed on a table is a photo of their second oldest son and his family, who are now located in Arizona. Photos of other children and grandchildren are in less prominent places. Mrs. Dawe gives the nurse a tour of the home, pointing out the large size of the rooms and explaining the candy in the dining room is not for her but for the visiting children. The nurse notes three boxes of cake mix in Mrs. Dawe's kitchen cupboards and a cake plate sitting out in the dining room. The home is larger than necessary for their present needs. The Dawes' previous lack of financial resources seems to have been surmounted.

Income for the family is derived mainly from Social Security benefits and two pensions from the medical center. Although the Dawes' income is limited, it does allow for travel; the previous summer they drove to Arizona to visit their son and his family. Limited financial help is received from their children in the form of home improvements and money for traveling. Recognizing the limitations of Medicare, Mr. and Mrs. Dawe paid for additional medical insurance; the premiums are a rather large expenditure for them.

Neighborhood and community resources are informal but supportive. Neighbors watch the homes of one another, and they all keep keys to one another's homes. In the summer and fall, the Dawes enjoy their neighbors' garden produce. The family faithfully attends a local Methodist church, because it is convenient and they like the parishioners, but both hastened to add that they are not members of the church. When questioned about involvement in community organizations, Mrs. Dawe speaks with pride of her work in the local school system when they were both employed. She tells the nurse about her initiation of an immunization program at a local elementary school. She remarks that she still had a feeling of accomplishment every time she saw the school. The family has informal and unstructured interface with community agencies and resources. In times of personal need, however, they obtain services from the church, which has also helped their daughter through some difficult times.

FAMILY EDUCATION, LIFESTYLES, AND BELIEFS
Education is highly valued by the family, especially Mrs. Dawe. She graduated from nurses' training program. She prides herself on keeping current with medical matters, gaining most of her knowledge from *Family Health* magazine, to which she subscribes. Mr. Dawe graduated from high school. All four of the Dawe children graduated from high school, and two completed college. Books, magazines, and newspapers are evident in the household.

The learning abilities of Mr. and Mrs. Dawe are adequate, although Mrs. Dawe cannot follow her ADA diet. The self-concept of this couple appears healthy. Together they express the view that they had worked hard in life "but had come through in good shape." As a couple, they both seemed to have achieved psychologist Erikson's various stages and were in the eighth developmental stage, completing the tasks of ego integrity (Erikson, 1993).

ADEQUACY OF FAMILY FUNCTIONING
The adequacy of family functioning is assessed on the basis of the self-report.

Mrs. Dawe appears to be viewed by her husband with fondness and warmth that developed during 47 years of a marriage marked by economic and personal tribulations. Mrs. Dawe is quick to say the marriage has been good and that they are happy together now. Mr. Dawe laughs in a somewhat embarrassed fashion, but nonverbal clues such as nods of agreement and appropriate smiles indicate that he agrees with her assessment. Relationships with their children seem healthy and supportive on the basis of Mr. and Mrs. Dawe's reports. Communication between husband and wife is adequate. Mr. Dawe is not as verbal as his wife, and he tends to let her finish his sentences for him. Support and encouragement for each other are communicated in important nonverbal ways, such as Mr. Dawe's willingness to take his wife to the outpatient clinic to talk with the nurses and his willingness to be available when the nurse arrives for the home visit. Another sign of mutual support and security is the fact that they still sleep in the same double bed together. Mr. and Mrs. Dawe maintain their emotional and financial resources carefully, sharing them mainly with their children.

The family's ability to accept help, especially in areas of health care, is limited. This is mainly because of Mrs. Dawe's background as a nurse; she must feel competent and self-sufficient in all medical areas. Other family members place demands on her that make it difficult for her to follow her health care plan. This area caused the greatest difficulty in patient and family education. Because Mrs. Dawe is not following her ADA diet, she is placed in a constant state of jeopardy—she knew what she should do but could not, or would not, comply. As a result, her weight continues to increase, and she is left in the rather untenable position of having to justify her situation by claiming she has "a strange case of diabetes." Unfortunately, her choices have negative outcomes for the family system.

Role flexibility is not of imminent importance to this family in its life cycle. The family has a traditional delineation of work: Mrs. Dawe did the household chores, and Mr. Dawe supervised a neighborhood teenager who did the yard work.

Decision-making in this family tends to fall primarily to Mrs. Dawe, as had discipline of the children in the past. Although some of the decisions are made in a de facto manner by Mrs. Dawe, there were also instances when decisions are made by the process of accommodation (such as, a process of begrudging compromise and a questionable commitment to the decisions).

In the Dawes' viewpoint, family status, goals, and relationships are not seriously impaired by chronic illness. Adjustments to Mrs. Dawe's diabetes and to Mr. Dawe's emphysema have been smooth. The concurrent onset of chronic illness and onset of aging has, perhaps, made acceptance of the illnesses easier.

Relationships have changed as the children grew up and moved out, but overall the family seems to have adjusted well.

With an immediate mobilization of energies, the Dawes respond to crisis situations, especially serious injury or death. Because of Mrs. Dawe's background as a nurse, she immediately was called on in times of illness or injury. Besides caring for the ill or injured family member, she also carried messages from the rest of the family. Mr. and Mrs. Dawe both indicate that although they became distressed in such situations, they felt they could respond appropriately.

FAMILY UNDERSTANDING AND THE PRESENT EVENT: CHRONIC ILLNESS

This family has a long association with diabetes through relatives on both sides of the family. The Dawe family genogram (Figure 7.5) shows the remarkably high incidence of diabetes and diabetes-related deaths on both sides of the family. Both partners seemed to accept diabetes philosophically, even fatalistically. When asked how he felt 17 years before about the diagnosis of his wife's diabetes, Mr. Dawe states, "It's just something that happens." He feels the only way her diabetes has affected him had been in her cooking: "it's not as good as it used to be."

This chronic illness was not diagnosed until late middle age, and relatively few restrictions were imposed on the family's ability to function at a pre-illness level, which probably accounts for the relative ease with which they had handled it. Although Mrs. Dawe had to contend with a limited menu and portions, insulin injection, blood glucose monitoring, and other medically prescribed guidelines, her role within the family was initially undisturbed. The complications of diabetes (retinopathies and hypertension) that were found in Mrs. Dawe are of concern to the family and interfere with daily activities. Mrs. Dawe cannot drive, which makes her more dependent on her husband. Based on this information, the nurse asks her to show how she performs her blood-glucose testing and insulin injection preparation. She is happy to do so, because she sees herself as "teaching" the visiting nurse. She draws up her insulin accurately with the assistance of a specially marked syringe. Her blood-glucose testing is done with a digital read-out designed for patients

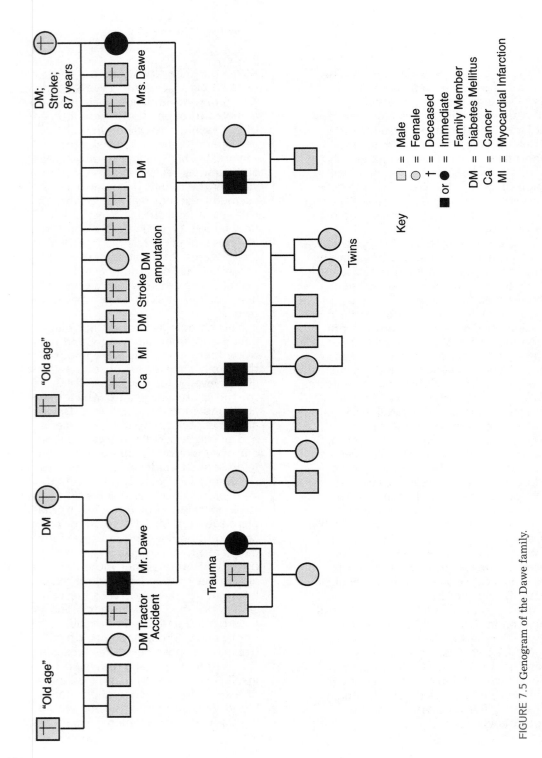

FIGURE 7.5 Genogram of the Dawe family.

184

with impaired vision. Her reading is 250 mg/dL, 2 hours after eating. This reading validated Mrs. Dawe's poor diabetic control. The nurse takes her blood pressure, which is 170/94 mm Hg, indicating hypertension. As her activity level declines and her weight increases, she cannot move around easily, which limits the mobility the couple enjoyed during the past few years. Mrs. Dawe's role as provider of nursing care and as child care provider for grandchildren and other family members is restricted.

The couple's children recognize the hereditary nature of diabetes and have their blood checked occasionally for glucose, Mrs. Dawe reported. As far as the parents knew, however, their children have no pervasive fear of diabetes.

HEALTH PROBLEM AND EDUCATIONAL NEEDS

Mrs. Dawe's educational background as an RN occasionally becomes a problem. Her self-concept involves an image of herself as one who should cope with diabetes management problems and, at times, she hesitates to ask for support or advice. "I just don't feel I can ask these young guys about things the way I used to when I knew them from working with them," she states. Further complicating the problem of daily diabetes management is her hypertension. The physiologic feedback she receives (headache, occasional nausea) is symptomatic for both conditions and therefore confusing.

The principles of diabetic self-care (diet, exercise, medication, response to hypoglycemic and hyperglycemic reactions, prevention of complications) are outlined for Mrs. Dawe by the nurse. She is proud of her medical knowledge and skills. It becomes clear, however, that in this case (as with many other

health professionals under medical care themselves), knowledge and skills are often not enough to promote healing behaviors. To assess Mrs. Dawe's learning needs accurately, the nurse encourages Mrs. Dawe to talk about problems with her treatment plan and her lifestyle. Mrs. Dawe's responses to questions defined the following areas that she saw as problems:

- Weight gain—diet is too restrictive; cannot eat "normally;" always hungry
- Cannot follow exercise program because of fatigue, shortness of breath
- Poor control of blood pressure because of an inability to follow low-sodium, low-fat diet; salt substitute "tastes awful;" husband likes salt used in cooking
- Poor control of diabetes, resulting in hyperglycemia, retinopathies

Mr. Dawe displays a lack of knowledge about diabetes and its management when questioned. He "left it up to her" to know what to do because she is a nurse. Mrs. Dawe did not talk about her diet with him, but he noticed that her "cooking had changed some."

The visiting nurse concludes the assessment for patient education by discussing and validating the problem areas with Mrs. Dawe.

CONCLUSION
- Altered Nutrition: More than body requirements related to nonadherence to diabetic low-salt, low-fat diet
- Educational Needs: Negotiate and coach behavior modification related to ADA diet
- Positive factors affecting behavioral change
  Patient is knowledgeable about health problems

Patient cooks

Patient makes decisions

- Negative factors affecting behavioral change

Self-concept is decreased

Environment includes availability of restricted foods

Patient feels hungry

Patient feels diet is too restrictive

Husband is not impressed with seriousness of health problem

Activity Intolerance related to decreased mobility and obesity

- Educational Needs: Negotiate and instruct to increase activity with consistent exercise program
- Positive factors affecting behavioral change

Interferes with role of caring for others, including grandchildren

Patient wants to be independent and more mobile

Symptoms bother patient

- Negative factors affecting behavioral change

Patient is obese

Patient's dependence on husband has increased

Patient cannot follow diet

SUMMARY

Patient education is an integral part of nursing care. Although the steps of the patient education process are always the same (assessment, planning, implementation, evaluation), the health care provider must tailor practice to meet the needs of patients and the constraints of the patient care setting. A detailed assessment guide helps health care providers understand the learner, so they can best individualize teaching. A good assessment helps health care providers focus on the most important information to teach, and provides insight into how best to present it. Consequently, they can use the available time to teach as efficiently as possible.

Two case studies illustrated how patient education begins in the hospital or clinic, but then must extend into the home, where learning is applied and internalized. Home visits can provide an opportunity to assess problems related to behavior management of chronic problems and build on family strengths. Even with limited time for assessment of a new patient, the educational needs identified in the hospital or clinic can later be refined as more detailed information is gathered.

In both cases, assessment highlighted problems commonly encountered by patients and families. An ongoing need exists for education of patients and families that extends beyond the walls of the hospital or the outpatient clinic. Every member of the health care team across the continuum of care must contribute to the process. First, the patient's and family's basic knowledge about the problem and its management must be assessed. Then, educational needs related to the treatment plan need to be identified, as well as the sorts of problems that may arise. The team must also assess the extended supports of family, friends, and community, and sources of continuing education, such as community classes, and clinical experts (such as dietitians and lactation consultants).

Patient education involves much more than simply sharing the medical information we have with the patient by communicating it in a vocabulary he or she can understand. It is important to assess patients to see them as they see themselves. Only then can we help patients to recognize and overcome obstacles that prevent the desired behaviors. This requires skill and practice. The next chapter guides the reader in applying the information gathered in the assessment, to develop a plan for teaching.

STRATEGIES FOR CRITICAL ANALYSIS AND APPLICATION

1. Using the Patient and Family Education Assessment Guide, conduct a home visit. Write a summary of your assessment simi-

lar to the summary of the Smith family or the Dawe family, illustrated in this chapter.

2. Have students role-play being a person with diabetes. Some students should be assigned the role of being a non-insulin-taking patient with diabetes who has to go onto a strict dietary regimen. The calories should be appropriate for the student; the idea is to follow a meal plan precisely for one week, adding no extra treats. Other students can be assigned roles with different levels of insulin therapy. For instance, a two-injection-per-day regimen, a three-injection-per-day regimen, and a four-injection-per-day regimen. They all need to perform self-monitoring of blood glucose, follow the diabetic meal plan, record all blood sugars and dietary intake, and inject saline in the appropriate doses per instructions. The sales product representatives from the various diabetes product companies will often provide the materials necessary for this exercise. Debriefing these experiences at the end of a week can add a great deal of insight into the problems of living with a chronic illness that requires self-management practices.

3. Have students play the roles of educator and patient. During the conversations, have some dyads use judgmental language asking why patients comply rarely or at all with suggestions. Have students practice asking questions to assess the personal meaning of the illness or condition to the individual. Compare the kinds of information received from the two types of communication used to assess patients and families.

4. Listen for references to "noncompliance" in your clinical practice setting. Use these reports in seminar discussions or post-clinical conferences to ask students to suggest other ways to describe the problem. Practice speaking up to other professionals in these circumstances, pointing out the need to consider the context in which the patient is functioning.

To find the latest information

Key search terms
assessment, learning needs, culture, interviewing, listening, motivation

Websites
- Patient Assessment Standard of Care (National Institutes of Health): http://www.cc.nih.gov/swd/pasc/assessment.html
- Comprehensive Geriatric Assessment: Home Visit Assessment (USCSD School of Medicine): http://meded.ucsd.edu/cga/Home_Visit.html

REFERENCES

Acton, G. J., & Malathum, P. (2000). Basic need status and health-promoting self-care behavior in adults. *Western Journal of Nursing Research, 22*(7), 796–811.

Bastable, S. (2003). *Nurse as educator: Principles of teaching and learning for nursing practice* (2nd ed.). Sudbury, MA: Jones and Bartlett Publishers.

Best, J. T. (2001). Effective teaching for the elderly: Back to basics. *Orthopaedic Nursing, 20*(3), 46–52.

Carpenito, L. (2002). *Nursing diagnosis: Application to clinical practice* (9th ed.). Philadelphia: Lippincott Williams & Wilkins.

Erikson, E. (1993). *Childhood and society.* New York: W. W. Norton.

Galloway, S., Bubela, N., McCay, E., McKibbon, A., Ross, E., & Nagle, L. (2003). Patient learning needs scale. In B. K. Redman (Ed.), *Measurement tools in patient education* (2nd ed.). New York: Springer Publishing Company.

Haynes, R. B., McDonald, H. P., & Garg, A. X. (2002). Helping patients follow prescribed treatment. *JAMA, 288*, 2880–2883.

Krumholz, H. M., Amatruda, J., Smith, G. L., Mattera, J. A., Roumanis, S. A., Radford, M. J., et al. (2002). Randomized trial of an education and support intervention to prevent readmission of patients with heart failure. *Journal of the American College of Cardiology, 39*(1), 83–89.

Leske, J. S. (2002). Interventions to decrease family anxiety. *Critical Care Nurse, 22*(6), 61–65.

London, F. (1999). *No time to teach.* Philadelphia: Lippincott Williams & Wilkins.

London, F. (2002). Wipe out learning barriers. *Health Care Education Association Newsletter, 4*(1), 6.

Maslow, A. H. (1987). *Motivation and personality* (3rd ed.). New York: Harper and Row.

O'Hara, D. (2002). *Given but not taken: When your patients don't take their medicines.* Retrieved July 14, 2004, from www.ama-assn.org/sci-pubs/amnews/2002/02/04/hlsa0204.htm

Rankin, S. H., & Fukuoka, Y. (2003). Predictors of quality of life in women 1 year after myocardial infarction. *Progressive Cardiovascular Nursing, 18*(1), 6–12.

Rowett, D. L. (2001). *Family life cycle.* Retrieved June 15, 2003, from http://www.laurushealth.com/library/healthguide/illnessconditions/topic.asp?hwid=ty6171

Smith, R. C. (2002). *Patient-centered interviewing: An evidence-based method* (2nd ed.). Philadelphia: Lippincott Williams & Wilkins.

Taliaferro, E. (2003). Screening and identification of intimate partner violence. *Clinics in Family Practice, 5*(1), 89.

Yeager, K., & Seid, A. (2002). Primary care and victims of domestic violence. *Primary Care, 29*(1), 125–150.

Planning: Shared Goals for Patient Education

LEARNING OBJECTIVES

After reading this chapter, the student should be able to:

1. List four characteristics of effective patient educators.

2. Describe three characteristics of the adult learner that are important to consider in planning patient education.

3. Discuss the importance of constructing learning objectives before developing learning interventions.

4. Briefly define cognitive learning, affective learning, and psychomotor learning.

5. List the key components of a learning contract and describe its benefits in goal setting with patients, family, and staff.

6. List two methods for increasing multidisciplinary collaboration in patient education.

INTRODUCTION

Goal Setting: Targeting Outcomes for Learning

A detailed assessment helps health care providers focus on the most important information to teach, and provides insight into how best to present it. Nurses organize this information, identify appropriate nursing diagnoses to apply, and validate them with the patient and family. If a computerized care planning system is used, a critical pathway is tailored to the patient, based on the problem or on the diagnosis-related group. The planning of teaching can now begin.

The health care team must look beyond the medical diagnosis and identify the actual or potential functional problems for this patient. Since a major purpose of teaching is to help the learner adapt behaviors to optimize health, patient education should address functional problems, not disease states. For example, not all patients with diabetes have the same functional problems; therefore, the information taught will not be the same for every patient with diabetes.

To identify teaching priorities, the health care provider should ask: "How does this diagnosis affect this patient?" "What is most critical to the safety of this patient?" Then, the learner should be asked his or her view on these issues, and short- and long-term goals should be negotiated. The health care team then works with the patient and family to define specific behavioral objectives for each, to make the learning experience outcome oriented and measurable. Care maps, which are discussed in Chapter 12, also help providers and patients to sequence learning goals within an estimated length of stay as part of the diagnosis-specific critical pathway. This dialogue integrates teaching with assessment. The patient and family gain a better understanding of the diagnosis and proposed treatment plan, while the health care providers assess readiness to learn.

This assessment of readiness to learn is essential. Patients who do not believe their health status is in jeopardy cannot participate in goal setting. A patient who denies there is a problem is not motivated to learn. When health care providers respond to the managed care environment by blindly applying a universal teaching schedule to every patient, teaching may proceed but leave the learner behind. Before a successful teaching plan can be developed, learning readiness must be assessed (Patient education: a handy guide for assessing needs, 2000).

Using Data from the Assessment

Chapter 7 discussed the process of assessment. The more comprehensive the assessment, the more the health care team knows about the patient's problems and needs. This awareness facilitates counseling and helps provide patients with learning experiences that give them the knowledge, attitudes, and skills to promote health.

Through assessment, health care providers gain information about what the patient and the family know, what they want or need to know, and how to prepare them to make informed choices. This assessment includes identifying barriers to behavior change, and expanding knowledge, attitudes, and skills related to diagnosis, complications, management, prognosis, prevention, and resources for assistance.

When patients and their families are actively involved in assessment, they articulate their perceptions of their needs and problems, and, in the process, begin to understand the impact of the illness on their lives. Participating in problem identification prepares them to participate in collaborative goal setting. Participating in goal setting prepares them to learn, because the goals of education are their own. Consequently, active involvement motivates them to learn, and apply what they learn, and improves outcomes.

Skills Needed

Although the health care team shares responsibility for patient education, planning is generally directed by the nurse. The nurse is ultimately responsible for determining priorities, sorting out need-to-know versus nice-to-know facts, and helping patients master skills critical to their future safety. Patients expect nurses to exhibit certain strengths in this process. The authors interviewed many patients to determine how they would describe a nurse who is an excellent teacher. Patients were articulate in accounting the teacher-learner relationship. The authors identified four characteristics of excellent nurse-teachers from these conversations (Box 8.1): confidence, competence, communication, caring.

Goals of Patient and Family Education

Goals for patient and family education must embrace the concerns of both the patient and the health care team. The health care team must be sensitive to the patient, yet they must provide direction and firm priorities for discharge teaching. Patients have told the authors they depend on nurses to do this. Therefore, goal setting is shared with the patient and family. Patient education goals are aimed at helping the patient and family develop decision-making skills, gain survival skills, and learn how to recognize problems and respond appropriately.

Goals are accomplished by mastering learning objectives that refer to the patient's ability to demonstrate or perform health behaviors. Setting goals is an important step in the patient education process, but it is too often ignored. Goals and objectives help the team focus on what is critical and keep patient teaching on track. Throughout this chapter, readers will learn how to work with the patient and family to negotiate goals. The authors demonstrate how learning objectives are constructed and how they direct the entire learning process. Components of a learning contract are outlined, and its use as a motiva-

tor for learning, a mechanism for communication, and a source of standards for evaluating the teaching and learning process is discussed. Strategies to promote planning with the interdisciplinary team are considered.

Learning About the Diagnosis

Every patient who enters the health care system should know why he is there at that time. This fact may seem obvious, but patients

---

BOX 8.1 The Four Characteristics of the Excellent Nurse-Teacher

Confidence
- Selects what to teach
- Alleviates the patient's anxiety
- Provides appropriate learning environment
- Prepares appropriate teaching plan and material

Competence
- Decides what is important to teach
- Ensures the patient's safety
- Provides individualized written instructions
- Teaches home management of special problems

Communication
- Gives clear directions
- Uses simple pictures or models
- Speaks the patient's language

Caring
- Has empathy
- Recognizes patient concerns
- Provides encouragement
- Ensures adequate time
- Shows sensitivity to patient's mood

often know their symptoms but not how the symptoms relate to a diagnosis. Patients often do not know how a group of symptoms relates to the current problem. By learning why they are "here, in this place, at this time," patients gain perspective on health management. Learning can be taken a step further by considering whether the presenting problem could have been prevented. If so, what might the patient and family do differently next time to avoid an acute episode of illness?

Patients and their families typically want simple explanations about the diagnosis, in terms they can remember and repeat to family and friends. Even before they are ready to engage in formal learning activities, they want to know what will be expected of them when they go home. Patients and families want to know about common trouble signs (such as difficulty breathing, bleeding after surgery, dizziness, fever, pain, or swelling) and how to get emergency care.

PATIENT-CENTERED GOALS FOR TEACHING AND LEARNING

Understanding Patient Concerns During Hospitalization

Although emphasis is on discharge teaching, health care providers must also be aware that patient concerns during hospitalization often interfere with discharge teaching. Health care providers must anticipate and address a patient's concerns during hospitalization. For example, a patient may be concerned with the following questions:

- Am I going to be all right?
- What is going on? What are they planning to do to me?
- Is this going to cost me my job? Will I be fired?
- Is my wife worried? Who is going to tell her what is going on?

- Do these doctors know what they are doing? My own doctor knows my condition, but what about all the other doctors?
- Am I going to be in a lot of pain after this surgery?
- There are so many staff members here. Who is really in charge of me?

Fear can be a barrier to learning, and lessening anxiety is always a goal of patient education. It is important to remember that the patient and family may interpret the seriousness of the illness differently from the nurse and may experience one or more of the concerns listed in Box 8.2.

When a patient is faced with altered body image, feelings of shame, anger, and grief commonly arise. Let patients know that these feelings are to be expected, even though they are difficult to confront. For example, adolescents who face surgery for inflammatory bowel disease may be concerned about appearance of the stoma, whether the pouch will be seen under clothes, how to empty the pouch, and how to deal with leaking or odor (O'Brien, 1999).

Patients and families may also feel guilty for how they have related to one another in the past. They may feel angry about becoming ill or the problems the illness brings to the family. They may feel helpless to cope with the illness. When family members have been caregivers, the experience of control (or lack thereof) in their stressful and complex lives brings an added dimension and additional

---

BOX 8.2 Potential Barriers to Learning

Patient Concerns During Hospitalization
- Fear of pain
- Fear that the illness cannot be cured
- Fear of scarring or deformity
- Fear of being a burden on others
- Fear of dying
- Fear of cost of hospitalization

needs to patient and family education. Health care providers should be attuned to language and behaviors of these caregivers to determine when interventions are needed, including possible support from community agencies (Szabo & Strang, 1999).

During the planning process, the nurse must attend to the issues causing greatest concern for the patient and family. Some questions addressed through patient education include what to expect, how to get help, and how to manage pain.

Critical Learning Needs: Preparing for Discharge

Patients must know many things and do them correctly to survive independently of the health care team, such as how to take medications, ambulate on crutches, or change a sterile dressing. These things must be learned before discharge. The health care team must determine what learning is critical by asking four key questions:

1. What potential problems are likely to prevent a safe discharge?
2. What potential problems are likely to cause complications or readmission?
3. What prior knowledge or experience does the patient and family have with this illness or surgical recovery?
4. What skills and equipment are needed to manage the illness or surgical recovery at home?

Ensuring patient safety through teaching is both an ethical necessity and a legal necessity.

Learning Overload

Health professionals often try to teach too much in a short time. This occurs most often in the inpatient setting, where patients are overwhelmed with instructions before discharge. Reinforcement and evaluation of learning are often neglected. Yet if a moment was taken to evaluate learning, it may become clear the information imparted is not being absorbed. This is an unfortunate waste of teaching time, since the quantity of information taught is less important than the quantity of information retained and applied.

Learning needs should be carefully prioritized and creatively met in various settings. Although teaching about chronic illness often occurs in the hospital setting, it must be followed-up and reinforced in the home, outpatient clinic, or physician's office. Telephone or written communication should be used to inform health care providers in health departments, offices, clinics, and nursing homes about the teaching plan and the patient's progress. Learning overload also occurs in outpatient settings, when patients are given many instructions related to self-care and prevention. Often, when the patient attempts to integrate the learning into daily life, review and reinforcement are not provided, and behaviors are not changed.

Considering the Patient's Needs

Health care providers who teach patients with diabetes struggle with priorities because so much content must be taught and skills must be learned in a short time. The patient's needs should be considered before beginning teaching. The nurse should not teach about the pathophysiology of diabetes when all the patient wants to know is whether he or she can return to work. Health care providers should concentrate on survival skills: the basics of glucose testing, medications, injection techniques, meal planning, hyperglycemia, hypoglycemia, sick day management, foot care, and the plan for continuing education (Ohio State University Medical Center, 2001). Further teaching can be done, as needed, in follow-up visits.

The nurse must always consider the patient's chief complaint or reason for admission. If the patient has a diabetic ulcer, wound management and healing are the teaching priorities. When we take into account the survival data for patients with diabetes who have lower extremity amputations, foot ulcer prevention and treatment of ulcers are considered survival skills (Valk et al., 2002).

Keep in mind that any patient, especially those of racial and ethnic minorities, elderly persons, and patients with chronic conditions, may have poor health literacy. Health literacy is a measure of patients' ability to read, comprehend, and act on medical instructions. One study found that among primary care patients with type 2 diabetes, inadequate health literacy is independently associated with worse glycemic control and higher rates of retinopathy (Schillinger et al., 2002). Consider the learner's abilities as well as available resources when setting goals for teaching with the patient and family.

Prioritizing Needs and Setting Realistic Goals

The following four points support the importance of prioritizing learning needs and setting attainable goals in each patient situation. They also highlight the need for cooperation among professionals in many health care settings.

Rising health care costs, bed and personnel shortages, improved technology, and prospective payment systems create a hospital environment in which patients are discharged when they are physiologically stable, rather than when teaching is completed. Patients are often acutely ill during most of the hospital stay and have physical and emotional restrictions that make learning difficult. They may leave the hospital having had little opportunity to practice skills, review information, or formulate questions to ask. Nurses are often informed of the patient's discharge with only a few hours' notice and not given enough time to ensure the patient can manage self-care.

Patients who are overloaded with learning materials and activities feel a sense of frustration and failure when they cannot perform all behaviors successfully. This makes them feel powerless, defeated, and dependent. Many adults would rather deny failure than admit to it, and they will revert to old behaviors instead of asking for assistance.

Patients need to know what self-care activities are most important in their individual situations. When time and energy are limited, they need to know what learning must be achieved for survival.

Setting priorities for teaching helps structure their time and ensures that acute learning needs are met. Health care professionals can discharge patients more confidently when they know that learning will be continued and reinforced.

The difficult task of assigning priority to learning needs is helped by considering the individual within the context of Maslow's hierarchy of needs (see Chapter 7). Because five different levels of needs exist, needs that are lower on the hierarchy must be at least partially met before needs on the next level can be satisfied. This approach helps health care providers prioritize learning needs and recognize the patient's reliance on others to help satisfy higher needs.

In acute and chronic illness, patient education is often limited to physiologic and survival needs (Box 8.3). To prioritize learning needs, the following questions should be asked: What are the most acute needs of the patient? What does the patient already know? What behaviors can the patient perform? What learning needs are unmet? Which problems are life-threatening? Box 8.4 provides a useful framework for assessing individual patient learning needs and educational goals.

One effective way to identify the topics about which patients desire to learn is to use the card sort method. In this method, the nurse interviews a group of patients with the same diagnosis to determine common questions, such as "what is wrong with me?" and "why do I need to take medicine?" She then chooses the top questions (up to a maximum of 12) and prints them on cards. The cards are presented to the patient and the patient is asked to stack the cards with the most important questions on top, and least important on the bottom. A blank card is provided on which the patient may write additional questions. The patient's card sort results are taken into consideration when prioritizing teaching topics (Luniewski, Reigle, & White, 1999).

BOX 8.3 Basic Needs of Patients

Physiologic and Survival Needs
Care and use of oxygen
Recognition of health problems, danger
    signs, and how to respond to them
Knowledge of nutrition and hydration
Comfort with sexuality
Management of pain
Recognition of depression and how to deal
    with it
Administration of insulin and other medica-
    tions or treatments
Care of ostomy or Foley catheter

Safety and Security Needs
Poison prevention for parents
Ability to hold job
Competence in handling hazards on job or in
    environment (eg, toxins, dangerous
    machinery, stress)
Ability to deal with family violence
Financial capabilities in meeting basic needs
    of food, shelter, medication

Affection and Belongingness Needs
Adaptation to peer pressure
Maintenance of family role
Ability to contribute to family, work group,
    community
Need to feel lovable and desirable despite ill-
    ness or problem
Ability to deal with body image, disfigurement

Esteem or Recognition Needs
Need to succeed
Need to make choices, control own destiny
Need to be recognized as a valuable individual
Need for privacy, dignity
Ability to deal with lack of respect, abuse, ill
    treatment on job or in family

Self-Actualization: Self-Determining Needs
Success through own definition of what is
    desirable
Ability to meet developmental milestones
Independence in meeting lower needs

Helping Adults Learn

Health care providers often ask how they can motivate patients to learn. They know from experience that the learners must play an active role in the teaching process.

Many health care providers teach patients and families in the way they were taught as children: the learner assumes a passive role, listening to lectures and watching demonstrations.

To understand why adult patients need a different environment, imagine yourself as an adult student seated in a fifth grade classroom. Imagine feeling anxious about what the teacher expects, concerned that the material may be repetitious and boring, the class schedule is rigid, and the chair uncomfortable. The learner knows not to speak without permission, thinks that past experience is not important, and that he or she may have to learn things that are not relevant to his or her interests.

Consider your own positive learning experiences as an adult, with an effective teacher or preceptor. You are likely to recall an environment of physical and psychological comfort in which you felt accepted, valued, and encouraged to contribute thoughts, ideas, and past experiences. The subject matter was useful and interesting. With help, you probably defined your own learning goals, and evaluated the result of the learning activities. You were offered opportunities for role playing or trying new behaviors. You felt free to ask questions without embarrassment. This review of your positive experience provides insight into the needs of adult patients as learners. Patients are motivated to learn through physical and emotional comfort, and

---

BOX 8.4 Scope of Patient Education Needs in Acute and Chronic Illness

1. Diagnosis: explained in ways understandable to patient
   a. Etiology
   b. Contagiousness, potentially fatal, heredity
   c. Anatomy, physiology involved (limit to basic facts)
2. Complications: provide meaning to patient symptoms or possible symptoms
   a. Causes
   b. Prevention
   c. Early signals
3. Management: "big picture" of treatment plan, including discussion of patient self-care behaviors needed after discharge
   a. Surgery
   b. Radiation
   c. Diet
   d. Exercise, relaxation programs
   e. Medication
   f. Behavior modification and controls
   g. Environmental control
   h. Counseling
   i. Appliances (e.g., pacemaker, braces, crutches, traction)
   j. Consultation and referral
   k. Soaks, hot packs, dressings, treatments
4. Aggravating factors
   a. Foods
   b. Tobacco
   c. Drugs, alcohol
   d. Schedule of work and rest
   e. Interpersonal relationships
   f. Environmental aspects
5. Prognosis
   a. Short-term
   b. Signs of trouble, complications
   c. Long-term
6. Prevention of recurrence of acute problems
7. Resources for assistance
   a. Continuing care plan
   b. Economic, transportation
   c. Self-help groups
   d. Printed patient education materials
   e. Patient videotapes, CAI, Internet sites
   f. Group or community classes

---

active participation in defining their own needs and goals.

Malcolm Knowles: Andragogy (Adult Learning)

Malcolm Knowles contributes four reasonable assumptions about adult learners that distinguish them from children. His book, *The Modern Practice of Adult Education*, provides detailed information on the role of the adult educator and on strategies for helping adults learn (Knowles, 1980).

Knowles' assumes that as a person matures:

1. His or her self-concept moves from dependency to self-direction. He or she feels capable of making decisions, taking responsibility for their consequences, and managing his or her own life.
2. He or she accumulates life experiences that are an increasing resource for learning.
3. His or her readiness to learn is increasingly oriented to developmental tasks and social roles.
4. His or her time perspective changes, and orientation to learning shifts. He or she needs immediate application (rather than postponed application) of knowledge, and learning is problem centered rather than subject centered.

Table 8.1 provides applications of each of the four assumptions to patient and family teaching. Knowles (Knowles, Swanson, & Holton,

1998) offers additional guidance in goal setting with the patient and family:

1. Adults see themselves as producers, or doers, and derive self-esteem from their contributions.
2. Adults need to be perceived by others as self-directing.
3. Adults respond in an informal and friendly environment, one in which they are known by name and valued as individuals.

To summarize, adults are performance centered and seek information that helps them in their daily lives. Patients listen for the bottom line and want health care professionals to tell them what they need to know, not what is nice to know. Patients rarely want a detailed description of anatomy and pathophysiology related to their body systems. They want to know how to perform a prescribed regimen of survival skills once they go home and how to adapt current lifestyles to include healthy behaviors.

Knowles suggests the adult's readiness to learn, thus, motivation to try new behaviors, is influenced by developmental tasks. Table 8.2 outlines the Erikson's eight stages of man (Erikson, 1993).

The Health Belief Model Applied to Goal Setting

The Health Belief Model is helpful in understanding patient motivation to adopt health behaviors and follow a treatment plan. As explained in Chapter 4, the Health Belief Model suggests that patient engagement in the patient education process can be promoted through understanding the patient's reasoning, and sequencing provider-patient interactions to support this reasoning. Table 8.3 outlines how the steps of the model can be applied to goal setting.

Before teaching, the health care provider gains the patient's commitment to learn healthy behaviors and incorporate them into daily life. She does not approach patients as passive learners who are obligated to change their behaviors based solely on direction. Patients calculate their perceptions of a return on investment. Performing health behaviors com-

---

TABLE 8.1 Application of Adult Learning Theory to Patient and Family Education

ASSUMPTIONS ABOUT LEARNER	APPLICATIONS
Self-concept moves from dependency toward self direction; sees self as capable of making own decisions, taking responsibility for consequences, managing own life.	Acknowledge learner's desire to articulate own needs, make choices, and gain respect for own ability to manage life; create psychological climate that communicates acceptance and support; help learner to feel comfortable taking chances, expressing thoughts and ideas without fear of shame or embarrassment; remember that adults are motivated to learn when they realize that they have a need to learn.
Growing reservoir of life experience is a resource for learning.	Use past experiences as a resource for learning; remember that adults experience positive feelings of support and recognition when their experience is acknowledged; relate new learning to old; have adults teach other adults in a group setting; be aware that negative past experiences may pose barriers for learner and teacher.
Readiness to learn is strongly influenced by social roles and developmental tasks.	Recognize social role of patient (eg, father, mother, husband, wife, worker) and developmental tasks; relate learning to ability to become, to succeed in these roles.
Time perspective changes; orientation to learning shifts; needs immediate application of new knowledge and problem-centered learning.	Give adults practical answers to their problems; help them to apply new knowledge immediately through role play or hands-on practice (eg, return demonstration); remember that adults are particularly motivated to learn at times of crisis or when problems arise; prioritize learning activities by immediacy of need and patient-family perception of need; reinforce learning and promote problem-solving skills.

TABLE 8.2 Erikson's Eight Stages of Man	
STAGE	**ISSUE**
Oral-sensory: birth to 1 yr of age	Trust vs. mistrust
Muscular-anal: ages 1-2 y	Autonomy vs. shame
Locomotion-genital: ages 3-5 y	Initiative vs. guilt
Latency: age 6 to puberty	Industry vs. inferiority
Puberty: adolescence: puberty to late teens	Identity vs. role confusion
Young adulthood: late teens to mid twenties	Intimacy vs. isolation
Adulthood: variable	Generativity vs. stagnation
Maturity: variable	Ego integrity vs. despair

monly involves cost, discomfort, shifting of time and priorities, breaking long-standing habits, and social isolation (for example, a person on a special diet may feel isolated from events focused on eating or food). By following the goal-setting process of the Health Belief Model, health care providers can help patients see how the benefits outweigh costs. Ongoing support from family and health care providers can help patients perform health-promoting behaviors.

The process will also reveal which behaviors the patient is unwilling to change or perform. Smoking is frequently a behavior that patients are unwilling to change, despite evidence presented by health care providers. By mutually agreeing upon goals before teaching begins, the nurse can focus on attainable outcomes.

A review of research testing the Health Belief Model suggests that the barriers and costs prevent individuals from engaging in preventive health behaviors or behaviors related to the recommended illness care (Koch, 2002). Susceptibility to, and severity of, an illness are not as powerful predictors of behavior as barriers and costs, except for persons who already have an illness, such as coronary artery disease. To achieve better outcomes, patients should be encouraged to discuss perceived barriers and identify possible resources to confront these barriers.

If a patient cannot afford to purchase the prescribed medication, financial assistance or a less costly medication is needed. If the patient has been unsuccessful with a therapeutic diet because it is too confining, negoti-ating the list of forbidden foods will set the stage for more successful outcomes (Holli & Calabrese, 1998). The family should be engaged in diet adaptation and taught how to prepare appropriate foods to suit their tastes, so they can make lasting lifestyle changes.

Challenges of Chronic Illness and Goal Setting

Another challenge in patient education is helping a patient who needs to change two or more behaviors simultaneously, such as diet, exercise, smoking cessation, taking medications, and maintaining treatments. Patients are often unsuccessful because they cannot make such profound changes, and may be inappropriately labeled as noncompliant. To enhance the potential for success, approach these situations realistically. Examine what the patient needs and wants to know at each stage of the illness. Connect learning goals and objectives to what is most important or applicable for the patient at that time. Take advantage of teachable moments and readiness to learn. Set priorities, sequence learning, and establish long-term plans for reinforcement, support, and follow-up across the continuum of care.

The importance of this long-term commitment to reinforcement and follow-up was demonstrated by a randomized, controlled study of asthma patients (Côté et al., 2001). They found a structured educational intervention emphasizing self-management (patient given choice of individual or small group

TABLE 8.3 The Health Belief Model Used in the Interview to Identify Patient Goals and Decisions

STEPS	APPLICATION
I. The patient perceives that he or she has a condition or is likely to contract it.	I. a. Discuss the problem and symptoms. b. Explore patient's prior knowledge and experience. c. Assess obstacles to understanding (anxiety, fear, misconceptions).
II. The patient perceives that the disease or condition is harmful and has serious consequences for him or her.	II. a. Patient's perception of consequences (includes lifestyle) b. Discuss prognosis. c. Discuss beliefs and attitudes; trust of providers and health care system. d. Discuss experiences of family/friends with similar problem.
III. The patient believes that the suggested health intervention is of value to him or her.	III. a. Understands proposed treatment plan (including medications). b. Discuss what may happen with or without proposed treatment. c. Is this a cure? d. Discuss financial costs, lifestyle changes, side effects.
IV. The patient believes that the effectiveness of the treatment is worth the cost and barriers he or she must confront.	IV. a. Contract (agreement) with the patient on the treatment plan. b. Outline provider responsibilities. c. Outline patient responsibilities. d. Outline patient education plan for developing needed knowledge, attitudes, and skills.

The Health Belief Model was constructed to predict health behaviors. It provides a tool for understanding the patient's perception of disease and his or her decision-making process in the consumption of health services. In each of the four steps, family members and significant others should be considered.

References
1. Hochbaum, G. M. (1958). *Public participation in medical screening programs* (U.S. Public Health Service Publication No. 572). Washington, DC: U.S. Government Printing Office.
2. Rosenstock, I. M. (1975). Patient's compliance with health regimens. *Journal of the American Medical Association, 234,* 402–403.
3. Rankin, S. H., Stallings, K. D. (1990). *Patient education: Issues, principles, and practices.* Philadelphia: J. B. Lippincott.

classes, involved in treatment decisions, and reinforcement provided in a 6-month follow-up visit) improves patient outcomes significantly more than a limited intervention (given an asthma action plan) or conventional treatment (taught to use inhaler). The authors noted that significant improvement in patient outcomes, such as urgent hospital visits, occurred only after six months because it takes time and reinforcement to change patient behavior.

Stating Goals

Adults are motivated to learn when they recognize a gap between what they know and what they want to know (Knowles, 1980). Assessment provides the health care provider with information about the patient's knowledge, attitudes, and skills for self-care. Goals are set when the patient educator comes to a mutual agreement with the patient for what he or she wants to accomplish (Osborne, 2002). Imposing your educational goals on the patient and family is not an effective method for teaching adults. Instead, meet the patient and family "on their own ground," encourage whatever participation the patient and family can make, and consider ways to support and reinforce the patient and family strengths.

MR. STANLEY

PHYSIOLOGIC DATA

A medical-surgical nurse begins to gather assessment information critical to the care of Mr. Stanley, a 60-year-old man admitted to the hospital with a medical diagnosis of asthma. His wife and daughter supply most of the assessment information, because Mr. Stanley is puffing and coughing. The initial assessment is conducted in approximately 30 minutes.

The patient was diagnosed with asthma 15 years ago. Questioning is focused toward self-care management: preventing acute episodes, using controlled breathing techniques, avoiding bronchial irritants, and using medications correctly. Asthma and chronic obstructive pulmonary disease are among the top diagnosis-related groups at the hospital, and a special patient education effort is aimed at improving the correct use of inhalers. It is estimated that more than 50% of patients who use inhalers experience therapeutic failure because of incorrect technique.

FAMILY PROFILE

The nurse learns that Mr. and Mrs. Stanley live in a ranch-style house. Their 38-year-old daughter lives 2 miles away. Mr. Stanley is a retired groundskeeper for the city and spends much of his time planning his home garden. He also likes to fish and is active in his church. Mrs. Stanley reports that, aside from discomfort from her arthritis, she is in good health.

UNDERSTANDING THE CURRENT EVENT

Mr. Stanley has had progressively worsening attacks of dyspnea for the last month, with occasional tachycardia. Today's episode occurred after working in his garden—"overdoing it," as Mrs. Stanley describes. Mr. Stanley reports a decrease in appetite and difficulty sleeping. The nurse notices that the Stanley's daughter completed Mr. Stanley's admission papers. All three family members appear anxious.

Mrs. Stanley reports that her husband worries her with his frequent use of his inhaler and increasing episodes of breathlessness. When asked to demonstrate controlled breathing techniques, Mrs. Stanley says that he has forgotten how to do them and that he just relies on his "trusty friend," his inhaler. Mrs. Stanley tells the nurse, "I've been trying to get him to go to the doctor for more than a week. It finally came to this!" Mr. Stanley's three prescribed asthma medications are inhalants. Because steroid inhalations can cause osteoporosis, Mr. Stanley also takes alendronate (Fosamax) every morning. Fosamax must be taken on an empty stomach 30 minutes before eating and the patient must stay upright after taking it. Mr. Stanley also takes calcium, three times daily, with meals.

Mr. Stanley admits to using albuterol on a daily basis against the orders of his physician. He admits to smoking "a few cigarettes" lately, despite having quit for 10 months after his last hospitalization.

Mr. Stanley is quickly fatigued. Therefore, the nurse completes an initial screening of systems and flags the assessment data base form so that additional information can be gathered in the following areas:

1. Observation of the patient's inhaler technique
2. Potential environmental irritants
3. Income and health insurance (which often prevents patients from obtaining needed medications)
4. Reading and writing abilities of the Stanleys (to determine appropriate written materials)

5. Typical diet and sleep patterns of the family
6. Daily schedule
7. Ability of family to handle crisis situations
8. Degree of limitation on the patient's and family's functioning
9. Family's desires and needs to know about the illness or problems associated with the illness

THE IDENTIFIED PATIENT, THE HEALTH PROBLEM, AND EDUCATIONAL NEEDS

Mr. Stanley summarizes his problems succinctly: frequent episodes of puffing and fatigue, sometimes with his heart beating too fast. Mrs. Stanley adds that her husband has had a poor appetite lately and that he has not been sleeping well. The nurse explains that poor appetite, rapid heart rate, and difficulty sleeping may be related to overuse or improper use of the inhaler. The nurse tells Mr. Stanley that the health care team will help him understand how to better manage his asthma at home.

NURSING DIAGNOSES AND EDUCATIONAL GOALS

Impaired Gas Exchange Related to Chronic Airway Obstruction
Educational goals. The patient will learn proper use of an inhaler; state the importance of eliminating smoking and other bronchial irritants, including stress; recognize warning signs and prevent exacerbations; and describe the danger of overuse of asthma medications.

Ineffective Airway Clearance Related to Reduced Cough Strength and Slowed Mucous Transport
Educational goals. The patient will perform coughing and breathing techniques; demonstrate ways to increase fluid intake; demonstrate proper use of inhaler; identify ways to avoid infection; and identify signs and symptoms of infection.

Activity Intolerance Related to Dyspnea
Educational goal. The patient can describe how to manage activity and prevent excessive breathlessness. Patient and family express feeling of helplessness; discuss how to handle acute episodes to increase confidence and gain support; suggest methods of relaxation.

Altered Nutrition: Less Than Body Requirements Related to Fatigue, Weakness, and Breathlessness
Educational goal. The patient and his wife will outline a plan of adequate fluid intake, small meals, and frequent snacks.

Risk for Noncompliance with Therapeutic Program Related to Chronic Nature of Disease
Educational goal. The patient will participate in the development of an individualized program to integrate all facets of management and consider referrals to a smoking cessation program and other resources that will help family cope with chronic illness.

Factors Influencing Mr. Stanley's Learning
The nurse identifies teaching priorities and organizes them so Mr. Stanley can learn according to his physical ability. She identifies both the positive and negative factors that will influence his learning. Positive factors affecting Mr. Stanley's behavioral change include that he has experience with this disease and its symptoms, that he was smoke-free for 10 months before resuming smoking, and that he wants to continue gardening. Negative factors affecting Mr. Stanley's behavioral change include that he tends to delay seeking treatment for dyspnea, that he resumed smoking, and that both patient and family exhibit anxiety.

Developing Behavioral Objectives

Patient education is a process of influencing behavior, not just giving information. Successful patient education must be directed toward accomplishing behavioral change. Setting specific behavioral objectives for patient education ensures that learning interventions will be tailored to the patient's unique situation and needs. Objectives describe the behaviors or actions the patient will perform to meet a goal (Figure 8.1).

When objectives are clearly stated, the learner knows what his or her role is and what is expected of him or her. The learner can organize his or her energy toward learning. Likewise, when goals and objectives are stated, the teacher knows his or her role. Both teacher and learner know how the results will be measured. Written documentation of learning objectives ensures the patient's straightforward communication with the health care team.

Learning connotes a change in knowledge, attitudes, or skills as a result of an educational experience. Behavioral objectives, also referred to as learning objectives, guide the planning of learning activities and the measurement of learning outcomes. These objectives should state what the learner will do as a result of patient teaching (see Figure 8.1). A common mistake is to define learning objectives in terms of the health care providers' behavior, rather than of the patient's behavior. For example, "Review the four signs of a hypoglycemic reaction with the patient" should be rephrased as, "The patient will describe or list four signs of a hypoglycemic reaction."

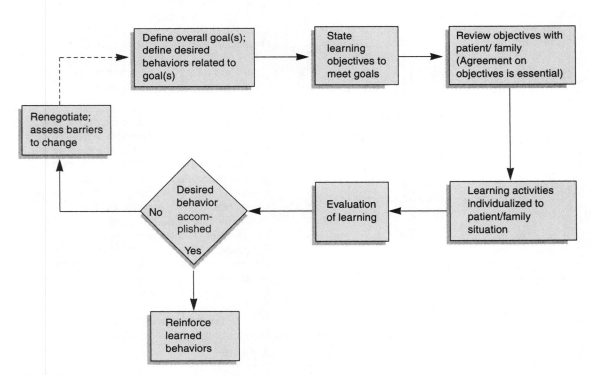

FIGURE 8.1 Using behavioral objectives in the learning process.

Types of Objectives

There are three types of learning objectives:

1. Cognitive objectives, which refer to knowledge
2. Affective objectives, which refer to attitudes
3. Psychomotor objectives, which refer to skills

Cognitive learning refers to rational thought, including basic facts and concepts. For example, cognitive learning is accomplished if the patient can describe his or her health problem in his or her own words, list signs and symptoms associated with the problem, and outline steps in a procedure. Cognitive learning moves from simple to complex concepts, so the patient can apply facts to different situations. Understanding basic anatomy and physiology addresses the cognitive domain of learning.

Affective learning refers to the patient's feelings and reactions to his or her illness, appreciation of the costs and benefits of treatment, and a willingness to change. The affective domain refers to beliefs, attitudes, and values (Maier-Lorentz, 1999). Helping patients explore their personal points of view, consider options, and gain support of significant others promotes affective learning.

Psychomotor learning refers to musculoskeletal movement, the ability to perform a procedure, skills, and the dexterity to manipulate objects or parts. Mastering psychomotor learning usually involves the need for demonstration, practice, and more practice until the skill is integrated. Periodic rehearsal or review is needed when skills are not required on a frequent basis.

Components of a Behavioral Objective

A behavioral objective has three components: performance, conditions, and criteria (Bastable, 2003).

Performance. The learning objective states any activity in which the patient will engage; it describes what the learner will do. The learning objective uses an action verb and denotes an activity that can be measured. The activity may be visible (such as writing a list) or invisible (such as solving a problem). Verbs such as believe, understand, value, and know are not measurable and should be avoided when describing performance in a learning objective.

When choosing an action verb, the nurse should ask: "Can I measure whether the learner can do this?" (Box 8.5) The verb should be simple enough that the learner can understand how he or she is expected to show competence, such as "writing" or "identifying." Each learning objective should reflect only one behavior.

Conditions. The learning objective states what constraints will be included when measuring the learner's performance. Conditions that may be part of a learning objective include time of day, sterile technique, equipment and tools, place, calorie restrictions, and specific symptoms. For example: Given a list of common foods, Mr. Jones will identify those high in sodium, which should be avoided.

Criteria offer a component of evaluation. They define how the teacher and learner will know when the learning has been accomplished. A criterion states how long or how well the behavior must be performed to be acceptable. It defines the level of competence to be achieved. Examples of criteria include score or speed, weight, quality, number of times, accuracy, and frequency. For example: Mrs. Harde will draw up and administer 22 units of insulin using sterile technique at 7:00 AM on 3 consecutive days. The criteria used in measurement include the number of units of insulin, the time, and the frequency of administration.

Criteria are especially important when teaching psychomotor objectives, such as walking with crutches. How many times does the nurse want to observe a return demonstration to be confident that the patient has mastered the skill? What degree of error or variation in performance is acceptable? For example, when teaching a

---

BOX 8.5 Suggested Verbs for the Three Domains of Learning

Cognitive domain: Developing Knowledge, Facts, and Concepts in Patient Education

*	Identify, define, list, match, name, record, repeat, show, state, select, tell, underline, choose, collect, locate, report
**	Describe, discuss, explain, outline, restate, review, summarize, give example, prepare, recognize
***	Apply, demonstrate, design, implement, measure, modify, prepare, schedule, solve, use, negotiate, compute, practice, write
****	Compare, contrast, diagram, differentiate, sort, test, debate

Affective domain: Developing Appreciation of Benefits and Value in Patient Education

*	Commit, describe, explain, defend, assist
**	Arrange, choose, combine, compare, explain, express, modify, relate
***	Disagree, help, join, initiate, propose, justify
****	Participate, perform, practice, state willingness, reply, try, label, attempt, answer
*****	Accept, accommodate, admit, heed, follow

Psychomotor domain: Developing Skills and Procedures in Patient Education

*	Choose, compare, describe, differentiate, identify, select, separate
**	Attempt, ask, copy, display, prepare, respond, show, start, volunteer
***	Apply, arrange, cleanse, count, connect, cut, demonstrate, examine, find, fold, grasp, guide, hold, insert, lift, locate, open, operate, place, pour, practice, pull, push, raise, remove, separate, shake, squeeze, stand, transfer, walk, wash, weigh, wipe
****	Adapt, modify, correct, rearrange, replace, substitute, vary

*to ***** notes increasing levels of complexity and competency.

---

patient to take his or her pulse, within how many beats of the nurse's measurement must the patient measure to be considered successful?

The teacher and the learner need to be able to answer these three questions about the behavioral objective:

1. **What can the learner do?** What does the learner have to do to show he or she has achieved the learning? (performance)
2. **Under what conditions will the learner do it?** Will he or she use special equipment? (condition)
3. **What is the performance standard?** How well must it be done? How will the learner know when it is done well enough? (criterion)

Each learning objective needs to be specific, measurable, and attainable. To accomplish this, understand what the patient wants to achieve. Although the learner's ability should not be doubted, it is important that goals are not set too high. Learning should be a positive, successful experience in which the learner gains confidence and self-esteem. Health care providers should begin learning with activities the patient can successfully accomplish, moving from simple behaviors to those that are more complex.

Learning objectives keep patient education focused on outcomes. The number of objectives should be based on what is feasible for the patient to learn in the time available. The nurse must identify three or four learning objectives that are critical for safety, and review and reinforce them often throughout the patient's stay.

Exhaustive lists of 30 or more objectives may look scholarly, but are useless to both health care providers and patients. Because so little time is available, these long lists were probably imposed by the health care provider, and not mutually established with the learner. Too many objectives also make it difficult to keep the teaching sessions interactive because long lists motivate health care providers to move into lecture mode to cover all the information in the time available.

Getting the Patient and the Family Involved

The involvement of the patient and family in setting learning goals affirms their willingness to participate. They need to understand, agree with, and want to meet the criteria for evaluation. Skipping this step can result in patients and families who are not invested in learning or adhering to the treatment plan, teaching efforts would be wasted, and health care outcomes would suffer.

Health care providers should encourage patients to talk about the changes they would like to make and help them state these in the form of objectives. Criteria should be defined in terms that make sense to and motivate the learner. For example, "working for one hour in the garden without breathlessness" or "caring for a toddler grandchild" may be more meaningful outcomes to a patient than "22 respirations per minute" or a "10-lb weight loss." The same behavioral change may be involved in these examples, and could satisfy both the provider and the patient.

Sometimes, negotiation and compromise are necessary to agree upon goals and objectives. The patient may understand the hazards of smoking but may not be willing to give up smoking cigarettes during the evening. The patient may understand the need for weight reduction and may want to lose weight, but may be unwilling to sacrifice ice cream. A measurable reduction in smoking or a measurable weight loss using a modified diet plan may be a workable compromise.

One way to involve the patient and the family is to ask them for their perceptions of the problems and what they would like to change. The nurse should share his or her view, and ask if the patient would like help in working on the identified problems. The nurse should then discuss the priority of needs, and write behavioral objectives with the patient, by working together, mutually agreeing upon what will be taught, what the patient will learn, and what the respective responsibilities will be. This information should be shared with the rest of the health care team through documentation, so they, too, may teach according to the plan.

CASE STUDY 8.2

MRS. DAWE

In Chapter 7, we introduced Mrs. Dawe, who was struggling with her daily management of hypertension and diabetes. Mrs. Dawe identified her greatest problems as her weight and her high blood pressure. She agreed that she would like to work on these problems. She stated that her shortness of breath would decrease if she lost weight and she felt that she could follow her exercise plan. She described the low-fat, diabetic ADA diet she had been prescribed 5 years ago as "too restrictive," but agreed to renegotiate an ADA diet that included one-half of a cup of ice cream each week and limited amounts of other favorite foods. She thought that her weight increase and blood pressure problem were closely related. She also saw her shortness of breath as a problem and stated, "I would be happy if I could keep my granddaughter for the day without getting sick."

The nurses involved in her care shared their perceptions with Mrs. Dawe. The nurses' perceived the same problems as Mrs. Dawe: her obesity, hypertension, and shortness of breath.

The nurses reinforced her knowledge of her health problems and her positive behaviors of checking her blood glucose and examining her feet regularly. The nurses complimented her dependability in keeping her appointments and in taking her medications. A meal plan was offered to help her lose weight and lower her blood pressure. She agreed with the nurses' suggestions. It was decided to continue a discussion of her diabetes management at her clinic visit scheduled for the next week. Mr. Dawe was present during the discussion but was silent.

The nurses stressed the importance of family support in improving the overall nutrition and health for both partners, because the recommendations for healthy eating and well-planned exercise are important for everyone. After a spouse or parent has a heart attack, it is critical that the family support healthful eating. When all family members make changes to lower calories, fat, and sodium in their diets, they show the patient that he or she is not alone. They demonstrate their commitment to help the patient stay alive. This kind of support helps the patient make necessary long-term changes. The Dawes were also advised to become members in the local chapter of the American Diabetes Association and to subscribe to the monthly newsletter *Diabetes News*, to help establish a new start to the treatment plan.

Learning goals and objectives related to obesity and hypertension were mutually negotiated. Mrs. Dawe's current intake was estimated at approximately 2,200 calories/day by 24-hour recall. She agreed to an appointment with the dietitian to learn about the new dietary guidelines and how to plan sample menus. She agreed to limit her use of salt and fat in cooking.

Nursing Diagnosis: Altered Nutrition: More Than Body Requirements Related to Nonadherence to Diabetic Low-fat Diet

Goal. Mrs. Dawe will follow a low-fat, diabetic meal plan by June 1.

Educational needs. With the dietitian, outline food suggestions for breakfast, lunch, and dinner using her meal planning guide. Describe how one-half of a cup of ice cream is worked into the weekly meal plan.

Behavioral objectives. Mrs. Dawe will record in notebook all foods eaten during the week. She will state why weight control is especially important in the management of diabetes. Mrs. Dawe will attend the patient with diabetes luncheon at the hospital.

Goal. Achieve systolic blood pressure below 160 mmHg and diastolic blood pressure below 90 mmHg by June 1.

Educational needs. Review high-sodium foods and ways to avoid them.

Behavioral objectives. Mrs. Dawe will omit salt in cooking, and name 10 high-sodium foods to avoid. Mrs. Dawe will eliminate canned foods from the diet during the week and substitute fresh fruits and vegetables, recording them in notebook.

Mrs. Dawe was willing to keep specific records in a notebook that she would bring to her next office visit. A contract was written up and signed, and Mrs. Dawe kept the contract at home. When the nurses returned to the office, they documented the agreement in the progress notes section of her chart and made an appointment for her with the dietitian; this had been suggested so she would have an opportunity to explore variations in her food choices and receive cooking suggestions. Mrs. Dawe would return to the family practice clinic for a visit 1 week later. Prioritizing problems was not difficult because the problems were closely interrelated physiologic needs. An effort to set achievable goals increased the probability of attaining success and developing a positive self-image. Mr. Dawe was willing to help by supporting Mrs. Dawe's renewed effort to follow her meal plan and to limit her salt intake. He remarked, "It would help me to cut down on my salt, too, and I can use some at the table."

THE LEARNING CONTRACT

The learning contract is a tool used to formalize the agreement between the teacher and learner. It clearly states learning behaviors, the responsibilities of the teacher and the learner, and the methods of follow-up and evaluation. As learning is accomplished and new goals are defined, the contract is renegotiated. If the patient changes his or her mind or finds the goals too difficult to achieve, the objectives can be revised. Learning contracts can be used in the hospital, home, and clinic settings (Figure 8.2).

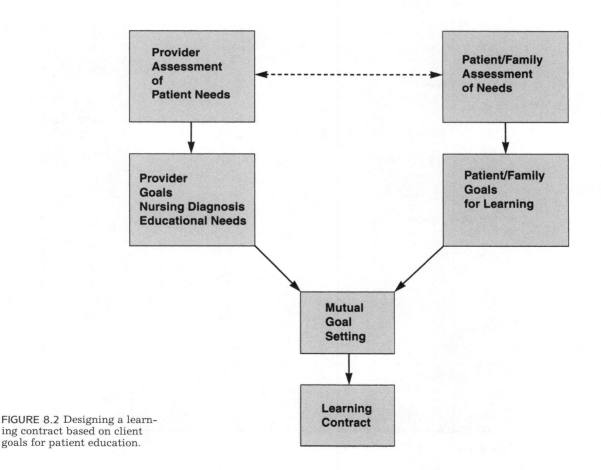

FIGURE 8.2 Designing a learning contract based on client goals for patient education.

Figure 8.3 illustrates the essential components of a learning contract for Mrs. Dawe. It is helpful to type a standard contract form on hospital or clinic stationery and complete it with the patient. A copy can be kept in the patient record and a copy should be given to the patient. A bonus clause has been used to denote additional resources available to the patient, such as self-help groups, classes, and other health professionals. As behaviors are accomplished and the contract is revised, include a reinforcement as an intervention to support the patient. The reinforcement may be weekly weight checks in the clinic, an

---

FAMILY MEDICINE CENTER

Learning Contract

Goals:
To lose 6 lb during the next 2 months.
To achieve systolic blood pressure below 160 mmHg, and diastolic blood pressure below 90 mmHg.

Learner Actions:
Record in notebook all foods eaten each day. Follow recommendations of American Diabetes Association (ADA) meal plan. Take medications daily and record in notebook. Eliminate canned foods this week. Return for clinic visit next week.

Teacher Actions:
Supply diet outline for ADA meal plan.
Check weight and BP weekly.
Label reading models—will review with Mrs. Dawe at clinic visit 4/7. Instruction in reading labels on canned foods done today in the home.

Method of Measurement:
Weight
BP
Patient record in notebook

Length of Contract:
2 months

Bonus Clause:
Diabetic luncheon at hospital
ADA diet plan and instructions for meal preparation and meal spacing
Booklet: "Your Diabetic Meal Plan"
Appointment with dietitian scheduled for 4/7

Signatures:

_____   _____

_____   _____

Date: 3/31

FIGURE 8.3 Learning contract for Mrs. Dawe.

occasional home visit, a telephone call, or a referral to the public health nurse or office nurse.

Mutually established learning contracts take advantage of the learner's readiness to change. One study (Haber, 2001) found that by engaging older adults in identifying their own goals for behavior change, 92% chose goals they were ready and willing to change. To enhance success, the goals were doable, and social support was solicited from a family member or friend. Patient readiness was increased by incorporating stress management and behavior management techniques into the behavior contract.

A learning contract provides purpose, structure, and coordination to patient teaching. It motivates patient, family, and health care providers to work together to improve outcomes. The contract provides specific, achievable, and clearly defined goals and objectives. Responsibilities, resources, and desired behaviors, conditions, and criteria are specified. Methods for measuring outcomes are identified. As a written tool, it enables the health care team across the continuum to work with the patient and family, without overwhelming the learners with too many goals, or conflicting messages.

CLINICAL RELEVANCE OF PLANNING

Motivating Patients

The best way to motivate patients to participate in their care and to follow the treatment plan is to find out what those patients value. It is different for every patient.

How can we motivate patients to learn? Recognizing what motivates a patient is probably the most important factor in having a patient successfully respond to patient education with the desired behavioral changes. Motivating factors can vary significantly. Some patients are motivated by feeling in control of their lives. Others are motivated by a desire to please the health care professionals.

Getting the Health Care Team Together

Coordinating patient education, just like coordinating patient care, involves the participation of all the disciplines on the health care team. To ensure the best care, everyone needs to share assessment information, collaborate on the plan, and coordinate efforts. For example, patients with newly diagnosed diabetes may be taught by nurses, registered dietitians, primary physicians, and sometimes endocrinologists, pharmacists, and social workers.

This team approach is supported by JCAHO standard PC.5.50: Care, treatment, and services are provided in an interdisciplinary, collaborative manner (Joint Commission on Accreditation of Healthcare Organizations, 2003). They encourage a collaborative, interdisciplinary approach to meeting the patient's needs and goals, to coordinate care, treatment, and services and achieve optimal outcomes.

One study of interdisciplinary cardiac preoperative patient education (van Weert et al., 2003) found that it is not always clear who was responsible for teaching what information and when to teach it. The health care providers were unaware that this caused overlaps and gaps in the education provided. Information was not tailored to the patient's needs; psychoeducational care, specifically attention to preoperative anxiety, was the greatest gap. The authors addressed this problem with an interdisciplinary information protocol list kept at the patient bedside, to facilitate communication between team members regarding the status of teaching. They also initiated an interdisciplinary team meeting, including the patient, to initiate planning and teaching a few weeks before the surgery.

A planning meeting can save time for everyone and minimize replication of efforts. It may be convenient to set this meeting for a time when the physician is scheduled to be on the unit or in the agency. The meeting should include all members of the health care team, including the patient and family. Goals should be planned collaboratively, agreed upon by all members of the team, and documented.

Logical progression of teaching, consistent messages, and continuity of care can be accomplished by having all health care team members use the same problem list, and document their teaching assessments and evaluations of understanding in one place in the chart. Using the team approach, communication is focused and concise, teaching efforts build on one another, time is not wasted through replication, and the entire health care team, especially the patient, benefits.

Physical Limitations and Environment: Effects on Patient Education

The environment provides the conditions for teaching and the conditions under which tasks are performed. In the hospital, the environment is sterile and clean, and supplies are readily available. However, the unnatural environment may make learners anxious. In the home learners may be more comfortable, but there may be distractions such as pets, or challenges such as no running water or electricity. Flexibility and creativity are essential to optimize use of given conditions.

The effects of pain, illness, and fatigue can affect patient education. Pain can be an all-encompassing experience. If the patient experiences severe pain, our only intervention should be alleviation of pain, either through medications or nonpharmacological techniques. Once pain has been lessened, teach relaxation and breathing techniques for use in the future. Necessary skills, such as using crutches or learning to cough, turn, and deep breathe, cannot be taught until pain is alleviated.

Illness and fatigue can deplete a patient's physical resources, leaving him or her little energy for learning. If the patient is not interacting or cannot retain simple information, stop teaching. Wait until the patient is more rested or until family members are present.

When appropriate, tell the patient's family when health care providers are available to teach, so they can be present and learn, too.

Pain experienced by older patients who have been discharged from acute care settings to long-term care facilities is underestimated, under-reported, and undertreated. If pain management in the long-term care facility is inadequate, the success of patient education in that setting is certainly affected. Assess the resident's perception of his or her pain. An effective pain management program can provide pain relief, improve sleep, promote independence in activities of daily living, increase participation in recreational activities, and heighten feelings of well-being and control over one's health (Loeb, 1999).

A review of the literature revealed that, in patients with cancer, pain education can improve pain control. Education helps patients manage side effects and improves adherence (Chelf et al., 2001).

Acute and chronic pain management is inadequate in all settings and within all age groups (Stieg, 2001). Those especially vulnerable to undertreatment of their pain are small children, older patients, patients who are intubated, people with mental disabilities, non-English-speaking patients, and patients with a history of substance abuse. Therefore, it is essential to consider pain management as a key component of the teaching plan with these populations.

Patient Education for Homeless Patients

Situations involving homeless patients with health problems are some of the most difficult in which to intervene. Consider the case of a man with insulin-dependent diabetes who lives on the street during the day and in a homeless shelter at night. Neuropathies make this patient more likely to develop skin breakdown and foot sores, and because of constant walking in poorly fitting shoes, major foot ulcers are more likely to develop than in a non-homeless person with diabetes. Additionally, self-monitoring of blood glucose is almost impossible to accomplish. Added to this are problems related to syringes, which on the streets are frequently shared or stolen for use in injecting intravenous drugs, thus increasing the risk of hepatitis B and human immunodeficiency virus (HIV) infection for a patient who has diabetes. Standard teaching regarding diabetes management is not realistic for these patients. At best, the patient should be encouraged to come to a health clinic in a shelter daily for insulin injection and occasional blood glucose monitoring.

Psychosocial problems are another factor when considering patient education in situations involving extreme conditions. For example, one nurse practitioner who works in a homeless shelter explained that circadian rhythms and sense of time quickly become confused by homeless people. Those who are newly homeless need constant reorientation to time and place and frequently state that they feel like they are losing it and going crazy. The nurse should provide some stability for the homeless patient and attempt to address some of the underlying problems related to homelessness, such as unemployment, alcohol and drug abuse, and mental illness.

Homeless women and children have many physical and psychological concerns and may underestimate the health care that is available to them. When asked to describe their health concerns, these women usually identify drug abuse, bipolar disorders, anxiety, depression, suicidal behaviors, self-mutilation, and domestic abuse. Shame, fear, need for information, and poverty influence attempts at patient education. Women and children may stay in homeless shelters for a long time, providing nurses an opportunity to intervene with health promotion and patient empowerment strategies (Walker, 1998).

Migrant workers and their families comprise a vast labor workforce for the American agriculture industry, which is constituted mostly of people of Hispanic, African, and Asian descent. The National Advisory Council on Migrant Health reports that nurses and nurse practitioners are the primary health care providers for these workers. In serving this population, nurses see disease transmission and domestic violence, resulting from cramped and unsanitary housing. The children of these workers receive interrupted schooling, which poses psychosocial and developmental risks.

Data indicate poor immunization rates, lack of dental care, and increased incidence of accidents and injury. The cohesive communities of migrant workers are based on language, music, food, and religion. When planning patient education, consider social interaction, folk health practices, and family structure. Teaching interventions must acknowledge cultural diversity and incorporate social supports.

One successful program, the North Carolina Maternal and Child Health Migrant Project, overcame barriers to health care, such as limited transportation, communication difficulties, and lack of child care, by training women in the migrant camps to serve as lay health advisors, providing health education, medication instruction, and first aid. They also targeted breast-feeding promotion among mothers, offering incentives for women to bring their friends and relatives to nutrition education appointments. Nurse practitioners work closely with this population to gather information about changes in family relationships and acculturation to be used in designing health programs to ensure that the health services match the needs of specific migrant cultures (Sandhaus, 1998.)

Patient Education in the Psychiatric Setting

Patient and family education has its own name in psychiatry: psychoeducation. Psychoeducation involves teaching patients and families about the problem, how to treat it, and how to recognize signs of relapse so they can get treatment before the difficulty worsens or occurs again. Family psychoeducation involves teaching coping strategies to families, friends, and caregivers to help them deal more effectively with the patient (PsychoEducational Counseling Services, 2003). Psychoeducation can be provided individually or in groups.

Note that patient education in psychiatry has the same goals as it does in medicine and surgery: informed consent, enhancing self-care skills, recognizing problems, and knowing how to respond. Psychoeducation is not therapy or treatment, but is used to enhance the effectiveness of treatments such as psychotherapy and medication. This is identical to the use of patient education in medicine and surgery. Family and caregivers are taught how to intervene at times when the patient is unable to provide self-care.

A Cochrane review of psychoeducation for schizophrenia showed psychoeducational interventions significantly decreased relapse or readmission rates at 9 to 18 months' follow-up, compared with standard care (Pekkala & Merinder, 2003). A review of the literature on the treatment of schizophrenia found psychoeducation is recommended as standard in most treatment guidelines (Joubert, 2003). Indeed, family psychoeducation is an evidence-based practice that has been shown to reduce relapse rates and facilitate recovery with a full range of mental illnesses (Dixon et al., 2001).

CASE STUDY 8.3

CINDY BENJAMIN, BIPOLAR ILLNESS

Cindy is a 32-year-old woman admitted to the acute care psychiatric unit because of a manic episode. She is loud, cannot sleep, and is impulsive. She resists limits set by the staff, and she responds with inappropriate and promiscuous behavior. The milieu is not therapeutic: other patients become angry and she responds with more aggression.

The patient care plan reflects the following approach to Cindy's care. The first step is to reduce the stimulation by confining Cindy to her room with hourly, supervised breaks. She is supervised to take care of basic grooming. A written contract is used to help her take responsibility for her own limits. She has to be reminded to follow the plan, but she does follow it. The plan is explained to the other patients at community meetings so they would reinforce the plan and understand that less stimulation helps Cindy focus on her behavior.

As the manic symptoms decrease, Cindy spends more time out of her room. Eventually the staff sees a mood shift to depression: less activity, loss of appetite, and neglected grooming. A new plan of care is initiated to support and encourage Cindy to spend more time out of her room.

Like most patients with bipolar illness, Cindy begins long-term drug therapy. Nursing diagnoses in her care plan included inappropriate aggression; manipulation; manic behavior; depressive behavior; alteration in thought process; and self-care deficit: feeding, hygiene.

As Cindy's nursing diagnoses are resolved, the care plan is altered to place priority on the nursing diagnosis of self-care deficit related to nature and management of bipolar disorder.

Goal. The patient will accept her illness and take responsibility for her own treatment, including ongoing drug therapy and outpatient psychotherapy.

Educational needs. Instruct Cindy about the nature of the illness, its course and symptoms, the treatment, and how to manage it. Include Cindy's fiancée and roommate in teaching.

Learning Objective: Survival Skills
Cindy will:

State the diagnosis and describe it in her own words.
Describe symptoms of manic and depressed states.
Outline the three components of the treatment plan she will follow after discharge.
Describe medications, including dose, schedule, and periodic blood level monitoring.

LEARNING OBJECTIVE: RECOGNIZING PROBLEMS
Cindy will:
State two situations for which she should contact her psychiatrist.
State the reason to avoid alcohol.

LEARNING OBJECTIVE: DECISION-MAKING
Cindy will:
Describe how she would recognize the early signs of relapse, and what she should do if any of the signs occur.
State the importance of notifying all health care providers about the medication she takes.

SUMMARY

Patient goals for patient education are derived from diagnoses and associated educational needs. The patient's concerns or fears and the pressing needs of the health care team members to ensure a safe discharge must be considered when making goals. Adult learning theory emphasizes the goal-directedness of adults and the importance of setting goals for patient education. Learning objectives related to goals were described for the three domains—cognitive (knowledge), affective (attitudes and understanding), and psychomotor (skills). For optimal efficiency and effectiveness, the health care provider should identify the three or four objectives that are critical to the safety of each patient, and have

every member of the health care team reinforce these in each encounter with the patient.

STRATEGIES FOR CRITICAL ANALYSIS AND APPLICATION

1. Imagine that you are diagnosed with a rare illness that will require treatment for the rest of your life. You are hospitalized after arriving in the emergency room after a fainting episode. What fears or concerns do you experience that may influence your readiness to learn? List your three most pressing questions.
2. You work as a nurse on the maternity unit of the hospital. Six years ago, when you began work on the unit, you participated in a patient education committee that developed the postpartum teaching plan. This plan was based on a 3-day length of stay. Your average patient stay after a routine vaginal delivery is now 24 hours. How can the patient learning objectives be reduced? Which three or four critical objectives could serve as a basis for teaching survival skills?
3. Using the case study of Mr. Stanley, write one learning objective for each of the three learning domains (cognitive, affective, and psychomotor).
4. Using the case study of Cindy, develop a learning contract using the format in Figure 8.3.

To find the latest information:

Key search terms
goals, objectives, cognitive, affective, psychomotor, Abraham Maslow, Malcolm Knowles, learning contract, psychoeducation

Websites
- Adapting Your Practice: Treatment and Recommendations for Homeless Patients (National Health Care for the Homeless Council):
http://www.nhchc.org/Network/index.htm#Adapting%20Your%20Practice. The

HCH Clinicians' Network has adapted six sets of clinical practice guidelines for homeless patients: diabetes mellitus; asthma; chlamydial and gonococcal infections; otitis media; reproductive health care; and HIV/AIDS

- Outreach to People Experiencing Homelessness: A Curriculum for Training Health Care for the Homeless Outreach Workers: http://www.nhchc.org/Curriculum/index.htm

REFERENCES

Bastable, S. (2003). *Nurse as educator: Principles of teaching and learning for nursing Practice* (2nd ed.). Sudbury, MA: Jones and Bartlett Publishers.

Chelf, J. H., Agre, P., Axelrod, A., Cheney, L., Cole, D. D., Conrad, K., et al. (2001). Cancer-related patient education: An overview of the last decade of evaluation and research. *CHELF, 28*(7), 1139–1147.

Côté, J., Bowie, D. M., Robichaud, P., Parent, J. G., Battisti, L., & Boulet, L. P. (2001). Evaluation of two different educational interventions for adult patients consulting with an acute asthma exacerbation. *American Journal of Respiratory & Critical Care Medicine, 163*(6), 1415–1419.

Dixon, L., McFarlane, W. R., Lefley, H., Luckstead, A., Cohen, M., Falloon, I., et al. (2001). Evidence-based practices for services to families for people with psychiatric disabilities. *Psychiatric Services, 52*(7), 903–910.

Erikson, E. H. (1993). *Childhood and society.* New York: W. W. Norton.

Haber, D. (2001). Promoting readiness to change behavior through health assessments. *Clinical Gerontologist, 23*(1/2), 152–158.

Holli, B. B., & Calabrese, R. J. (1998). *Communication and education skills for dietetics professionals* (3rd ed.). Media, PA: Williams & Wilkins.

Joint Commission on Accreditation of Healthcare Organizations (JCAHO). (2003). *2004 hospital accreditation program standards.* Retrieved June 17, 2003, from http://www.jcaho.org/accredited+organizations/2004+standards.htm

Joubert, A. F. (2003). Providing quality care to patients with schizophrenia. *Psychiatric Clinics of North America, 26*(1), 213–230.

Knowles, M., Swanson, R., & Holton, E. (1998). *Adult learner: The definitive classic in adult education and human resource development.* Houston, TX: Gulf Publishing Company.

Knowles, M. S. (1980). *The modern practice of adult education* (revised and updated ed.). Englewood Cliffs, NJ: Prentice Hall Regents.

Koch, J. (2002). The role of exercise in the African-American woman with type 2 diabetes mellitus: Application of the health belief model. *Journal of the American Academy of Nurse Practitioners, 14*(3), 126–129.

Loeb, J. (1999). Pain management in long-term care. *American Journal of Nursing, 99*(2), 48–52.

Luniewski, M., Reigle, J., & White, B. (1999). Card sort: An assessment tool for the educational needs of patients with heart failure. *American Journal of Critical Care, 8*(5), 297–302.

Maier-Lorentz, M. M. (1999). Writing objectives and evaluating learning in the affective domain. *Journal for Nurses in Staff Development, 15*(4), 167–171.

O'Brien, B. (1999). Coming of age with an ostomy. *American Journal of Nursing, 99*(8), 71–73.

Ohio State University Medical Center. (2001). *Diabetes survival skills.* Retrieved June 23, 2003, from www.acs.ohio-state.edu/units/osuhosp/patedu/Materials/PDFDocs/tguides/flow-sheet/diab-surv.pdf

Osborne, H. (2002). *Partnering with patients to improve health outcomes.* Gaithersburg, MD: Aspen Publishers.

Patient education: A handy guide for assessing needs. (2000). *Health Care Food & Nutrition Focus, 17*(3), 5–7.

Pekkala, E., & Merinder, L. (2003). *Psychoeducation for schizophrenia.* Retrieved July 3, 2003, from www.medscape.com

PsychoEducational Counseling Services. (2003). *PsychoEducational counseling services.* Retrieved July 4, 2003, from http://www.psychoeducation.com/

Sandhaus, S. (1998). Migrant health: A harvest of poverty. *American Journal of Nursing, 98*(9), 52–54.

Schillinger, D., Grumbach, K., Piette, J., Wang, F., Daher, C., Palacios, J., et al. (2002). Association of health literacy with diabetes outcomes. *JAMA, 288*(4), 475–482.

Stieg, R. L. (2001). *Roadblocks to effective pain treatment in the United States*. Retrieved July 2, 2003, from http://www.painconnec-tion.org/cm/CMDisplayArticle.asp?ArticleId =151

Szabo, V., & Strang, V. (1999). Experiencing control in caregiving. *Image—The Journal of Nursing Scholarship 31*(1), 71–75.

Valk, G. D., Kriegsman, D. M. W., & Assendelft, W. J. J. (2002). Patient education for preventing diabetic foot ulceration: A systematic review. *Endocrinology and Metabolism Clinics, 31*(3), 633–658.

van Weert, J., van Dulmen, S., Bar, P., & Venus, E. (2003). Interdisciplinary preoperative patient education in cardiac surgery. *Patient Education and Counseling, 49*(2), 105–114.

Walker, C. (1998). Homeless people and mental health: A nursing concern. *American Journal of Nursing, 98*(11), 26–32.

Educational Interventions for Patients and Families

After reading this chapter, the student should be able to:

1. List the benefits and drawbacks for individual teaching and group teaching.

2. Discuss how a variety of instructional methods (such as lecture, discussion, demonstration, role-play, tests, programmed instruction) can be used to achieve learning objectives.

3. Describe how to effectively use patient education videos.

4. List guidelines for developing effective written patient teaching handouts and discharge instructions.

5. Describe strategies that encourage active patient involvement in patient education interventions for both individual and group teaching programs.

6. Discuss how family roles and expectations can affect learning.

INTRODUCTION

Interventions for Patient Education

Individualized goals set the course for patient education interventions. After goals are agreed on and before learning activities begin, decisions must be made about content, methods, tools, and who will teach. The nurse often coordinates this planning through team conferences, contact with the patient's family, and community resources. A case manager or other health care team member may promote patient education as an integral part of the total care plan.

This chapter offers practical advice and frameworks for designing and implementing educational interventions. Characteristics of a positive learning environment are outlined, teaching and learning styles as they relate to program design are discussed, and the selection of instructional methods and media is explored. There is an emphasis on making patient education realistic, basing it on the patient's length of stay and the survival skills needed. Suggestions for developing and evaluating both printed patient education materials and educational videotapes are included. This chapter discusses interventions for individual patients and groups and includes case studies to illustrate practical applications.

Scope of Teaching Programs

Planning interventions involves making decisions about the patient education setting, content, resources, and instructors. Interventions must be tailored to each patient, based on the assessment findings.

On a larger scale, when creating an organizational environment that supports patient and family education, it is helpful to identify the target populations with highest volume (such as asthma) and greatest risk (such as tracheostomy care). Resources should then be focused on these target populations to opti-

mize effectiveness and efficiency of patient education efforts, house-wide.

Interdisciplinary teams, including patients and families, can develop the content and tools for these teaching programs, linking standards for care, learning needs, community resources, and quality improvement systems. A patient education coordinator, hospital-based educator, clinical nurse specialist, or other health care provider may organize interdisciplinary task forces, to coordinate teaching resources for special groups. Organization-based programs often provide teaching tools, such as care maps, to meet the needs of a variety of learning styles, and teaching guides for health professionals (see Chapter 12). By including patients, families, and all health care disciplines involved, this approach to developing patient education programs optimizes collaboration by enhancing team support and helping everyone feel confident about the quality of the interventions and the preparation and knowledge of the staff.

The range of teaching programs spans:

- Coordinated resources for one-on-one teaching
- Development and delivery of group teaching classes
- Comprehensive disease management programs

Teaching programs also facilitate measurement of the effectiveness of patient education. Patient teaching programs must be continually evaluated to assure effectiveness, through outcome measurement. Dramatically changing delivery patterns for health care can outdate patient education programs within months of their development. For example, the program of a large academic medical center to teach parents of pediatric bone marrow transplant patients became outdated within months of development, when care shifted from the hospital to the outpatient setting. To minimize this, health care providers must develop flexible programs that include providers across the continuum, address patient needs in all settings, and focus on patient outcomes. These programs are often called product-line models.

There are many resources to tap when developing a teaching program including:

- Other health care agencies
- Organizations and associations, such as the American Hospital Association, the National Institutes of Health, the American Cancer Society, and the American Diabetes Association
- Summaries of evidence-based practice, such as those developed by the Canadian Task Force on Preventive Health Care (CTFPHC) or the Agency for Healthcare Research and Quality (AHRQ)
- Clinical Practice Guidelines such as those developed by the Agency for Healthcare Research and Quality (AHRQ)

Clinical Practice Guidelines can be especially helpful because they help practitioners in the prevention, diagnosis, treatment, and management of clinical conditions, with a focus on patient outcomes. For each clinical practice guideline developed under the sponsorship of AHRQ, several documents are produced to meet different needs. These guidelines contain background information, research findings, a literature review, and bibliography. A patient's guide (or parent guide for pediatric problems) is also available in English and Spanish, providing information to increase patient involvement in health care decision-making. A strong feature of the AHRQ guidelines is their recommendation for patient education (Agency for Healthcare Research and Quality, 2003).

SETTING THE STAGE FOR TEACHING AND LEARNING

Health care providers know how to care for patients with acute and chronic illnesses. However, they may be unclear about the needs for care outside of the health care environment. What survival skills are needed?

What challenges may arise or what could go wrong, and how should the learner respond? Consequently, essential content may be missed, incorrect information may be given, or learning activities may be inappropriate. Some health care providers may react to this lack of preparation by avoiding teaching, hoping someone else will meet the patient's learning needs.

Administration and management can ensure the quality of patient education in the organization by creating and maintaining an environment that supports practice. All disciplines need to participate in the development of patient care standards that include patient education. Performance evaluations need to consider competencies in teaching skills. Coaching and modeling need to be made available to ensure continual improvement of skills. Patients and families should be consulted to ensure the teaching tools provided by the organization and the teaching skills of the health care providers meet the needs of the learners.

Teaching tools, such as handouts, videos, and models, are helpful reinforcers of teaching. The right educational materials are accurate, age-specific, easily accessible, and appropriate to learner needs. Management and organization of such teaching tools may be centralized or decentralized. A centralized system is recommended for maintaining adequate supplies, ensuring quality control, and monitoring costs. Written materials may be uploaded to the organization's computer system to be printed on demand, so everyone has access to the same materials. A data base of other teaching tools, such as pamphlets, models, and posters, may be available in printed or computerized form to inform staff of what is available and how to access it. The data base should itemize the date the material was developed, the learning outcomes addressed, the literacy level, the languages in which it is available, the target population, and the cost of producing or purchasing it. Videos may be offered through that system, or through a closed-circuit television system that can play selections on demand.

Setting Priorities

To set teaching priorities, the health care provider returns to the results of the team's assessments (see Chapter 7 for details) and considers the patient's ability and readiness to learn. If pain management issues preoccupy a patient's attention, addressing this topic is an educational priority. It is important to consider what the patient and the family view as priorities, the level of their anxiety about the topic or skill, the level of need, and the time available for implementing teaching activities.

In general, learning should progress from familiar to unfamiliar and from simple to complex. The three or four most important learning objectives should be selected, remembering that the three goals of patient education are to help patients (1) gain survival skills, (2) learn to recognize problems, and (3) have the confidence to make appropriate decisions that benefit health status. (See Chapter 8 for details.)

Selecting Instructional Media and Methods

Health professionals sometimes justify their lack of teaching because there is a shortage of funds to purchase CDs, videotapes, television equipment, and computers. They miss the point. Instructional media do not teach. They are tools used by the teacher to help the learner to retain, compare, visualize, and reinforce learning. "Modern technologies provide tools that can enhance, but not substitute for, skilled and dedicated teachers" (Gaba, 2002).

Although the effectiveness of instructional media in patient education is emphasized in the literature, the specific tools used need to be chosen to fit the needs of individual learners. When too much emphasis is placed on media, instruction is insufficiently personalized. One-on-one teaching using a clear list of instructions can often result in better patient outcomes than when patients are overwhelmed with information from various formats, and possibly conflicting content, in a short timeframe.

Instructional methods should be chosen and aligned with the teaching format (such as self-directed, individual, small group, large group) and the learning activity (such as lecture, demonstration, discussion, roleplay).

Creating a Climate for Adult Learning

As indicated in Chapter 8, adults are performance-centered and seek information that helps them in their daily lives. Patients listen for the bottom line and want health care professionals to tell them what they need to know, not what is nice to know. Patients want to know how to perform survival skills at home, and how to adapt current lifestyles to include healthy behaviors. When these needs are met, learning becomes satisfying and effective. If the teacher fails to acknowledge the patient's needs, barriers arise that slow down or prevent the learning of new behaviors.

A climate that promotes adult learning considers the physical and emotional needs of the learner. It uses problem-centered learning, in which the material is related to the patient's life situation and concerns. The learning activities include interactive opportunities for an exchange of ideas between the teacher and learner, and for applications of learning in simulated or real exercises.

Physical Comfort

Pain or anxiety interferes with the exchange of ideas or the ability to listen. Patients who are in the hospital or bedridden may depend on others to assist them with bathing, elimination, dressing changes, medication, and ambulating. A thoughtful teacher is sensitive to these needs and helps the patient achieve as much comfort as possible. The teacher should consider whether the patient can physically tolerate a lengthy teaching session or can participate in group learning and encourage the patient's participation by making certain he or she has eyeglasses or dentures and is positioned comfortably. It is important to watch for signs of hunger, thirst, restlessness, or discomfort.

The health care provider should also capitalize on the time spent helping patients to meet their basic needs by teaching content and skills related to their care and taking full advantage of teachable moments. For example, the patient and family members could be taught about medication while it is being administered. The next time that medicine is administered they could be asked to repeat the information they learned about it earlier. Alternatively, a health care provider could talk through the procedure while changing a patient's dressing. The next time he changes the dressing, he could ask the learner to tell him what to do next. The function of insulin could be discussed with the patient at the time he or she administers it, or insulin reactions could be discussed with the patient after he or she experiences a reaction.

Ability

A major determinant in identifying appropriate teaching methods and content is the learner's health literacy, which is the ability to obtain, process, and understand basic health information and services needed to make appropriate health decisions (Williams et al., 2002). A good assessment provides data about what the learner already knows, allowing the health care provider to present new information in the context of known information. To optimize teaching efforts, it is essential to individualize teaching methods and content to the needs and abilities of the learner, and evaluate understanding to ensure the methods were effective.

Emotional Needs

Many patients attribute a mystique to the roles of physicians and nurses. Especially in times of illness or change, patients often want to be cared for or to find someone who will perform magical acts to restore a previous state of health, erase pain, or remove conflict. Health care personnel have frequently perpetuated this desire by encouraging dependence, or by not taking the time to encourage patient participation in medical management. Patients may hesitate to participate later, feeling incapable of managing self-care or of learning necessary skills. They may worry that if they become more independent, they may be deprived of necessary help and unable to meet their own needs.

Each patient's anxiety about learning new health behaviors and his or her support needs should be acknowledged. Patients should know that medical personnel will support them, and they will receive necessary help and teaching until new skills are mastered. Patients may be afraid to disclose their lack of knowledge or to make mistakes. Learning should be structured to proceed from simple to complex, so the patient will experience success. Support and advice should be provided as the patient tries out newly learned behaviors. In times of crisis or stress, the patient may need greater support and may test the health care provider's willingness to help.

Patients and families frequently feel ill-prepared for discharge after a short hospital stay. Some report that they were given "too little information, too late." Others report that they were given "too much information, too soon," causing them to be overwhelmed, insecure, and unable to manage. The key to successful patient education is to focus on three or four critical learning objectives relating to survival skills. All patients should know how to recognize problems and how to reach help after their hospital discharge.

The following are two examples that illustrate emotional needs in patient education:

CASE STUDY 9.1

MR. BENTON'S DIABETES

Mr. Benton is a 53-year-old man who has had insulin-dependent diabetes for 6 years. He makes frequent visits to the clinic with various minor complaints and leaves the clinic much improved after each visit. He lives alone and depends on the clinic staff for support. He calls the nurse station almost daily, occasionally stating, "I just can't seem to get going, give myself my insulin, and get to work." Through the teaching and review, the staff members knew he had mastered the necessary skills to do so. The clinic's social worker is called to help Mr. Benton get involved in the local chapter of the American Diabetes Association, thus increasing his support system. In addition, the clinic's nurses schedule regular, monthly, 30-minute visits, during which they support Mr. Benton and occasionally ask him to share his expertise in insulin injection with patients who had newly diagnosed diabetes.

CASE STUDY 9.2

MRS. HESTER'S BABY

Mrs. Hester receives prenatal care at the clinic and looks forward to breast-feeding her baby. She reads books on infant care and attends prenatal classes. Although the classes stressed the importance of being flexible in planning labor and delivery, Mrs. Hester plans to have a vaginal delivery. A breech presentation, however, necessitates cesarean section. Mrs. Hester successfully nurses her baby in the hospital and has good support and teaching from the hospital staff.

Two days after discharge, Mrs. Hester calls the clinic's nurse. She cries, stating that she feels like a failure because the baby "will not take her milk." After supporting her on the telephone, the nurse suggests that Mrs. Hester come to the clinic and feed her baby in the examination room where the nurse can offer assistance. Mrs. Hester happily agrees. When she arrives, the nurse realizes that Mrs. Hester's anxiety and fatigue were causing her difficulty with nursing. Together they review the progressive muscle relaxation exercises done in prenatal classes. Mrs. Hester then relaxes before nursing the baby, and the baby nurses successfully. The nurse compliments Mrs. Hester on how well she cares for the baby. She points out signs of effective nursing, such as the jaw movement back to the baby's ears with sucking, audible sucking, and the number of wet diapers the mother reported changing in the last day.

The nurse weighs the baby so the patient can verify that the baby is gaining weight. The nurse also offers additional visits of this nature if needed. She reminds Mrs. Hester to nap when the baby naps, and to drink plenty of fluids. The patient agrees to call the nurse the next day and let her know how the breast-feeding is progressing. When she did, the report was a positive one. Mrs. Hester remarks, "It is just so good to know I can call you if I need help."

Problem-Centered Learning

Learning activities should be centered on potential problems the patient may face, such as an asthma episode, or a hypoglycemic reaction. The teacher will want to help the learner recognize the problem, know what to do, and feel competent in performing the necessary behavior. Patients should describe their diagnosis or health problem and how their symptoms relate to it.

Patient education should help the patient who experiences an acute episode to answer the following questions: Why am I here at this time? What could I have done to prevent it? Patients often bring problems or concerns with them to the learning session. Breast-feeding problems are a good example. Similarly, expectant parents may express the following concerns:

- How can I deal with the pain of labor?
- How will I know if the baby is sick?
- What do I do if the baby does not stop crying?

Preoperative patients also want information:

- What will it be like in surgery?
- What will they do to me?
- Will I be in pain?
- What will it be like when I wake up?

Patients with diabetes and their family members also often have questions:

- Why are insulin shots needed?
- How difficult will it be to give myself shots?
- What is an insulin reaction?

Some patients mention their problems and concerns freely, whereas others hesitate to do so. Occasionally, patients with newly diagnosed problems do not know what to ask. The nurse should encourage the patient to verbalize concerns and then address these concerns in learning activities. If the patient and the family need help describing concerns, teachers may begin, for example, by saying: "Patients who are pregnant often have questions about labor and delivery and want to know what to expect. I wonder if you might have concerns about that?"

Application of Learning

New information is internalized through learning activities that provide opportunities to apply it. After new information is provided to the learner, the health care provider should pose problems and give the learner a chance to respond, applying the new information. Exposure to the new information and its application should occur in the same teaching session.

Participative Learning

Alternating instruction with return demonstration is an effective strategy. This approach allows the patient to see incremental learning, receive immediate feedback, and learn through repetition. Participation should be encouraged at the onset of learning activities, so patients build confidence. Some patients are comfortable in voicing concerns and attempting new skills; others are reluctant and anxious, and may need special attention. With adequate support and realistic learning goals, participation can be gained from even the most reluctant learner.

Health care providers evaluate the learner's understanding during this active involvement process. Demonstration of skills ("show me how you would ...") and solutions offered to hypothetical problems ("what would you do if ...") offer insights into the learner's ability to problem-solve and provide safe self-care.

Teaching through interaction also gives the teacher constant feedback on the effectiveness of teaching, minimizing the time that may be wasted by misunderstandings or information overload. Communication problems can be identified quickly, and corrected.

The Teacher–Learner Relationship

Learning is a shared experience, requiring openness from both the teacher and the learner. The health care provider must be willing to establish a relationship with the learner. The health care provider must be dependable, must encourage the learner until goals are met, must be flexible enough to negotiate, and must provide support and reinforcement. The health care provider commits herself in an agreement—a learning contract (described in Chapter 8)—whether verbal or written. The health care provider must be willing to admit when she does not have an answer and be eager to seek additional information.

As in all therapeutic relationships, the teacher–learner relationship takes time to develop. By giving the patient an opportunity to tell his or her story, the teacher and patient become acquainted. Assessment and problem identification begins. The learner begins a testing phase, in which he or she considers the willingness and ability of the health care provider to understand his or her needs, to help and support him or her, and to commit to mutual goals. Eventually, the teacher and learner establish a working relationship and engage in activities together. The teacher respects the patient's cultural and religious beliefs and acknowledges the patient's right to make choices. The teacher also provides experiences through which the learner tries new behaviors. The teacher must instill in the patient the confidence that he or she can learn to participate in his or her health care and perform survival skills. To do this, the teacher focuses on few priorities, uses repetition, and helps the patient relate teaching to everyday life.

Styles of Learners

Patients approach learning in various ways determined by individual lifestyle, personality, and past experience. The patient educator should identify characteristics of the learner's style to help plan teaching interventions. Some patients may read extensively about the health problem and may vocalize many questions; others may want to know only the basic facts. Some patients are comfortable in group learning situations, and others are not. Some patients may be enthusiastic to return demonstrate a procedure taught by the nurse, whereas others may hesitate and ask the nurse to review the procedure several times. Some patients may freely discuss difficulty and confusion, but others may deny problems unless they know they are observed. Some patients may play the informed expert and offer the nurse a challenge during a learning needs assessment; other patients may hold back what they know, wishing to be taken care of rather than to assume responsibility

in health management. Patients also learn at different rates, depending on age, intelligence, motor skills, degree of impairment, anxiety, and past experience. Each teaching and learning activity must be adapted to the style and need of the learner.

Styles of Teachers

Each health care provider has a personal teaching style. Some teachers are comfortable with an expert role in telling or showing; others encourage constant involvement through discussion. Some teachers have difficulty dealing with the patient who sees himself or herself as an expert; others may feel comfortable letting the patient direct the teaching while they clarify, correct, and supplement knowledge. Some health care providers have difficulty teaching a passive, dependent, or depressed patient. The teacher should be aware of his or her own teaching style, and the patients he or she is most comfortable working with. It is important for the teacher to stretch and learn how to teach in situations outside of his or her comfort zone. It is the responsibility of the health care provider to individualize teaching to the style of the learner, despite the fact that he or she may have a preferred style of teaching.

It is not always possible to consider the compatibility of the teacher with the learner when selecting members of the health care team. For example, a nurse with high control needs as a teacher may compete with the expert patient, creating a frustrating and unproductive teaching session. Frustration is a cue to return back to the assessment data, to identify how to better individualize teaching to optimize success. If a passive, dependent patient is only taught according to the needs he or she verbalizes, little will be learned. Again, the teacher must return to the assessment and plan, and tailor teaching to the learner's needs.

When teaching is not individualized, therapeutic relationships suffer and valuable teaching time is wasted. For example, we are familiar with a case in which a nurse who communicated little empathy was assigned to teach tracheostomy suctioning to a patient who had a radical neck dissection and glossectomy. The patient attempted to control his environment in response to his multiple losses and refused to accept any teaching from the nurse. His discharge from the hospital was delayed until another nurse, who understood his attempts to exert control, was assigned as his primary nurse.

Preparing Staff to Teach

A planned, consistent approach in patient education presents the material in an organized manner and avoids unnecessary repetition. It gives the patient and family ample opportunity for review and practice, ensuring they are not overwhelmed with content.

Collaboration by interdisciplinary team members to provide patient and family education does not require that every member of every discipline teach every patient. The team should collaborate to identify the overall key learning needs, based on the prognosis, and distill these into one set of discharge instructions. Teaching can then be organized to prepare the patient for discharge throughout the hospitalization. One way to involve the team is to collaborate to develop teaching protocols, and then individualize them to specific patient situations. Protocols may be in the form of a clinical pathway, targeted toward specific patient groups (Gorski, 2002). These protocols outline provider responsibilities, saving time and alleviating confusion.

Although everyone on the health care team is responsible for contributing to patient and family education, this may be difficult to coordinate when the hospital stay is short. In these situations, patient education may be more effective when one or two professionals are responsible for the entire teaching plan.

Staff development efforts should support interdisciplinary involvement in patient teaching, eliminating perceived barriers, such as inadequate knowledge of the content to be taught. Chapter 5 addresses how to prepare staff to teach patients and families.

STRATEGIC USE OF INSTRUCTIONAL METHODS

Chapter 8 reviewed three types of learning behavior: cognitive (knowledge and information), affective (attitudes and values), and psychomotor (skills and performance). Learning in each of these three areas contributes to behavior change. For example, for educating a patient with newly diagnosed diabetes, the following behaviors are desirable:

1. **Cognitive learning.** The patient can describe what diabetes is and name three things a patient with diabetes should do to manage his or her care. The patient can state that insulin reactions may be caused by the wrong amount or kind of medication, late or omitted meals or snacks, failure to follow diet plan, and increased activity.
2. **Affective learning.** The patient can discuss why it is important for him or her, the family, the physician, and other health care professionals to work together in medical management. The patient can state why he or she should tell friends and coworkers that he or she has diabetes, explain to them the signs and symptoms of insulin reactions, and tell them how to help if reactions occur.
3. **Psychomotor learning.** The patient can make food choices to plan one breakfast, one lunch, and one dinner within guidelines of an ADA meal plan. The patient can demonstrate proper technique for daily washing and checking of feet.

Categorizing learning objectives into these three areas facilitates the selection of teaching and learning formats, methods, and media best suited to patient education needs. In many cases, a combination of formats can be used to provide learning experiences, add variety, and meet different types of objectives.

Individual Teaching

Often called one-on-one teaching, individual instruction is ideal for continued assessment of the learner and technical skill training (such as urine testing, insulin injection, or self-catheterization). One-on-one teaching facilitates sharing of confidential information and problems. It is easiest to individualize teaching to adapt to learners with poor health literacy skills, physical impairment, or emotional difficulties. Teaching is often begun with individual teaching, to improve basic knowledge and skills and increase the patient's confidence in self-care. Advantages of this format include an active learner role that builds motivation, an opportunity for consistent and frequent feedback, and flexibility to immediately adapt teaching to learner's needs in an unstructured, informal atmosphere.

The best response to a teachable moment is immediate one-on-one teaching. By responding to the learner's problems and needs as they arise, teaching is done when the learner is most open to assimilating the new information, and build problem-solving skills.

One-on-one teaching is often most productive because it is intensive, highly individualized to the learner's needs, and can occur spontaneously during every patient encounter. Preoperative teaching, initial diabetic teaching, and diet teaching are often performed using the individual format. The obvious disadvantages of individual teaching are a lack of sharing with, and support from, other patients and their families and the high cost of staff time for instruction.

Another form of individual teaching is telephone calls initiated by the patient, a family member, or health care provider. Nurse advice lines provide answers to questions, reassurance, clarification, and assistance. They provide a safety net for follow-up after discharge from the hospital. Telephones can be used to accomplish individual preoperative assessment and teaching and are invaluable for reaching learners who live in rural communities or who are homebound. Telephone teaching is also effective for many learners with low literacy skills (London, 1999).

Group Teaching

Group learning takes advantage of adult learning principles when participants learn from one another and teach one another through their own experiences. It helps learners feel less alone, and fosters positive attitude development. The group format is ideal for teaching patients and their families together.

Because the most effective adult education involves active involvement, and group classes allow participants to share knowledge and experiences with one another, group teaching is better used to help learners process and integrate information with behaviors, rather than to cover a great deal of data in a short amount of time.

However, before health care providers can offer group classes, they need to have a group of learners who need to learn the same content at the same time. This is often only possible with large populations of learners, such as childbirth preparation, CPR, and nutrition for cardiac patients.

Group classes also take preparation time that makes them cost-effective only when the same program can be offered repeatedly, over time. Since all teaching needs to be individualized to the needs of the learner, it is essential to involve patients and families in determining class content. Although group members have slightly different learning goals, they may share a few universal concerns and questions. These shared learning needs are best addressed in a group. Even when the content is derived from focus groups with the patient population, it is important to confirm its appropriateness with the participants at the beginning of each class.

It is easiest to individualize group teaching when all the participants share knowledge base, culture, and literacy skills. Physiologically or emotionally unstable learners are poor candidates for group teaching. When the group consists of learners with a variety of skills or abilities, it is more difficult to meet the needs of all, equally.

It is also often difficult to evaluate, in the group context, each participant's ability to apply the information. Classes need to be followed-up with individual education sessions, to answer questions, evaluate understanding, and help the learner apply the information to his or her specific situation.

Small groups (2 to 5 learners) are ideal for skill training. The key to leading small groups is promoting active participation and the ready expression of ideas. The leader determines with the learners what they want to learn or achieve, they identify learning outcomes, determine the tasks that will deliver those outcomes (such as a problem to solve), and then the leader organizes and monitors the group to meet those objectives (Jaques, 2003).

The leader guides the group by giving the learners responsibility to learn through interaction, rather than by hand-feeding information. This method can be applied in a variety of settings. Nurses in psychiatric acute care offer small groups to teach about medications and coping with their side effects, conduct discussions about organizing activities of daily living, and to share post-discharge concerns. Older outpatients can discuss approaches to managing functional problems and strategies for health promotion in small groups.

Medium-sized groups (6 to 30 learners) also involve promoting active participation and the ready expression of ideas. It may be necessary to break out into smaller groups to do work, and have each report back to the whole group. Because more than five learners make learner–teacher feedback difficult, groups are not appropriate for skill training. Medium-sized groups may be used effectively for prenatal care, child care, stress reduction, safety, diabetes review, or self-help and support groups.

Large groups (30 or more learners) are appropriate for community education of health promotion or illness prevention, rather than preparing patients for self-care after discharge. Large group sessions are most effective when brief lectures and videos are interspersed with small group experiences or discussion, to enable active involvement (Cantillon, 2003). It is difficult in these groups to evaluate whether individual learning goals have been met.

Support Groups, Self-Help Groups, and Self-Management Groups

Some groups are designed so patients with common health-related problems can come together for learning, sharing, and mutual support. These groups range widely in purpose, structure, leadership, membership, and how they meet. They may meet in person, on-line, or both. The booklet, "Now You Have a Diagnosis: What's Next? Using health care information to help make treatment decisions" (Agency for Healthcare Research and Quality, 2000), suggests readers join a support group because research shows they often help people cope better with their conditions.

Self-Help and Support Groups

Lay persons who recognize the need for mutual support in dealing with prevention, management, and adaptation to chronic illnesses begin some self-help groups themselves. These groups are organized and led by patients or family members. They may meet in places such as houses of worship, senior centers, library meeting rooms, or members' homes.

Other groups may be sponsored by disease-related organizations, community agencies, or hospitals. The agencies or organizations provide a place to meet, and some administrative support, such as paying for mailings. Sometimes they take a greater role, and provide leadership, facilitators, speakers, and educational materials. Because of public interest and demand, many hospitals now sponsor self-help groups open to the community on a range of topics. These groups may be offered at no cost, or a small fee.

Self-help and support groups exist for nearly every chronic illness, some acute illnesses, and situations where support is needed, such as grief or caregiving. They offer information, inspiration from the courage of others, role models, and hope (Johnson, 2000).

Support groups for patients with various types of cancer, and their families, are readily available. Researchers are now looking at who participates in these groups, and how to make them more accessible (Bui et al., 2002, and Katz et al., 2002). Twelve-step programs for substance abuse have been shown to improve outcomes of treatment and decrease health care costs (Humphreys & Moos, 2001). Support groups have also helped patients cope through difficult transitions, such as menopause (Boggs & Rosenthal, 2000) and pregnancies that require hospitalized bed rest (Maloni & Kutil, 2000).

Support groups that meet electronically have been effective, too. A web-based support group has been shown to be useful in women with primary breast carcinoma, by reducing depression, cancer-related trauma, and perceived stress (Winzelberg et al., 2003). A randomized controlled trial of a closed, moderated e-mail discussion group for patients with chronic back pain was found to positively affect health status and possibly health care utilization (Lorig et al., 2002). Patients with mood disorders use Internet support groups to discuss the impact of their illness on daily life, discuss benefits and drawbacks of treatments, review new research, and encourage one another (Lamberg, 2003).

To learn more about self-help and support groups, see the self-help group sourcebook online (White & Madara, 2004). This site (http://www.mentalhelp.net/selfhelp/) offers a searchable data base of North American contacts.

Self-Management Groups

Chronic illness requires chronic care that, at each moment, adapts to the needs of the learner at that time. Self-management, like other patient education, begins with the patient's perceived problems. Research has shown patterns to patients' needs (Lorig, 2001). People with chronic illness need to deal with the medical management of the disease, including medication, activity, and diet. People with chronic illnesses want to know how to maintain their roles in life. They also need to deal with the emotional sequelae of the disease, including fear, frustration, depression and anger.

Self-management programs guide groups of patients dealing with the same chronic illness through the process of learning how to best take care of themselves. Each program runs from 4 to 7 weeks, with sessions from 2 to 2½ hours per week. Content is determined by assessment of patients' needs; every patient gets a detailed manual. Every session has the same structure: It begins with feedback, they learn something, they take a break, they learn two more things, they make action plans, and they go home. Skills mastery, modeling, and social persuasion help the participants enhance self-efficacy (Lorig, 2001).

Controlled clinical trials suggest that programs teaching self-management skills can reduce costs, and are more effective at improving clinical outcomes than providing information alone (Bodenheimer et al., 2002). A two-year health status follow-up of patients who completed a Chronic Disease Self-Management Program (CDSMP) determined the low-cost program improved perceived self-efficacy, lowered health distress, and reduced ambulatory health care and emergency room use, thus reducing health care costs (Lorig et al., 2001).

Care Maps

Many hospitals and health care agencies have developed systematic patient care maps for educating patients with specific diseases or problems. These care maps use individual and group teaching interventions, including self-directed learning. Patients and their families are taught through use of a standard outline, including basic information components that are tailored to the learner. The care map is individualized through deletions and additions.

Care maps generally include teaching about pathophysiology, treatments, medications, diet, diagnostic tests, procedures, recommended activity, and self-care skills. With care maps, patient instruction can be tailored to be relevant to the patient's experience in that institution or facility. Patient learning outcomes are tied to each phase of the patient's course, based on an estimated length of stay, thus improving efficiency, quality, and potentially decreasing inpatient days. Staff members are trained to use the teaching formats and strategies through classes and tutors. The roles of various providers are outlined according to subject matter and areas of expertise. Specific provider responsibilities are identified. Nurses often perform the initial assessment, and other members of the health care team intervene, evaluate, and document teaching and learning.

The patient's interests, abilities, and cultural background determine which teaching materials are selected. The time required for teaching segments of the content is estimated, and resources are suggested to help patients meet the learning goals. Content, teaching strategies, and activities suitable to meet the goals are provided by a planning committee when the care map is established. The care plan may include individual teaching, group teaching, and referral to community resources for support after discharge. Teaching aids, such as audiovisuals and printed matter, may be purchased or developed by the health care institution to enhance patient teaching. In addition, the care map specifies what types of information should be documented in the medical record and where it will be located. Measures for evaluation of patient learning are specified. (See Chapter 12 for more information about patient care maps.)

To evaluate if care maps are being used appropriately, the health care provider should compare the charts of several patients taught using the same care map. If documentation on all the charts looks identical, it should be considered a red flag. Most likely the patients were not identical, and each had different concerns, learning abilities, and learning needs. Identical charting indicates the patients may not have been adequately assessed, and teaching may not have been individualized. Consequently, what may appear to be documented teaching according to plan may actually be evidence of inefficient and ineffective teaching.

STRATEGIC USE OF LEARNING ACTIVITIES

Whether the format for teaching is individual or group, the principle of patient inclusion applies. At the outset, the teacher should collaborate with the patient to determine the three or four critical skills he or she needs to learn. By providing this big picture or bottom line, the patient acknowledges the need to participate actively in the process of patient education.

Knowing how to use various learning activities to meet educational objectives can make patient education more interesting, challenging, and effective for both the teacher and the learner. The patient educator will want to choose learning activities thoughtfully, so that they will be suitable for particular patient objectives. Box 9.1 offers a guide for selecting activities conducive to cognitive, affective, and psychomotor changes. Some learning activities are appropriate for more than one type of learning objective. Brief descriptions of the major types of learning activities are offered with suggestions for effective and appropriate application.

Self-Directed Learning

Computer-assisted instruction (CAI) and self-directed learning workbooks have become popular resources for patient education. The use of the Internet for patient education is also increasing in popularity (see Chapter 10). A growing trend in health care settings is the creation of patient and family education resource centers—small libraries containing books, videotapes, and pamphlets that discuss

BOX 9.1 Selecting Learning Activities for Patient Education

I. Cognitive (Knowledge)
　Learning Facts
　　Lecture
　　Demonstration
　　Independent study format
　　Tests
　Discussion-Questions and Answers
　　Practice
　　Simulation
　Visual Identification
　　Demonstration
　　Simulation
　　Tests
　　Practice
　　Independent study
　Understanding and Applying Knowledge
　　Demonstration
　　Practice
　　Role-play
　Discussion-Questions and Answers
　　Independent study
　　Simulation
　　Tests

II. Affective (Attitudes and Appreciations)
　　Discussion-Questions and Answers
　　Role Play
　　Simulation

III. Psychomotor (Skills and Performance)
　　Practice
　　Role Play
　　Simulation
　　Demonstration
　　Tests
　　Independent study

support groups, and tips on coping with cancer treatment. When patients are first diagnosed with cancer, they usually have many questions about the illness, treatment, and prognosis. They are concerned about their insurance, how surgery or treatment will affect them, and how to talk to their children about the disease. But most important, they want to know that as their questions continue they will have somewhere to turn for answers.

A resource center offers assistance based on the patient's expressed needs and information about support groups in which experienced facilitators can help patients learn about treatment options, nutrition, coping with cancer, survivorship, and insurance. It even offers a program that pairs newly diagnosed patients with other patients who have the same diagnosis. These resource centers are responsive when patients are ready to learn, and they bridge the gaps often experienced by patients as they receive care in multiple settings from multiple providers. Resource centers are viewed as especially valuable by patients and families who cope with chronic health problems.

Lecture

Lecture can teach cognitive information, but it is not the best method for teaching adults (see Chapter 8 for adult learning principles). Lecture is most effective when used with discussion, and enhanced by use of handouts, pictures, and visual aids (overheads and slides) that involve the learner. Learners may be eager to contribute or to try out or apply knowledge; this eagerness may be stifled by a formal lecture approach in which the teacher is the expert. Material presented in a lecture should be prepared to the learner's level of understanding, and learners should have an opportunity to ask questions during, not after, the presentation. Lengthy lectures may cause loss of attention; learners become bored, distracted, or anxious about the material presented. Lectures may also create the impression that the patient's problem is so complicated that he or she cannot manage it.

health and illness topics. For example, a hospital-based Cancer Resource Center serves patients and families by providing answers to questions about cancer, information about

Although lectures can effectively influence cognitive behaviors, they are not effective in achieving affective or psychomotor learning objectives. For example, a lecture is often used to give initial knowledge about pathophysiology to patients with diabetes, but is ineffective when used alone to teach insulin injection. Lectures may be given in person, televised, or audiotaped. The amount of total teaching time should include a minimum of lecture because the focus of teaching is on building survival skills needed to ensure patient safety after discharge.

Group Discussion

Discussion requires two or more people to exchange ideas. It differs from lecture in that it is an excellent method of involving patients in the learning process. This learning activity promotes understanding and application of knowledge (cognitive behaviors) and development of certain attitudes (affective behaviors). The teacher, who asks specific questions or proposes problem situations, frequently directs it. Discussion facilitates learning from the experience of others, fosters a feeling of belongingness, and reinforces previous learning.

Demonstration

Demonstration is useful for cognitive and psychomotor learning. It is most often used to teach skills and to present performance standards. Demonstration may be done in person or in videotaped programs. The sense of sight is used in learning from demonstration, but hearing, smell, and taste may also be stimulated. The teacher should demonstrate slowly, and be certain the learner can see and hear well. This strategy shows the learner that the behavior is possible and increases confidence that he or she can perform it. For example, when teaching insulin injection, the nurse may demonstrate injection using sterile water before the patient actually performs an insulin injection. When demonstration is used to teach discharge skills, the actual type of equipment or supplies to be used at home should be used for teaching. Repetition and return demonstration are needed for teaching procedures with multiple steps.

Role-Play and Return Demonstration

Learners can practice or do with either role-play or return demonstration. These activities help the learner apply knowledge or skills, usually after the teacher demonstrates. During role-play or return demonstration, the teacher offers guidance and feedback and tailors the learning to the patient's past or present life experiences.

In role-play, the learner acts out his own situation or that of another person. This is highly effective in meeting affective objectives. Return demonstration begins with watching the teacher perform the skill, then the learner doing it himself or herself, one or more times. In both cases, clear instruction must be given to the learner about what to do and how to do it. Enough practice time should be allowed for the learner to repeat the skill until he or she has mastered it. Role-play and return demonstration are effective strategies for teaching cognitive, affective, and psychomotor behaviors. Role-playing helps patients learn to recognize and handle problem situations, such as a hypoglycemic reaction or a cardiac arrest, with which they have no first-hand experience.

For patients with complications or readmission, return demonstration can be used to assess skills that may have contributed to exacerbations of a chronic condition. For example, nurses in one rural community hospital assessed through return demonstration that there was a high readmission rate for patients with chronic obstructive pulmonary disease who were previously discharged with metered-dose inhalers. Although the patients were taught during hospitalization, the return demonstration identified improper inhaler technique that prevented patients from getting the prescribed doses of medication at home. Priority in patient teaching was placed on practice and coaching to develop proper technique for using inhalers.

Tests

Tests are effective in meeting cognitive and psychomotor objectives, but are inappropriate for affective learning, since attitudes and values are personal, and cannot be considered right or wrong. Tests reveal current knowledge and what the patient needs to learn or master, but they may not be the best assessment tool. Patients may become anxious about testing. Before you present a test, assess the learner to make sure this test would be appropriate for this person at this time. Tests are helpful when used to guide patients and give feedback. They may be used to determine the patient's initial level of understanding or skill, either as assessment (before teaching) or evaluation of understanding (after teaching). Introduce tests in a nonthreatening way, and use the results to reinforce progress toward the learning goal. Tests may use a written, oral, or skill format.

Programmed Instruction

Patients can learn by independent study using specially prepared workbooks, textbooks, audiotape, videotape, and computer programs. Many commercially prepared programs are available, or you may prepare your own. Programmed self-study units allow learners to work at their own pace to master cognitive and psychomotor behaviors. Frequent testing and review are offered during instruction. Knowledge about chronic illness and management, preventive health topics, and diet teaching are commonly offered in programmed instruction packets. The teacher should be aware of the level of motivation or readiness of the learners, their literacy levels, and visual and hearing abilities. These factors are crucial in evaluating the appropriateness of such programs for individual patients. When programmed instruction is used, it must be suited to patient needs and situations. The teacher should set the stage by

introducing the three or four critical things the patient needs to learn, and then follow-up teaching with review to ensure that the patient has achieved those outcomes. Patient readiness, physical ability, intellectual and language ability, and interest should be considered before programmed instruction is selected for teaching.

STRATEGIC USE OF EDUCATIONAL MEDIA

Media, such as videotapes, audiotapes, and computer programs, are usually used to enhance the previously mentioned learning activities. Research shows media cannot be used in place of the teacher (Clark & Lester, 2000), but can effectively promote all three types of learning when used in combination with other teaching interventions. A health care professional needs to discuss, demonstrate, and clarify concepts introduced by media, and evaluate understanding. When professionals skip these steps, teaching is less effective. Media should be carefully selected and should be consistent with instructional objectives.

General Guidelines for Media Use: Prepare, Present, Review

Having cautioned our readers that media should not be used carelessly in patient education, one may ask: What then is the advantage in using media? Media help to deliver a message. Media can be used creatively to help patients learn more, to help them retain better what they have learned, and to encourage the development of skills. To avoid some of the common pitfalls of inappropriate or unsuccessful use of media, the teacher should faithfully follow three steps: preparation, presentation, and review.

To prepare, it is necessary to preview the media to be used. A plan for using a medium is constructed, including how it will be introduced, followed-up, and related to other learning experiences. The environment also must be prepared. This includes obtaining physical facilities and equipment needed to display the medium. The learner must be informed of what to expect from the medium (such as what will be taught, or upcoming discussion). Presentation of media requires care, so that projection and materials are clear, sound is adjusted, and, in general, the message can be received. Review involves follow-up of the learning experience and evaluation of whether learning objectives were met. Box 9.2 details several generalized principles that can be applied to all types of media.

Posters, Displays, Flipcharts, and Bulletin Boards

Visual displays using drawings and illustrations do not have to be works of art to deliver a message. They should be aesthetically appealing, using contrasting colors, and large lettering. Posters, displays, flipcharts, and bulletin boards are inexpensive, require little time to prepare, and attract interest. They clarify information, simplify concepts, and summarize teaching. Contributions from participants can be written on flipcharts or chalkboards during a teaching session. Bulletin boards in waiting rooms or hospital corridors can spark curiosity about health care issues and problems.

Posters, displays, flipcharts, and bulletin boards are inappropriate for use with large groups unless the displays are enlarged. They are not well suited to teaching in which movement needs to be demonstrated.

Graphics

Graphics include graphs, charts, diagrams, cartoons, and maps. They emphasize the most important points of a presentation. They can show proportions and relationships that are difficult to understand when presented only by spoken or written material. Drawings and cartoons can deliver a message to patients with limited reading and vocabulary levels,

---

BOX 9.2 General Principles for Using Instructional Media

1. **No one medium is best suited to all purposes.** For example, in some cases, visual identification is best accomplished with a picture, cartoon, or slide; in others, three-dimensional images, such as films or videotapes, are most effective.

2. **The application of media should be consistent with learning objectives.** Just as learning activities promote certain types of behaviors, media are also chosen to coincide with objectives.

3. **The teacher must be familiar with the content of the media.** A common mistake made by nurses is to use materials that are inappropriate in message, presentation, or educational level. Media must be previewed and evaluated.

4. **Media must be compatible with learning formats.** Videotapes and DVDs may be used in a large group (provided that they can be projected adequately), but audiocassettes should not.

5. **Media must be selected with the capabilities and learning styles of the audience in mind.** Printed booklets with few illustrations are poorly suited to the patient who cannot read or who dislikes reading, and the message will fail to reach him or her.

6. **Physical conditions influence the effectiveness of media.** Improper acoustics, lighting, seating, distractions, and room temperature may interfere with the delivery of the message.

---

and to children. For example, picture pages are often used to teach insulin injection techniques to newly diagnosed patients with diabetes. Cartoons can make learning fun and present thoughts in a humorous but effective fashion (London, 1999). Graphics highlight sequence and also convey general information and key concepts. Graphics can attract attention and deliver information economically.

Overhead Projection and Slides

Overhead transparencies and slides are popular for teaching both large and small groups. They require a projector and a screen or white wall. They encourage verbal and visual creativity and allow the teacher to control the materials shown in order and timing. They can present ideas in a colorful sequence and help the learner focus on thoughts and ideas. Overhead transparencies are easy to make and can be prepared ahead of time by hand, copy machine, or computer printer. Computer-generated slides can also be generated and edited quickly with programs such as PowerPoint. PowerPoint is a software program produced by Microsoft that can be used to make four different kinds of presentations:

- **Overhead transparencies:** Design the content in PowerPoint, print them on blank transparencies on your printer, and use them with an overhead projector. The document can also be saved to disk, taken to a printing center, and professionally produced. Overheads can be used in a well-lit room as long as there is dimmed light near the screen. This makes overheads more desirable than slides for keeping learners awake and attentive.
- **Slide presentations:** Design the content in PowerPoint, and e-mail or send a disk with the file to a large commercial copy center that can convert the presentation to 35-mm slides.
- **Computerized slide show:** Design the content in PowerPoint, define slide show timing and transitions, and add sound or movie clips. The slide show can be saved and shown on computer screen, or, with special equipment, projected onto a screen.
- **Web slide show:** Upload and run the PowerPoint presentation from a website.

This lets others view the program from an Internet-connected computer (Concordia University, 2003).

There is much information on the Internet on how to use PowerPoint most effectively, as well as commentaries on how it is overused and misused. For example, each overhead or slide should present one idea or topic with a limited word count. Print should be large and details kept to a minimum. Be careful not to present too much material. It is most helpful to use a few overheads or slides to bring out the main points and provide review.

Photographs and Drawings

Patients enjoy pictures and learn from them. Visual images promote understanding of facts and ideas by helping the learner to imagine real situations and reflect on past experiences. Pictures may be presented in printed matter, on slides, or on videos. To initiate discussion, ask the learner to describe what he or she sees.

Pictures can attract and maintain the patient's interest. They also help the patient to remember what has been said. In general, color pictures appeal to learners more than black and white pictures do, but black and white line drawings may illustrate behaviors more clearly, without distractions. Images should be relevant to the learners, reflecting a familiar environment, similar age of patients, various gender and cultural backgrounds, and familiar geographic locations (Doak, Doak, & Root, 1996).

Slide-tape or slide-voice programs have a recorded message that explains the picture and adds content. A synchronized program of still pictures and speech can be made available as a web-based computer program or with a cassette tape player and a slide projector. These programs may be used for self-instruction and for group teaching. They can be purchased, or produced by the teacher, and can be used to teach patients with low literacy skills if the text is concise, simple, and clear, with vocabulary restricted to one- and two-syllable words.

Audio Materials

Cassette tapes offer a distinct advantage for some patient teaching occasions. They are small and easy to transport, and they play on inexpensive, readily available equipment. Audiotapes can be made by the teacher and tailored to the individual situation to reinforce facts, directions, and support. For example, when teaching is done with a learner with low vision, the session can be audiotaped. The tape is then given to the learner to review at home, when needed. Commercially produced cassette tapes are available on various topics, are economical, and can be used almost anywhere. Patients may use them in the home, car, office, hospital, or clinic. Study kits with printed text or pictures may accompany the audio component.

Audio materials help deliver a message to patients who enjoy radio and who benefit from repetition and reinforcement. Relaxation and stress reduction exercises also are well suited to delivery by audiotape. For patients who have poor vision, patients with low literacy skills, and patients who do not speak the English language, audiocassettes may be the only practical medium. Doak, Doak, and Root (1996) offer detailed instructions on preparing an audiotape.

Videotapes and Closed Circuit Television (CCTV)

Television's popularity and pervasive use in American households promotes learning in many spheres, and influences knowledge, attitudes, and skills. It is entertaining and educational. Videotapes present experiences, places, and situations that can recreate life situations, thus encouraging patients to explore attitudes and understandings. Videotaped programs also teach basic facts and how to handle problems. They may be effective for patients with limited reading abilities.

The use of television and videotaped recordings has become an attractive teaching and learning activity in the school, office, and health care setting. Many organizations have made significant investments for the purchase of programs (software) and equipment (hardware). Videocassette recorders (VCRs) are now used in all types of health care settings and in patients' homes.

Video is best used when the program is carefully selected, introduced, and integrated into patient teaching. Watching a video is a passive activity. Its effectiveness is greatly enhanced when it is used as part of an interactive learning experience, including a worksheet the learner uses during the video, and discussion with evaluation of understanding after (Doak, Doak, & Root, 1996).

Hospitals with cable distribution systems may wish to provide video programs because they can be broadcast throughout the hospital and reach more people. Videotapes may be purchased commercially or prepared by teachers and their organizations' audiovisual departments.

It takes time to preview and select an appropriate video. It is important to evaluate the film, not just for accuracy and content that is consistent with your practice, but its appropriateness for the needs and abilities of the learner. The video should be suited to learning objectives, and cover key points. Films 15 minutes to 20 minutes in length are ideal for most situations; those longer than 30 minutes may be too long to hold a patient's attention. When offering a video, plan to meet with the learner immediately after it is done to discuss the interactive activity, reinforce the content, evaluate understanding, and clarify misunderstandings.

Since the focus of teaching is the provision of survival skills, videos have a limited role. They can provide information and model appropriate behaviors, but must be balanced with skill practice and return demonstrations to be effective teaching tools.

Making and duplicating videos has become a common strategy to combat the pressures of early discharge by supplementing teaching in the patient's home. Sending a video home with the patient may be one of the best applications for this medium, because it can continue coaching, provide for continued affective learning, and prevent feelings of isolation (Engelke, 1999). Also, many situations that patients are instructed to handle may not be experienced until the patient goes home. For example, baby care and feeding are often learned best after discharge with the help of a video, provided the patient has a VCR and an interest in using it. Many hospitals also use videotapes for preadmission teaching and preoperative teaching. A video may offer self-care instructions by health professionals and realistic accounts by patients with the same diagnosis. These videotapes may demonstrate self-care, outline warning signs that necessitate physician contact, and answer commonly asked questions. Patients and family members can review a demonstration of self-care procedures as often as needed. When sending a patient home with a video, communicate this to the continuing care provider, so he or she can integrate this into patient education provided.

The use of patient education videos has been associated with increased patient satisfaction; increased physician satisfaction; assistance with meeting the requirements of the Joint Commission on the Accreditation of Healthcare Organizations; reduced risk of malpractice, negligent discharge, and inappropriate readmissions; and enhanced community image and cost savings.

Electronic Media

Computer-assisted instruction is available in hospitals, physician offices, and homes, on the Internet. Many software programs are available to help patients learn how to adopt healthier lifestyles and manage health problems. There are six types of CAI: drill and practice, tutorials, problem-solving, simulation, gaming, and testing. Printed material, such as workbooks, frequently accompanies CAI.

Drill and practice lessons help patients learn or review facts and offer question-and-answer formats to assess understanding. Tutorials use branching options to individu-

alize lessons to the knowledge and needs of the patient. Problem solving, simulations, and gaming help patients gather information and make decisions in hypothetical situations. Testing can be done with CAI as part of tutorials, simulations, and practice to assess knowledge and attitudes, and feedback can also be provided.

CAI programs can be purchased, or a skilled designer can develop the software. The program should be compatible with hardware, and evaluated based on each program's instructional objectives and how well the objectives can be met by the CAI lesson. Just as with other media, electronic media lessons should be previewed and evaluated, giving consideration to patient needs, the patient's actual life situations, level of understanding, and literacy. Patients vary in comfort and experience with computers, and some may be anxious about or uninterested in CAI. Other patients, especially teenagers and young adults, may be reached effectively with CAI lessons on topics such as pregnancy prevention, birth control, drug abuse prevention, and wellness.

As with videos, when offering a CAI, plan to meet with the learner upon completion to discuss the interactive activity, reinforce the key points, evaluate understanding, and clarify misunderstandings.

Experts expect computers will be used much more creatively for patient education. Computer programs already help patients with diabetes to adjust insulin dosages and plan meals, track data about glucose levels, offer self-paced instruction about knowledge of diabetes, and offer nutritional analysis of foods. Many health insurance providers offer their members CAI activities on their websites.

Objects, Models, and Demonstrations

Teaching a patient using an object or model actively involves the learner and encourages immediate application of knowledge and skills. The patient may observe, handle, manipulate, display, discuss, assemble, and disassemble objects while the teacher provides feedback. For example, breast models are often used to teach patients to examine their breasts. The teacher usually demonstrates the use of the objects or models, and the patient repeats the performance. Some models are expensive, such as the resuscitation manikin used to teach cardiopulmonary resuscitation (CPR). Pharmaceutical companies may supply others free of charge, such as a plastic female pelvic area. Through creative experimentation, health care providers can make their own models for teaching various skills. One nurse, who was unable to purchase an expensive breast model, made her own from a nylon stocking stuffed with cotton socks. She simulated a breast mass in another stocking by adding Styrofoam particles and used the two models to teach breast self-examination.

Displays can be used to encourage patient participation. For example, teaching about infant safety becomes more effective when it is accompanied by actual infant car seats. Demonstration and return demonstration may also be performed by the patient without the use of models. Examples include blood glucose monitoring, breast examinations performed in the privacy of the patient's room, dressing changes, and baby bathing. These teaching and learning opportunities can occur even if funding for teaching aids is lacking.

Community Resources

Health departments and agencies, businesses, and professional groups such as fire and police departments offer learning experiences for patients. Valuable support and information can be gained through such resources as groups with diabetes, ostomy clubs, first aid classes, bicycle safety programs, and infant car seat programs.

The patient educator can benefit from knowledge of and referrals to teaching programs that offer skills training. In one outpatient clinic, the staff saw many patients and

their families in the rehabilitation phase after myocardial infarction. The authors wanted to give family members CPR training but were unable to do so because there was not enough staff to offer the teaching or the finances to purchase equipment. Many of the family members were unable to pay registration fees for CPR classes at local schools. The authors discovered that a local fire department offered CPR classes free of charge, and the patients were referred to them.

Games and Simulations

Instructional games can involve the patient, provide information, and offer practice in simulated situations. They are often used with pediatric patients for preoperative parties that introduce them to hospital procedures, environment, and staff before elective surgery. During a game, the patient can take a course of action and view the consequences in a nonthreatening way. Problem solving can be incorporated into the game.

The patient should succeed, yet be challenged, in the exercise. Games may use flash cards, pictures, or computer programs. They may be modifications of popular games, such as Bingo or crossword puzzles. With the exception of computer games, most games are relatively inexpensive to purchase or to make. Simulations include planning low-fat meals, using food models, and shopping for low-sodium foods in a mock supermarket. Before introducing a game, evaluate its appropriateness for each specific learner.

Printed Materials

Pamphlets and information sheets are among the most common teaching tools. As a home reference, they can outline details of self-care, list how to recognize problems, and indicate how to respond. The individualized teaching plan, incorporating patient assessment data, will guide educators in the appropriate use of books, pamphlets, and information sheets.

Printed materials can describe health issues and their management, and make the public more aware of health risks and prevention. For example, printed materials can be especially helpful in contraceptive counseling. After receiving basic teaching in the office, patients may take a booklet home to consider the various methods of contraception. Patients then return for the next visit prepared to ask questions and willing to take responsibility for choosing a method. Although many patients initially come to an office visit with a particular birth control method in mind, we have discovered, through assessment, that the decision is usually based on experience or the advice of friends. A combined approach of one-on-one counseling and written patient education materials promotes enlightened choices.

If specific information needs to be taught, it is essential to evaluate understanding and share your findings with the rest of the health care team through documentation. Pamphlets and information sheets don't teach; people do. Pamphlets and information sheets are tools that can facilitate interaction and reinforce information. Research repeatedly shows that printed information is not effective when the contents are not discussed with a health care provider (Moore et al., 2002; Webber, Higgins, & Baker, 2001). The mere distribution of printed materials does not change health behaviors, and may not even transfer knowledge. Patients may be anxious about the information in the pamphlet, may not retain what they read, may not learn by reading, or may not be able to understand the new information. Unless a health care provider discusses the content, evaluates understanding, answers questions, and clarifies misunderstandings, there is little chance a pamphlet will have any impact on health outcomes. Good communication is the basis of effective patient and family education.

Kessels (2003) reports most patients immediately forget as much as 80% of what their doctor tells them, and nearly half the information they say they remember, they remember incorrectly. The more information presented, the lower the proportion correctly recalled. This ability to obtain, process, and understand basic health information and services needed to make appropriate health decisions is referred to as functional health literacy (Williams et al., 2002). Fortunately, an accurate assessment and individualized teaching enable the teacher to effectively teach learners with poor health literacy skills. Strategies include the following: emphasize benefits, involve the senses, emphasize key points, instruct in small steps, seek frequent feedback, link known information to new, and personalize the message (Schultz, 2002). Teaching is best done with simple, specific instructions that give the most important facts first, backed up with written or visual material (Kessels, 2003).

To optimize reinforcement of teaching, the qualities of the most effective printed materials have been identified and operationally defined by Doak, Doak, and Root (1996). They have created a tool to assess the suitability of materials, designed for printed materials, but that can also be applied to video- and audiotapes. This validated tool, the Suitability Assessment of Materials (SAM), is provided in Box 9.3. It takes into account content, literacy demand, graphics, layout, typography, learning stimulation, motivation, and cultural appropriateness. The Fry Readability Formula, used to determine the reading grade level, is provided in Box 9.4. Word processing software also measures reading levels of text.

When using SAM to evaluate a teaching tool, you obtain a numerical score, in percent, that rates the materials as superior, adequate, or not suitable. Despite the overall score, if the reading level is not suitable, the teaching tool may not be understood. If the cultural appropriateness is not suitable, the teaching tool may not be accepted. Consequently, reading level and cultural appropriateness are two factors that must be rated adequate or superior.

BOX 9.3 Suitability Assessment of Materials (SAM)

A dilemma facing many health care providers is how to systematically assess the suitability of a health care instruction for a given patient population, and do it in the short time available. The authors recognize that an ideal way is to evaluate the instruction with a sample of the intended audience, but often there is neither time nor resources for that. The assessment must be made analytically "at your desk."

Our response to this dilemma was to develop and validate SAM: a suitability assessment of materials instrument.[14] Validation was conducted with 172 health care providers from several cultures.[15] The cultures included Southeast Asians, Native Americans, and African Americans as well as students and faculty from the University of North Carolina School of Public Health and Johns Hopkins School of Medicine.

SAM was originally designed for use with print material and illustrations, but it has also been applied successfully to video- and audiotaped instructions. For each material, SAM provides a numerical score (in percent) that may fall in one of three categories: superior, adequate, or not suitable.

There is a continuing need for more comprehensive evaluation instruments. For instance, one can expect that in the near future a computer program will be developed that will evaluate instructions in text, visuals, audio/verbal, interactive television, multimedia, and combinations of these. Until such a program is developed, SAM is a logical step toward meeting that need.

The application of SAM can pinpoint specific deficiencies in an instruction that reduce its suitability. If the material is still in its developmental stage, these deficiencies can be corrected. If the material is already in use, the deficiencies indicate what supplemental instructions (perhaps verbal explanations) are needed.

Using SAM to evaluate a health care instruction

To use SAM for the first time, follow the six steps below:

1. Read through the SAM factor list and the evaluation criteria.
2. Read the material (or view the video) you wish to evaluate and write brief statements as to its purpose(s) and key points.
3. For short instructions, evaluate the entire piece. For long instructions, select samples to evaluate.
4. Evaluate and score each of the 22 SAM factors.
5. Calculate total suitability score.
6. Decide on the impact of deficiencies and what action to take.

The entire process to evaluate your instructional material should take 30 to 45 minutes the first time through. For subsequent applications of SAM, you may skip the first step because the SAM factors and criteria will be already familiar to you.

For a first-time use of SAM, we suggest you test a simple, short material that has only a few illustrations.

1. **Read the SAM instrument and the evaluation criteria.**
2. **Read the material to be assessed.** Read (or view) the material you plan to evaluate. It will help if you write brief statements as to its purpose(s) and its key points. Refer to these as you evaluate each SAM factor. Use a note pad to jot down comments and observations as you read the material, view the video, or listen to the audiotape.
3. **The sampling process for SAM is somewhat similar to that described earlier for selecting samples to apply a readability formula.** If you are applying SAM to a short material such as a single-page

(continued)

BOX 9.3 Suitability Assessment of Materials (SAM) *(Continued)*

instruction or a typical pamphlet (twofold or threefold), assess the entire instruction. Similarly, for audio- and videotaped instructions of less than 10 minutes, evaluate the entire instruction.

To apply SAM to a longer text, such as a booklet, select three pages that deal with topics central to the purpose of the booklet. For booklets of more than 50 pages, increase the sample size to six pages. For video- or audiotaped instructions exceeding 10 minutes, select topics in 2-minute blocks from the beginning, middle, and end sections of the video or audio presentation.

4. **Evaluate material vs. criteria for each factor, decide on its rating, and record it on the score sheet.** As you seek to evaluate your material against each factor, you are likely to find wide variation among different parts of your material. For any one factor, some parts may rate high (superior) while other parts of the same material rate low (unsuitable). For example, some illustrations may include captions while others do not. Resolve this dilemma by giving most weight to the part of your material that includes the key points that you previously identified in step 2 above.

Materials that meet the superior criteria for a factor are scored 2 points for that factor; adequate receives 1 point; not suitable receives a zero. For factors that do not apply, write N/A. Use the SAM scoring sheet shown in Figure 9-1 to record your score for each of the 22 factors and to guide you in calculating the overall rating in percent.

5. **Calculate the total suitability score.** When you have evaluated all the factors, and written a score for each one on the score sheet, add up the scores to obtain a total score. Spaces to do this are provided

on the score sheet. The maximum possible total score is 44 points (100 percent)-a perfect rating, which almost never happens. A more typical example: if the total score for your material is 34, your percent score is 34/44 or 77 percent.

For some instructional materials, one or more of the 22 SAM factors may not apply. For example, for an audiotape or a videotape, the text readability level (factor 2a) does not apply. To account for SAM factors that occasionally may not apply to a particular material, subtract 2 points for each N/A from the 44 total. Let's do that using the example from the paragraph above. If you arrived at a total score of 34 as noted above, but had one N/A factor, subtract 2 points from 44 to a revised maximum score of 42. Thus, the percent rating would become 34/42, for a rating of 81 percent.

Interpretation of SAM
percentage ratings:
70-100 percent   superior material
40-69 percent   adequate material
0-39 percent   not suitable material

6. **Evaluate the impact of deficiencies; decide on revisions.** A deficiency, especially an "unsuitable" rating, in any of the 22 factors is significant. Many of these can be readily overcome by revising a draft material or by adding a supplemental instruction to a material already published. However, factors in two of the groups, the readability level and cultural appropriateness, must be considered as potential go-no/go signals for suitability regardless of the overall rating.

For example, except in the rare cases where an instruction contains a set of illustrations that replicate the entire message given in the text, a written instruction with

(continued)

BOX 9.3 Suitability Assessment of Materials (SAM) *(Continued)*

a very high readability level will not be understood and is unsuitable. Similarly, a material that portrays an ethnic group in an inappropriate way is almost surely unsuitable because it is likely to be rejected by members of that ethnic group.

SAM evaluation criteria

1. Content

   A. PURPOSE

   Explanation: It is important that readers/clients readily understand the intended purpose of the instruction for them. If they don't clearly perceive the purpose, they may not pay attention or may miss the main point.

Superior	Purpose is explicitly stated in title, or cover illustration, or introduction.
Adequate	Purpose is not explicit. It is implied, or multiple purposes are stated.
Not suitable	No purpose is stated in the title, cover illustration, or introduction.

   B. CONTENT TOPICS

   Explanation: Since adult patients usually want to solve their immediate health problem rather than learn a series of medical facts (that may only *imply* a solution), the content of greatest interest and use to clients is likely to be behavior information to help solve their problem.

Superior	Thrust of the material is application of knowledge/skills aimed at desirable reader behavior rather than nonbehavior facts.
Adequate	At least 40 percent of content topics focus on desirable behaviors or actions.

Not suitable	Nearly all topics are focused on nonbehavior facts.

   C. SCOPE

   Explanation: Scope is limited to purpose or objective(s). Scope is also limited to what the patient can reasonably learn in the time allowed.

Superior	Scope is limited to essential information directly related to the purpose. Experience shows it can be learned in time allowed.
Adequate	Scope is expanded beyond the purpose; no more than 40 percent is nonessential information. Key points can be learned in time allowed.
Not suitable	Scope is far out of proportion to the purpose and time allowed.

   D. SUMMARY AND REVIEW

   Explanation: A review offers the readers/viewers a chance to see or hear the key points of the instruction in other words, examples, or visuals. Reviews are important; readers often miss the key points upon first exposure.

Superior	A summary is included and retells the key messages in different words and examples.
Adequate	Some key ideas are reviewed.
Not suitable	No summary or review is included.

2. Literacy demand

   A. READING GRADE LEVEL(FRY FORMULA)

   Explanation: Unless the instruction presents the topics completely without text (via visual, demonstrations, and/or

(continued)

BOX 9.3 Suitability Assessment of Materials (SAM) *(Continued)*

audio), the text reading level may be a critical factor in patient comprehension. Reading formulas can provide a reasonably accurate measure of reading difficulty.

Superior	5th-grade level or lower (5 years of schooling level).
Adequate	6th-, 7th-, or 8th-grade level (6-8 years of schooling level).
Not suitable	9th-grade level and above (9 years or more of schooling level).

B. WRITING STYLE

Explanation: Conversational style and active voice lead to easy-to-understand text. Example: "Take your medicine every day." Passive voice is less effective. Example: "Patients should be advised to take their medicine every day." Embedded information, the long or multiple phrases included in a sentence, slows down the reading process and generally makes comprehension more difficult.

Superior	Both factors: (1) Mostly conversational style and active voice. (2) Simple sentences are used extensively; few sentences contain embedded information.
Adequate	(1) About 50 percent of the text uses conversational style and active voice. (2) Less than half the sentences have embedded information.
Not suitable	(1) Passive voice throughout. (2) Over half the sentences have extensive embedded information.

C. VOCABULARY

Explanation: Common, explicit words are used (for example, doctor vs. physician). The instruction uses few or no words that express general terms such as categories (for example, legumes vs. beans), concepts (for example, normal range vs. 15 to 70), and value judgments (for example, excessive pain vs. pain lasts more than 5 minutes). Imagery words are used because these are words people can "see" (for example, whole wheat bread vs. dietary fiber; a runny nose vs. excess mucus).

Superior	All three factors: (1) Common words are used nearly all of the time. (2) Technical, concept, category, value judgment (CCVJ) words are explained by examples. (3) Imagery words are used as appropriate for content.
Adequate	(1) Common words are frequently used. (2) Technical and CCVJ words are sometimes explained by examples. (3) Some jargon or math symbols are included.
Not suitable	Two or more factors: (1) Uncommon words are frequently used in lieu of common words. (2) No examples are given for technical and CCVJ words. (3) Extensive jargon.

D. IN SENTENCE CONSTRUCTION, THE CONTEXT IS GIVEN BEFORE NEW INFORMATION

Explanation: We learn new facts/behaviors more quickly when told the context first. Good example: "To find out

(continued)

BOX 9.3 Suitability Assessment of Materials (SAM) *(Continued)*

what's wrong with you (the context first), the doctor will take a sample of your blood for lab tests" (new information).

Superior Consistently provides context before presenting new information.

Adequate Provides context before new information about 50 percent of the time.

Not suitable Context is provided last or no context is provided.

E. LEARNING ENHANCEMENT BY ADVANCE ORGANIZERS (ROAD SIGNS)
Explanation: Headers or topic captions should be used to tell very briefly what's coming up next. These "road signs" make the text look less formidable, and also prepare the reader's thought process to expect the announced topic.

Superior Nearly all topics are preceded by an advance organizer (a statement that tells what is coming next).

Adequate About 50 percent of the topics are preceded by advance organizers.

Not suitable Few or no advance organizers are used.

3. Graphics (illustrations, lists, tables, charts, graphs)

A. COVER GRAPHIC
Explanation: People *do* judge a booklet by its cover. The cover image often is the deciding factor in a patient's attitude toward, and interest in, the instruction.

Superior The cover graphic is (1) friendly, (2) attracts attention, (3) clearly portrays the purpose of the material to the intended audience.

Adequate The cover graphic has one or two of the superior criteria.

Not suitable The cover graphic has none of the superior criteria.

B. TYPE OF ILLUSTRATIONS
Explanation: Simple line drawings can promote realism without including distracting details. (Photographs often include unwanted details.) Visuals are accepted and remembered better when they portray what is familiar and easily recognized. Viewers may not recognize the meaning of medical textbook drawings or abstract art/symbols.

Superior Both factors: (1) Simple, adult-appropriate, line drawings/sketches are used. (2) Illustrations are likely to be familiar to the viewers.

Adequate One of the superior factors is missing.

Not suitable None of the superior factors are present.

C. RELEVANCE OF ILLUSTRATIONS
Explanation: Nonessential details such as room background, elaborate borders, unneeded color can distract the viewer. The viewer's eyes may be "captured" by these details. The illustrations should tell the key points visually.

Superior Illustrations present key messages visually so the reader/viewer can grasp the key ideas from the illustrations alone. No distractions.

Adequate (1) Illustrations include some distractions. (2)

(continued)

BOX 9.3 Suitability Assessment of Materials (SAM) *(Continued)*

Insufficient use of illustrations.

Not suitable One factor: (1) Confusing or technical illustrations (nonbehavior related). (2) No illustrations, or an overload of illustrations.

D. GRAPHICS: LISTS, TABLES, GRAPHS, CHARTS, GEOMETRIC FORMS

Explanation: Many readers do not understand the author's purpose for the lists, charts, and graphs. Explanations and directions are essential.

Superior Step-by-step directions, with an example, are provided that will build comprehension and self-efficacy.

Adequate "How-to" directions are too brief for reader to understand and use the graphic without additional counseling.

Not suitable Graphics are presented without explanation.

E. Captions are used to "ANNOUNCE"/EXPLAIN GRAPHICS

Explanation: Captions can quickly tell the reader what the graphic is all about, where to focus within the graphic. A graphic without a caption is usually an inferior instruction and represents a missed learning opportunity.

Superior Explanatory captions with all or nearly all illustrations and graphics.

Adequate Brief captions used for some illustrations and graphics.

Not suitable Captions are not used.

4. Layout and typography

A. LAYOUT

Explanation: Layout has a substantial influence on the suitability of materials.

Superior At least five of the following eight factors are present:

1. Illustrations are on the same page adjacent to the related text.
2. Layout and sequence of information are consistent, making it easy for the patient to predict the flow of information.
3. Visual cuing devices (shading, boxes, arrows) are used to direct attention to specific points or key content.
4. Adequate white space is used to reduce appearance of clutter.
5. Use of color supports and is not distracting to the message. Viewers need not learn color codes to understand and use the message.
6. Line length is 30-50 characters and spaces.
7. There is high contrast between type and paper.
8. Paper has nongloss or low-gloss surface.

Adequate At least three of the superior factors are present.

Not suitable (1) Two (or less) of the superior factors are present. (2) Looks uninviting or discouragingly hard to read.

B. TYPOGRAPHY

Explanation: Type size and fonts can make text easy or difficult for readers at all skill levels. For example, type in ALL CAPS slows everybody's reading comprehension. Also, when too many (six or more) type fonts and sizes are used on a page, the appearance becomes confusing and the focus uncertain.

(continued)

BOX 9.3 Suitability Assessment of Materials (SAM) *(Continued)*

Superior   The following four factors are present:
1. Text type is in uppercase and lowercase serif (best) or sans-serif.
2. Type size is at least 12 point.
3. Typographic cues (bold, size, color) emphasize key points.
4. No ALL CAPS for long headers or running text.

Adequate   Two of the superior factors are present.

Not suitable   One or none of the superior factors are present. Or, six or more type styles and sizes are used on a page.

C. SUBHEADINGS OR "CHUNKING"
Explanation: Few people can remember more than seven independent items. For adults with low literacy skills the limit may be three- to five-item lists. Longer lists need to be partitioned into smaller "chunks."

Superior   (1) Lists are grouped under descriptive subheadings or "chunks." (2) No more than five items are presented without a subheading.

Adequate   No more than seven items are presented without a subheading.

Not suitable   More than seven items are presented without a subheading.

5. Learning stimulation and motivation

A. INTERACTION INCLUDED IN TEXT AND/OR GRAPHIC
Explanation: When the patient responds to the instruction-that is, does something to reply to a problem or question-chemical changes take place in the brain that enhance retention in long-term memory. Readers/viewers should be asked to solve problems, to make choices, to demonstrate, etc.

Superior   Problems or questions presented for reader responses.

Adequate   Question-and-answer format used to discuss problems and solutions (passive interaction).

Not suitable   No interactive learning stimulation provided.

B. DESIRED BEHAVIOR PATTERNS ARE MODELED, SHOWN IN SPECIFIC TERMS
Explanation: People often learn more readily by observation and by doing it themselves rather than by reading or being told. They also learn more readily when specific, familiar instances are used rather than the abstract or general.

Superior   Instruction models specific behaviors or skills. (For example, for nutrition instruction, emphasis is given to changes in eating patterns or shopping or food preparation/cooking tips; tips to read labels.)

Adequate   Information is a mix of technical and common language that the reader may not easily interpret in terms of daily living (for example: *Technical:* Starches—80 calories per serving; High Fiber—1-4 grams of fiber in a serving).

Not suitable   Information is presented in nonspecific or category terms such as the food groups.

(continued)

BOX 9.3 Suitability Assessment of Materials (SAM) *(Continued)*

c. Motivation
Explanation: People are more motivated to learn when they believe the tasks/behaviors are doable by them.

Superior	Complex topics are subdivided into small parts so that readers may experience small successes in understanding or problem solving, leading to self-efficacy.
Adequate	Some topics are subdivided to improve the readers' self-efficacy.
Not suitable	No partitioning is provided to create opportunities for small successes.

6. Cultural appropriateness

A. Cultural match: logic, language, experience (LLE)
Explanation: A valid measure of cultural appropriateness of an instruction is how well its logic, language, and experience (inherent in the instruction) match the LLE of the intended audience. For example, a nutrition instruction is a poor cultural match if it tells readers to eat asparagus and romaine lettuce if these vegetables are rarely eaten by people in that culture and are not sold in the readers' neighborhood markets.

Superior	Central concepts/ideas of the material appear to be culturally similar to the LLE of the target culture.
Adequate	Significant match in LLE for 50 percent of the central concepts.
Not suitable	Clearly a cultural mismatch in LLE.

B. Cultural image and examples
Explanation: To be accepted, an instruction must present cultural images and examples in realistic and positive ways.

Superior	Images and examples present the culture in positive ways.
Adequate	Neutral presentation of cultural images or foods.
Not suitable	Negative image such as exaggerated or caricatured cultural characteristics, actions, or examples.

In summary, the SAM offers a systematic method to assess suitability of materials. In about 30 minutes you can obtain a numerical suitability score that you can use to decide whether or not a material is suitable for your patient population.

When making an evaluation using SAM, or using the checklist presented earlier in this chapter, you may have uncovered one or more specific deficiencies. If so, decide on how critical the deficiencies are to patient comprehension and acceptance of the key messages of your material. Guidance for making this decision may be found in Chapters 2 and 5. To overcome the deficiencies, you will find specific details related to each instructional media in the following chapters: Chapter 6 for written materials, Chapter 7 for visuals and graphics, and Chapter 8 for videotapes, audiotapes, and multimedia.

Summary
The health care "culture" relies heavily on written instructions. These may be assessed by using a checklist of attributes that define easy-to-read materials. Another assessment worth making is to test the material using a readability

(continued)

BOX 9.3 Suitability Assessment of Materials (SAM) *(Continued)*

formula. If you assess the readability and suitability of your health care instructions, you are more likely to provide instructions your patients will understand.

Materials that have readability levels of 9th grade or higher need to be rewritten to make them understandable by most Americans. If the materials are not rewritten, supplemental instruction will be needed by most patients when the material is used.

The suitability of a written material depends on many factors. Although readability formulas measure only a few of these characteristics, the reading level is usually a "go-no/go" criterion to predict patient comprehension of the material.

Consider using the SAM instrument to obtain a numerical rating that covers the many other suitability factors not included in readability formulas. SAM addresses suitability in terms of content, literacy demand, graphics, layout, learning stimulation/motivation, and culture of the intended audience.

It is important to note that the assessment methods presented in this chapter use analytical methods exclusively. Another method of assessment-using patients to test the suitability of the material-is presented in Chapter 10, Learner Verification and Revision (LVR) of Materials.

Actions you can take during the next 90 days
- Use the checklist to screen three of your frequently used health care instructions.
- Test the readability of 10 of your written health care materials and record the grade level on the back of each piece. Share this with your colleagues.
- Compare the readability levels of the 10 materials with the reading levels of the adult population of the United States by referring to literacy data in Figure 1-1. Determine how many of the 10 instructions are "over the heads" of at least half the U.S. adult population in terms of reading skills.
- Use the SAM instrument to evaluate the suitability of one of your frequently used health care instructions.

Source: From Doak, C. C., Doak, L. G., & Root, J. H., (1996). *Teaching patients with low literacy skills* (2nd ed., pp 49–59), Philadelphia: J. B. Lippincott.

Research demonstrates that people with good reading skills are not offended by clearly written materials (Doak, Doak, & Root, 1996). Because the stress of a new diagnosis, side effects of medication, or symptoms of illness may make it difficult to focus and lower a person's functional literacy, patients and families generally welcome clear, easy-to-understand instructions. The teacher optimizes investment in resources by using the SAM criteria to choose all of the printed, audio, and video tools purchased or created.

The Home Care Instruction Sheet

Patients should always be given written discharge instructions that outline medications, treatments, follow-up appointments, and emergency guidelines. Patients benefit from instructions that use short, nontechnical words of two syllables or fewer, that give simple definitions, that use no medical abbreviations (such as "P.O." or "Q.D."), and that are written in active voice. The instructions should tell readers only what they need to know and do.

SAM (Suitability Assessment of Materials)

	Superior	Adequate	Not Suitable
CONTENT			
Content focused on a specific patient issue			
Scope limited to what can be absorbed			
Directed towards behaviors - not information			
Keypoints are reiterated and summarized			
LITERACY LEVEL			
Appropriate reading level (9th grade or below)			
Conversational writing style using active voice			
Common word vocabulary, no jargon			
Advanced Organizers (topic statements) precede new content			
GRAPHICS and MULTIMEDIA			
Illustrations and multimedia presentations are simple and relate to content			
No distracting elements are present			
All graphics and multimedia elements are explained by text			
Audio tones are of appropriate pitch and quality			
Video is of appropriate resolution and clarity			
Audio/video elements are brief and realistic			
LAYOUT			
Illustrations are adjacent to text			
Limited scrolling (two pages) occurs			
Layout compliments and does not distract from text			
White space is prevalent			
Hypertext is limited if used at all			
Type size is suitable for easy viewing			
Type is sufficiently varied to divide information into small, discrete sections			
LEARNING STIMULATION and MOTIVATION			
Opportunities for interaction are included			
Behavioral activities are modeled and subdivided into small "doable" segments			
CULTURAL APPROPRIATENESS			
Logic, language, experience present match patient			
Realistic portrayal of cultural images			
TOTALS			
SAM PERCENTAGE RATINGS			
35 to 50 points (70% - 100%)	X		
20 to 34 points (40% - 69%)		X	
0 to 19 points (0% - 39%)			X

FIGURE 9.1 Suitability assessment of materials (SAM) tool. Adapted from SAM, Suitability of Materials by C. Doak, L. Doak, and J. Root, (1996) *Teaching patients with low literacy skills*. Philadelphia,: Lippincott.

BOX 9.4 Fry Readability Formula

Assessing Readability Using the Fry Formula

Nearly all the 40+ readability formulas provide a reasonably accurate grade level (typically plus or minus one grade level with a 68-percent confidence factor). Among these formulas, the authors recommend the Fry formula. The Fry is widely accepted in the reading literature and among reading professionals and is not copyrighted. This formula applies from grade 1 through grade 17, and compared to some formulas, the Fry does not require as extensive a test sample.

It is not necessary to test the readability of every word and sentence. This would be especially tedious in a long booklet. Instead, test three samples from different parts of the instruction. For a very long text, such as a book of 50 pages or more, double the number to six samples.

Select a piece of material that you customarily use with your patients/clients and follow the five steps given below to determine its reading level using the Fry formula.[9]

Detailed Directions

1. **Select three 100-word passages from the material you wish to test.** Count out exactly 100 words for each passage, starting with the first word of a sentence. (Omit headings.) If you are testing a very short pamphlet that may have only a few hundred words, select a single 100-word sample to test.

   Readability levels may vary considerably from one part of your material to another. Therefore, select the three samples from different content topics, if possible. For example, if a pamphlet includes such topics as the disease process, treatment options, and actions the patient should take, select one sample from each of these topics.

Additional information:
   - Count proper nouns. Hyphenated words count as one word.
   - A word is defined as a group of symbols with a space on either side; thus "IRA," "1994," and "&" are each one word.

2. **Count the number of *sentences* in each 100 words, estimating the fractional length of the last sentence to the nearest** $\frac{1}{10}$. For example, if the 100th word occurs 5 words into a 15-word sentence, the fraction of the sentence is $\frac{5}{15}$ or $\frac{1}{3}$ or 0.3.

3. **Count the total number of *syllables* in each 100-word passage.** You can count by making a small check mark over each syllable. For initializations (e.g., IRA) and numerals (e.g., 1994), count 1 syllable for each symbol. So "IRA" = 3 syllables and "1994" = 4 syllables.

   There is a short cut to counting the syllables. Since each 100-word sample must have at least 100 syllables, skip the first syllable in each word. Don't count it; just add 100 after you finish the count. Count only the remaining syllables (that are greater than one) in the 100-word sample. Thus, you don't put check marks over any of the one-syllable words; you put only one check over each two-syllable word, two checks over three-syllable words, and so forth.

   Occasionally you may be in doubt as to the number of syllables in a word. Resolve the doubt by placing a finger under your chin, say the word aloud, and count the number of times your chin drops. Each chin drop counts as a syllable.

4. **Calculate the average number of sentences and the average number of syllables from the three passages.** This is done by dividing the totals obtained from the three samples by 3 as shown in the example below.

(continued)

BOX 9.4 Fry Readability Formula *(Continued)*

Example:

	NUMBER OF SENTENCES	NUMBER OF SYLLABLES
1st 100 words	5.9	124
2nd 100 words	4.8	141
3rd 100 words	6.1	158
Totals	16.8	423
Divide Totals by 3:	5.6 Average	141 Average

5. **Refer to the Fry graph.** On the horizontal axis, find the line for the *average number of syllables* (141 for above example). On the vertical axis find the line for the *average number of sentences* (5.6 for the example). The readability grade level of the material is found at the point where the two lines intersect.

In the example above, the Fry chart shows the readability level at the 8th grade (see dot at the intersection in Figure 9-2). The curved line through the center of the Fry graph shows the locus of greatest accuracy. With a little practice, the five-step process will become much easier. You will soon be able to determine a readability level in less than 10 minutes.

Source: From London F. (1999). *No time to teach* (pp. 227–229). Philadelphia: Lippincott Williams & Wilkins.

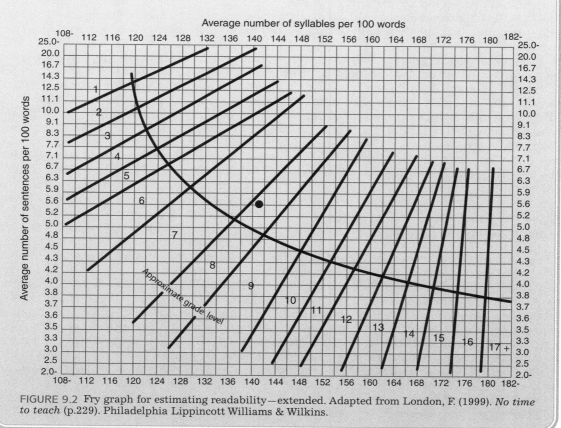

FIGURE 9.2 Fry graph for estimating readability—extended. Adapted from London, F. (1999). *No time to teach* (p.229). Philadelphia Lippincott Williams & Wilkins.

It may be helpful to organize instructions chronologically, outlining what to do before breakfast, before leaving for work, at lunch, and before bed. Often instructions are given to both the patient and another family member. The health care provider should always review the instructions before discharge, having the learner state what he or she is going to do. It is common hospital policy to have the patient or family member sign at the bottom of the instruction sheet, indicating that he or she received the information. A duplicate copy is placed in the patient record.

With the widespread use of computerization, it may be helpful to prepare basic instructions for patients with a particular diagnosis-related group. These standard instructions can be individualized for each patient and printed out on the unit. Only the most pertinent information should be given, and instruction lists should be only as long as necessary.

Brief patient emergency instructions can be printed on refrigerator magnets with a telephone number. Also, encourage patients to post their one-page instructions at one or all of the following locations: on the refrigerator, by the telephone, and at the workplace. Instructions are ineffective if the patient cannot find them or has difficulty remembering the self-care regimen when he or she is away from home.

Special Challenges: Patients with Low Literacy Skills

One component of poor health literacy is low literacy skills. Nearly 20% of Americans are functionally illiterate; that is, they are unable to read and understand enough to benefit from even the simplest handouts or videotaped programs. Patients who are functionally illiterate may be difficult to reach in patient education encounters. Even when printed materials are clarified and presented at a sixth-grade level, the patient with low literacy skills is still lost.

The classic book *Teaching Patients with Low Literacy Skills* (Doak, Doak, & Root, 1996) should be read, if not owned, by every health care provider. The authors provide insights into how these patients think and function. The book describes how to test learners' ability to read and understand, how to write and rewrite materials, and how to develop and incorporate audio and visual aids in patient education.

Kessels (2003) reports that existing evidence shows that visual communication aids are especially effective with patients with low literacy skills, but video and multimedia techniques do not improve memory or adherence to therapy. Doak, Doak, & Root (1996) explain why: Illiteracy is not just the inability to read. Adults with low literacy skills process information differently than do readers. They may have average IQs and speak articulately. However, they may also have limited vocabulary, may not understand abbreviations, and usually do not ask questions. Identifying learners with poor literacy skills can be difficult because they have learned to cope and can hide their limitations from others. Some secretly ask friends or family members to read things to them, as needed.

A patient with limited reading skills often has a short attention span; thus, the message should be short, direct, and specific. The patient may depend on visual cues to clarify or interpret words; therefore pictures, illustrations, and graphics must be combined with words. A patient with low literacy skills also has difficulty understanding complex ideas. Information should be condensed into basic points with examples that apply the information to real-life situations the learner is likely to encounter.

For teaching patients with low literacy skills, guidelines are offered to help adapt existing methods and materials for these adults (Box 9.5). These tips may successfully be applied to any learner, not just those with low literacy skills. For example, what is critical when the patient is given a medication prescription? Should he or she know how to spell the name of the medication? Is it more important that he or she knows the medication's purpose, what it looks like, when to

---

BOX 9.5 Guidelines for Teaching Patients with Low Literacy Skills

- Focus information on the core of knowledge and skills patients need to survive and to cope with problems.
- Teach the smallest amount possible.
- Make points vivid. Put important information either first or last.
- Sequence information logically, for example, step-by-step (1, 2, 3...), chronological (a time line), or topical (using 3 or 4 main topics).
- Have the patient restate and demonstrate.
- Review.

- Keep do's and don'ts separate; don't mix them together in a list. This may confuse patients.
- When giving instructions for medications, list the exact times the patient will take the medicine; don't say, "take three times a day."
- For PRN medicine, list each medicine separately with the instruction "take for _____," using the learner's terms for the symptom that medicine treats. Also, mention how often it can be taken, how long between doses, and how many times in 24 hours it can be taken. Indicate what the patient should do if the symptom is not relieved.
- Provide a list of signs and symptoms for which the patient needs to "Call the doctor right away if ..."

take it, and possible side effects? To keep instructions as simple as possible, ask the following questions:

- What should the patient do?
- What should the patient change or do differently?
- Which one or two points are most important for the patient to understand?

We may consider it critical that an older patient take his or her diuretic medication at the beginning of the day to avoid sleep disturbance from increased urination. The patient should weigh himself or herself daily, record weight, and report dizziness, falls, rapid weight loss or gain, swelling in ankles or fingers, bleeding, bruising, or muscle cramping.

The patient educator should use simple messages, familiar words, and pictures, and organize text in small sections with headings such as, "Your fluid pill," and "Every morning."

Other suggestions for providing useful instructions include:

- Always list the most important information first.
- Always list first what the patient should do. Limit the number of don'ts.

Writing and Reviewing Instructions

Table 9.1 provides tips for writing medication instruction sheets. A safety hint for all patients: Give a complete list of all medications to be taken after discharge, with the times each was last given to the patient. Patients may have old prescriptions at home or PRN medications that should not be part of the current treatment plan. The instructions must be clear. This list helps reinforce the medication plan.

Every printed teaching material given to patients should be evaluated using the SAM tool, without using materials with total scores of "not suitable." Then, the teacher should have each printed teaching material reviewed by actual patients, followed by an assessment of their comprehension of the material and suggestions for making the content more "patient friendly." This can be done as a separate step, in a focus group, or incorporated into care with the first learners who get the materials. The teacher may ask the learner to read a portion aloud and explain what it means in his or her own words; this is the final and most critical test for readability.

TABLE 9.1 Medication Instructions

USE	RATHER THAN
Take once a day	Take daily
Take at or near 8 AM and 8 PM	Take twice daily
	Take every 12 h
Take at or near 8 AM, 2 PM, and 10 PM	Take 3 times daily
	Take every 8 h
Take at or near 8 AM, 1 PM, 6 PM, and 10 PM	Take 4 times daily
	Take every 6 h
Take 30 min before meals when the stomach is empty	Take before meals
Take 3 times a day at breakfast, lunch, & dinner	Take with meals
Take every _____ h as needed for (symptom)	Take as needed for (symptom)
Do not take more than _____ in a 24-h period	

Do Not Use

Take for (symptom)
Take as directed

If the learner cannot read, the teacher should still provide the printed material because the learner may have a friend or family member who can read it when needed for reference. Patients who cannot or will not read written material include patients who are illiterate, those with physical handicaps, and those who do not speak the language. Teachers should teach verbally, using a language interpreter if necessary, and use graphics and illustrations to reinforce the message. The learner's understanding and memory of critical details should be evaluated through discussion, involving family members, significant others, and community members, as appropriate.

DESIGNING PATIENT EDUCATION PROGRAMS

Health care providers have a choice of teaching individually, in groups, or using a self-management program. Health care providers have a choice of determining the teaching plan for each learner independently, or collaborating with the team to create a general template of patient education for all patients with a specific diagnosis or treatment, to be individualized for each learner.

These choices are influenced by such variables as patient population, the number of different diagnoses treated or treatments provided, the setting, the availability of resources (such as handouts and audiovisual equipment), and the availability of experts to develop classes.

Designing Patient Education Interventions: Variables to Consider

Individual Teaching

Each patient must have some one-on-one teaching, to ensure individual needs are met, and to evaluate understanding, and answer questions. Every patient in every setting should know why he or she is there, what he or she can contribute to managing his or her health, and what he or she can expect to learn from health care providers to do this. All patients need some individual teaching to help them understand and accept their diagnoses and understand their own role in the management of their health.

Individual patient teaching is more effective than group teaching (whether with a family group or a large, unrelated group) in the following situations:

- **When the health professional has little knowledge of the patient and learning needs assessment has not been completed.** It is difficult, if not impossible to assess individual knowledge in a group, because most learners do not want to reveal their knowledge deficits to a group. Readiness to learn needs to be assessed individually.
- **When family members or friends try to dominate teaching sessions.** Some family members may use teaching sessions to make the patient feel guilty for not following a medical regimen, or to attract attention to themselves and their roles as caregivers.
- **When the information to be taught provokes a great deal of anxiety** (such as teaching related to cardiac surgery), or when the information is sensitive (such as sexual function, reproduction, or bowel function).

Group Teaching

Group teaching may be appropriate in settings where there are enough patients with the same cognitive or affective learning needs, available to teach at the same time (such as a group of pregnant women). Important considerations in offering group classes include whether transportation and time are convenient, and whether patients and their families can attend.

Group teaching sessions help patients with acute and chronic conditions feel less alienated. Patients frequently remark after a group teaching session that it was helpful to hear other people express the same problems and feelings. Groups in which patients are encouraged to formulate their own agenda and conduct the group session seem to be even more motivated to learn. Groups also

encourage patient sharing of coping techniques and useful hints. For example, it may be difficult for health professionals who have never had to struggle with an ileostomy or with asthma to understand or be aware of the many problems of daily existence involved with these conditions. The sharing and social support in group sessions can be augmented by technical assistance from health professionals.

Group teaching also helps families gain added support from health professionals and other patients and their families. Families gaining support from one another is especially evident in pediatric settings, and is one of the reasons for the success of the Ronald McDonald Houses for parents of critically ill children. This sharing and support transfers to more structured settings, such as group teaching classes where spouses of patients with heart disease share recipes with one another. The feeling that "we're all in this together" is especially gratifying to family members, who are frequently more overwhelmed than the patient with the magnitude of the problem.

Group teaching can be used to persuade patients to perform health behaviors. Information and facts are presented to help them understand the need to perform certain health behaviors; then, examples are given to help patients understand how they can accomplish this. These principles apply equally to health promotion or self-management classes.

Advanced preparation and coaching are important before teaching a group. Teachers need a strong understanding of the health problem being addressed in the patient education session. The instructor should review the professional literature and the AHRQ guidelines. Presenting information persuasively requires a confident teacher, with a lively affect, who can keep the attention of the learners. It is important to observe others who are experienced in group teaching and witness first-hand group teaching techniques.

Another benefit of group teaching is the decreased costs because once a class is developed, more learners can be taught with less health care provider time. However, groups cannot be used for all teaching, in as much as one-on-one time is still needed for assessment of learning needs and abilities, teaching physical self-care skills, and evaluation of understanding.

Teaching Protocols

Sometimes, the health care team members collaborate to create a general template of patient education for all patients with a specific diagnosis or treatment, to be individualized for each learner. These may be expressed in the forms of critical pathways or care maps. Although they are typically used in hospitals, they can also be effective in an outpatient clinic or home health setting.

These systems direct the coordination of the health care team through teaching protocols. Statistics, either computer-generated or collected from clinical experiences, can be used to identify high-volume or high-risk groups of specific patient populations that require ongoing teaching. Further research can identify common learning needs. For example, using a log-keeping method in an outpatient clinic, we discovered several situations ideal for teaching protocols: weight reduction, hypertension, diabetes, prenatal care, and neonatal care.

Matching Teaching Activities to Content and Situation

In general, a combination of learning activities works best, by involving a range of senses and learning pathways. There are several ways to help the patient and family assume active roles in learning, and enjoy patient education:

- **Match learning activities with learning objectives.**
- **Keep the patient and the family involved through discussion, role-play, games, and media.**

- **Incorporate a variety of methods to teach skills and develop the patient's attitude. Never use lecture alone.**
- **Build success and reinforcement into the teaching process. Test the patient's new abilities to help him or her feel a sense of accomplishment.**
- **Make learning fun.** Humor and support decrease patients' anxiety and help them learn at their own pace.
- **Provide enough time to practice skills.** Put skill-building exercises in the middle, not at the end of the session. This skill practice often determines how safely the patient can perform new skills at home.

Applying Theory to Practice to Optimize Impact

Patient education is much more than transmitting facts. It is the process of collaborating with the learner to identify and reach mutually agreed upon goals to optimize self-care and, ultimately, health or quality of life. Part of this process includes coaching the learner to modify attitudes and opinions that get in the way of achieving these goals. A good assessment of learning needs and abilities includes identifying the learner's perceptions, beliefs, and attitudes. Effective interventions apply the Health Belief Model (see Chapter 6) to prepare the learner to see how behavior changes would facilitate reaching goals, and help motivate the learner to commit to making the effort to make those changes. Table 9.2 shows how teaching can be organized to apply this theory to practice.

The Health Belief Model can be used as a guide in designing a group class. First, patients must believe they have been, or are likely to be, affected by a particular health problem. The instructor can provide evidence that the patient has hypertension or diabetes, or is at risk for these conditions. Patients should understand in their own words a simple definition of the health

TABLE 9.2 The Health Belief Model Used in Planning Patient Education Interventions

The Health Belief Model was constructed to predict health behaviors. It provides a tool for understanding the patient's perception of disease and his decision-making process in the consumption of health services. In each of the four steps, consider family members and significant others.

STEPS	APPLICATION
I. The patient perceives that he or she has a condition or is likely to contract it.	I. a. Discuss problem and symptoms (to be prevented or treated). b. Explore prior knowledge and experience of audience. c. Address obstacles to understanding (anxiety, fear, misconceptions, denial).
II. The patient perceives that the disease or condition is harmful and has serious consequences for him or her.	II. a. Describe potential consequences of the problem. b. Discuss prognosis. c. Explore common beliefs and attitudes. d. Describe experiences of individuals with similar problem (including lifestyle).
III. The patient believes that the suggested health intervention is of value to him or her.	III. a. Describe proposed treatment plan, health promotion activities, proposed behavior changes (includes medications). b. Discuss what may happen with or without proposed treatment. c. Is this a cure? d. Financial costs, lifestyle changes, side effects discussed.
IV. The patient believes that the effectiveness of the treatment is worth the cost and barriers he or she must confront.	IV. a. Outline provider responsibilities. b. Outline patient responsibilities. c. Outline needed knowledge, attitudes, and skills. d. Suggest and provide resources for knowledge and skills development.

problem. Second, the patients must believe the condition discussed is harmful and has adverse consequences. Patients frequently wish to talk about how this problem has affected or may affect their lives, families, work, and social roles. Third, the patients need to understand the proposed treatment plan or health promotion plan, and what behaviors the patient is asked to consider integrating into his or her life. These behaviors should be stated clearly, with practical suggestions to help patients overcome barriers they might encounter, including learning skills, finding ongoing support, and perhaps acquiring financial assistance. Fourth, patients weigh the perceived costs and benefits of the proposed health interventions and make decisions about their commitment to act.

CASE STUDY 9.3

MRS. FOX'S FRACTURE

Mrs. Fox is 70 years old. She is well known on the medical-surgical unit of the small community hospital. She was admitted 3 months ago because of her poor dietary habits, her blood sugar was dangerously high, and her diabetes was out of control. She is physically inactive, watches television and plays bridge for entertainment, and smokes two packs of cigarettes daily.

Her current admission is the result of a fall down the front stairs of her home. Mrs. Fox has a fractured tibia. A cast is applied in the emergency room.

Because of poor circulation and immobility, Mrs. Fox is admitted overnight for evaluation. Her physician plans to discharge her within 2 days.

ASSESSMENT AND NURSING DIAGNOSES
During the admission assessment, her nurse notes the following important information:

The Foxes live in a one-story ranch home with wood floors and area rugs. Mr. Fox works the evening shift as a security guard for the local shopping mall. Mrs. Fox has not followed her diabetic meal plan. Mr. Fox found Mrs. Fox asleep on the couch with a burning cigarette in her hand last week and is worried about a fire in the home while he is at work.

The nursing staff has a conference to discuss a patient care plan for Mrs. Fox. Considering the short time she will be hospitalized, the nurses are overwhelmed by the behavior changes Mrs. Fox needs to make to safely manage her own care. Should they immediately get a dietitian involved to repeat diet teaching? What about the smoking and its hazards? The nurses list all her nursing diagnoses, and then work together to set priorities. Mrs. Fox's nursing diagnoses are:

1. Altered tissue perfusion in peripheral system
2. Impaired tissue integrity
3. Risk for injury
4. Impaired physical mobility
5. Altered nutrition: more than body requirements
6. Impaired home maintenance management
7. Activity intolerance
8. Pain

GOALS AND IMPLEMENTATION
After careful consideration of survival skills, safety issues, and Mrs. Fox's priorities, the nursing staff decides the most important issues are impaired physical mobility, risk for injury, and altered tissue perfusion. The survival skills Mrs. Fox needs are the ability to walk on crutches and the ability to check circulation on her affected leg. The goals for Mrs. Fox and her family are then:

- Properly maintain the cast with adequate circulation.
- Assess the cast and the skin under the cast edges to determine skin condition (four times daily).
- Assess foot and leg for circulatory and neurologic impairment (four times daily).
- Walk safely with the use of crutches and appropriate gait.
- Prevent axillary skin breakdown.
- Administer medication as ordered.
- Adapt home environment to prevent injury caused by falls.
- Provide at-home assistance with activities of daily living.

Skills such as cast care and crutch walking must be taught with active learner involvement and repeated practice. Health care team members need to accurately assess and document the patient's abilities in these areas.

The staff members caring for Mrs. Fox decide to focus their immediate efforts on the problems posed by her broken bone injury, and address diabetes management and smoking cessation with post-hospital referrals. They call an interdisciplinary team conference. The physical therapist will teach crutch-walking skills, the dietary department will reinforce appropriate eating, and the hospital social worker will discuss with the Foxes a referral to home health and at-home assistance to assure safety.

Every nurse who enters Mrs. Fox's room for the next 24 hours carries out the teaching plan by reinforcing and evaluating her ability to perform circulation checks and crutch-walking skills. Mr. Fox also is involved in teaching. A one-page instruction sheet is created, with specific instructions regarding ambulation and circulation.

Discharge and Home Health Care Services

As a result of economic pressures, patients are often discharged while still needing some level of professional health care. All health care team members must be aware of continuing care services, such as home health care, to best help patients with discharge planning. Anticipate the needs patients will have at home, what kinds of resources are already available, and what types of services they will need. The case study of Mrs. Fox illustrates critical needs, including patient teaching and safety measures, which remain after discharge. The health care team works with the family to assess the physical layout of the home, how to adapt it if necessary, and how to add needed equipment. They help the family assess whether the principal caregiver will need other helpers to assist, pick up medications, and run errands. The health care team must also help the patient determine what insurance will cover. Third-party payment may reimburse for at least part of home health care services. To facilitate home health care referral and authorization, clearly communicate through documentation:

1. The homebound status of the patient. The patient's condition prevents him or her from leaving home without help from others; therefore, leaving home is rarely feasible. Stress functional limitations.
2. Emphasize acute episodes or acute exacerbation of the condition.
3. Reflect the level of current need. For example, document the size and appearance of wound, rather than stating,

"wound healing well." Provide specific measurements whenever possible.
4. Emphasize the need for reinstruction rather than for reinforced teaching. If the family's ability to master learning is limited, this should be noted.
5. Document whether the patient's condition is unstable. Skilled nursing care to monitor medications or vital signs may not be reimbursed unless the patient's condition is unstable.

Many acute care nurses are unaware that home care nurses must also focus on discharge planning at the time of admission and must skillfully achieve patient learning outcomes. As in acute care, there is a limit on the number of visits allotted for follow-up by home health nurses.

Clinical Relevance: Prenatal Education Program

Two of the authors of this book developed a prenatal education program, first as a pilot program, and then as an established component of prenatal care for all patients enrolled in the obstetrical practice at the family medicine center. One author (KS) was head nurse in the family medicine center and the other (SR) was a faculty member from the school of nursing.

A program of prenatal education was originally developed as an advanced practice nursing student doing a clinical practicum at a university family medicine practice. The classes evolved in response to an informal needs assessment conducted at the outpatient clinic of a university's family medicine residency training program. Faculty, residents, and nurses designated prenatal classes as the outstanding patient education need for clinic patients.

The clinic served a group of prenatal families who were socioeconomically and culturally diverse. Teenage parents, single mothers, and international patients were not well served by traditional couple-oriented approaches to childbirth education. The involvement of childbirth coaches, including mothers, sisters, friends, and spouses, was strongly supported. After a successful pilot program developed by the APN student, the Family Practice Clinic assumed the leadership of the prenatal classes and established the following philosophy about the delivery of prenatal education.

Education is an essential ingredient in the health care delivered to prenatal patients. The family medicine center made a commitment to offer prenatal classes to all of our patients on a regular basis.

Prenatal classes should be attended as early as possible in pregnancy. There are many advantages to the patient, her family, the physician, and the nurse.

1. The mother's participation in her own care is essential, especially in the areas of nutrition and care of her body. The classes give parents and significant others the information they need to work in partnership with the physician and nurse.
2. Classes that address the labor and delivery processes give expectant parents an opportunity to verbalize anxieties or fears about childbirth.
3. Expectant parents enter a supportive relationship with other expectant parents.
4. Relaxation and breathing techniques make both routine obstetric examinations and the labor and delivery better experiences.
5. Expectant mothers and fathers and significant others are encouraged to communicate their feelings effectively with one another and to consider ways to keep the communication lines open during stressful events surrounding the birth of their child.
6. Parents gain knowledge about newborn care and helpful suggestions for dealing with the new baby's siblings and other family members.
7. The prenatal care curriculum offers a blend of general childbirth education and Lamaze techniques. No single approach to

the birth experience or child care is promoted. Instead, the aim is to provide expectant parents with information that enables them to consider their own needs and wishes. Most important is openness and flexibility in planning for labor and delivery and in considering each family's special circumstances.

8. Expectant parents learn from the health care providers and from each other. Health care providers also learn a great deal from the patients in an informal group, in which all members are supported and encouraged to share their thoughts and feelings with one another.
9. A commitment to patient education is demonstrated by the willingness to become team members in health care with patients. It is a statement of the nurse's respect for patients as consumers. Finally, offering an attractive prenatal care package is an important step toward enrolling new families in the practice (Duke-Watts Family Medicine Program, Durham, NC).

This philosophy articulated the benefits to the prenatal patient and her support system, as well as the agency. Care was taken to ensure continuity of the prenatal classes regardless of changes in clinic staff and residents. Guidelines and standards were developed to help staff nurses who would serve as a prenatal class coordinator handle the logistics of the classes, and allay anxiety they might have about the program.

After guidelines were developed, objectives were written for each class (Box 9.6). During the first of four class meetings, each patient and her significant other filled out a learning needs assessment. These assessment data were then put into the general schema of classes. Thus, the prenatal patients set their own agenda. The class is taught to meet the needs of the learners, not those of the health care professionals. Data from the learning needs assessment were transferred to the patient's chart, with her knowledge, so during office visits the physician could discuss her stated concerns. The learning needs assessment included questions about previous pregnancies, who would attend classes and delivery with the patient, previous prenatal education, and what the patient was hoping to learn in the classes.

Group discussions and demonstrations enlivened classes. During the first class, a couple who attended the previous set of classes was enlisted to bring their infant. The expectant parents had many questions for the parent visitors, and seeing the outcome of the prenatal period (the healthy baby) focused the class for everyone. Participants were divided into smaller groups of five or six to discuss topics (such as sexual activity during pregnancy) and to play educational games related to nutrition.

During the fourth class, which discussed the care of the newborn, a family nurse practitioner or a family medicine resident demonstrated physical assessment of a neonate. The couples were invariably amazed to see the newborn's

---

BOX 9.6 Objectives for Prenatal Classes

Class I: Nutrition During Pregnancy
At the close of Class I, each participant will be able to do the following:

A. Answer the following questions correctly:
   1. How much weight do you plan to gain during your pregnancy?
   2. Now that you are pregnant, how many more calories do you think you need: 2 times normal, 3 times normal, only 300 calories more, only 100 calories more?
   3. Which of the following foods do pregnant women especially need: dairy products, sweets, fatty foods, fresh vegetables, protein foods?
   4. Which of the following items might be dangerous to eat or use while you are pregnant: alcoholic beverages, salt, sugar, nicotine, caffeine?
   5. In which of the following situations would a pregnant woman be wise to lose weight: if the woman were overweight before pregnancy, if the woman has diabetes and is overweight, if the woman suddenly gains 10 lb that is primarily fluid?
B. List three advantages of breast-feeding.
C. State three advantages of exercise during pregnancy.

D. Choose one type of exercise and describe where and how often it will be done.

Prenatal Class II: Physiologic and Psychological Changes of Pregnancy
By the close of Class II, each participant will be able to do the following:
A. Describe breast changes and care of the breasts during pregnancy.
B. Describe recommendations for the following during pregnancy:
   1. Rest and sleep
   2. Smoking and alcohol
   3. Dental care
   4. Travel and work
C. Name two common discomforts of pregnancy and recommended treatments.
D. State why the doctor should be consulted before *any* medication is taken during pregnancy.
E. Identify three warning signs for which the doctor should be notified immediately.
F. Demonstrate the Kegel exercise for toning pelvic musculature, demonstrate slow, deep chest breathing used during the initial stage of labor.

(continued)

BOX 9.6 Objectives for Prenatal Classes *(Continued)*

Prenatal Class III: Labor and Delivery
At the close of Class III, each participant will be able to do the following:
A. Describe the work of the uterus in labor.
B. Describe the changes of the cervix in labor.
C. Describe three signs of labor.
D. Demonstrate the timing of contractions.
E. Describe how and when to contact the doctor when there has been a sign of labor.
F. Describe three stages of labor.
G. Consider own plans for labor and delivery (e.g., birthing room, rooming-in arrangements, early discharge).
H. Describe some variables that make cesarean section necessary.

Prenatal Class IV: The Newborn
At the close of Class IV, each participant/couple will be able to do the following:
A. Describe why fatigue is a problem that most new parents face.
B. Discuss two ways new parents can minimize unnecessary fatigue.
C. Consider which helpers might be staying with patients when they come home from the hospital and describe what helpers can do.
D. Describe three infant care problems for which the doctor should be notified.
E. Describe three needs for which babies depend on their parents.
F. Describe two issues that new parents often confront as a couple.

Prenatal Class V: The Postpartum Period
At the end of Class V, each participant will be able to do the following:
A. Identify two common postpartum discomforts and describe how to initiate relief measures.
B. Identify two symptoms or problems for which the doctor should be notified.
C. Consider a method of contraception that is acceptable to them.
D. Demonstrate the following in a mock labor and delivery:
1. Deep chest breathing
2. Shallow breathing
3. Panting
4. Pushing

---

range of behaviors and could anticipate their forthcoming infant, laying the foundation for infant stimulation practices. Demonstration segments allow the participants an opportunity to become acquainted with one another.

At the end of the last class, each participant completed an evaluation form rating the classes and teachers and offering suggestions for improvement. Evaluations were useful in planning future classes and in giving specific teachers feedback on their performance. Another evaluation format, a confidence survey, was used during the first class series to obtain information related to the participants' growth in confidence levels during the five class meetings. One of the purposes of any type

of prenatal education is to instill confidence in the couple so that they are able to manage self-care practices related to pregnancy and to care for the neonate. Confidence levels on 19 different items were determined on pre- and post-tests (that is, at the beginning of the class series and after the last class).

The confidence level survey used in the classes is shown in Figure 9.3. Another method of evaluation and feedback used was to ask patients to write a summary of their birth experiences. Patients were given a guide for writing the report (Box 9.7). This is a keepsake for the family and a process to help the mother work through feelings about such a powerful experience. Although not all patients are willing to write a report, most are eager to discuss the birth experience. This provided us with valuable pointers about how to improve childbirth classes to better prepare patients for labor and delivery.

Evaluations of the prenatal classes prompted additional classes at the clinic. More in-depth classes were offered on breast preparation and breast-feeding for patients in the seventh to eighth month of pregnancy. A room at the clinic was also equipped for patients to view videotapes on cesarean delivery, basics of baby care, and postpartum fatigue and depression. A daily baby care "call-in" telephone hour was proposed to provide information and answer patient questions before the first return visit to the clinic.

To achieve successful outcomes of group teaching, incorporate assessment, preparation, and individualized approaches for non-English speaking patients from different cultural backgrounds.

INSTRUCTIONS

We are interested in knowing how confident you feel about your knowledge associated with pregnancy, labor, and delivery. Please answer these questions carefully by circling the response that refers to your confidence level.
A sample question will help you understand how to fill out the questionnaire.
I know how to fill out this questionnaire.

VC C ? I VI

VC — I feel very confident and secure in my knowledge of this material.
 C — I feel confident that I can deal adequately with this material.
 ? — I have no particular feelings about this material; I do not know what this material means.
 I — I feel insecure, knowing that I would have a difficult time dealing with this material.
VI — I feel very insecure, knowing that I definitely could not deal with this material at this time.

1. I know which foods a pregnant woman should eat and why.

  VC   C   ?   I   VI

2. I understand the changes in my breasts.

  VC   C   ?   I   VI

3. I know about the possible effects of alcohol on my baby.

  VC   C   ?   I   VI

4. I know how many pounds I can gain during my pregnancy.

  VC   C   ?   I   VI

5. I understand restrictions placed on me because of my job.

  VC   C   ?   I   VI

FIGURE 9.3 Prenatal confidence level survey. *(continues on page 262)*

6. I know how to do a pelvic tilt.

| VC | C | ? | I | VI |

7. I understand the reasons for frequent urination during pregnancy.

| VC | C | ? | I | VI |

8. I know the danger signs to watch for during pregnancy.

| VC | C | ? | I | VI |

9. I understand the fear—tension—pain cycle.

| VC | C | ? | I | VI |

10. I know how to do breathing exercises to be used during labor.

| VC | C | ? | I | VI |

11. I know what to expect from a newborn baby.

| VC | C | ? | I | VI |

12. I understand the differences between bottle-feeding and breast-feeding for the mother and baby.

| VC | C | ? | I | VI |

13. I know how to give a baby bath.

| VC | C | ? | I | VI |

14. I know what kind of birth control to use while nursing.

| VC | C | ? | I | VI |

15. I know what kinds of pain medications are available during labor.

| VC | C | ? | I | VI |

16. I know at least three signs of beginning labor.

| VC | C | ? | I | VI |

17. I know how to get my body into shape after delivery.

| VC | C | ? | I | VI |

18. I understand the various forms of birth control and the ones best suited for me.

| VC | C | ? | I | VI |

19. I know the types of equipment and clothing necessary for me and my baby.

| VC | C | ? | I | VI |

FIGURE 9.3 *(Continued)*

BOX 9.7 Suggestions for Writing About the Birth Experience

Beginning of Labor
How and when did it begin? What did you do? How did you feel?

Admission to the Hospital
When were you admitted? What was it like?

Stages of Labor
How long did each stage last? Did you feel that the nurses kept you informed on your progress? Which tools helped the most? Which helped the least? Did you receive medication? If so, what kind, when, how effective was it? What kind of emotional support did you have?

Birth
What did the baby look like? How did you feel during and immediately after birth?

Postpartum
How long did you stay in the hospital? Describe how you felt during the first week you were at home after delivery. What problems did you have? What people or things were most helpful to you?

CASE STUDY 9.4

THE VUONG FAMILY

GENERAL CONSIDERATIONS: CULTURAL PRACTICES AND PRENATAL CARE

Childbirth is an important event in the lives of families, and cultural practices affect how prenatal care is provided. Health care providers need to respect each patient's background, and through patient education help families form partnerships in prenatal care. Freda

(2002) suggests the best and most direct way to learn about members of the cultural group you want to reach is to ask questions, such as what are their culture's pregnancy beliefs or customs.

CASE PRESENTATION

Mai Vuong, a Vietnamese woman, comes for her first clinic visit when she is 12 weeks pregnant. She comes alone, is quiet, and seems withdrawn. The assessment of her learning needs about the pregnancy is difficult. Also, time is limited during an outpatient encounter. A nursing student working at the clinic that day offered to conduct two home visits to help compose a family assessment and identify Mai's needs.

FAMILY ASSESSMENT

The family unit is composed of the husband, Tran, age 38, who works in a print shop; Mai, age 28, the wife, who works full-time as a seamstress and is pregnant with their first child; and Li, age 28, who is Tran's sister and works in the same print shop as her brother. Mai states she knows nothing about pregnancy, labor, delivery, or caring for a newborn child and denies having had any role model in these areas.

Mai and Tran are both Vietnamese and emigrated legally from Vietnam. Li has always lived with them. Before leaving Vietnam, Tran was a farmer. This was a difficult life, physically and economically. He came to the United States in hopes of a better and prosperous life. Mai did not complete high school; she left school to work and support her family. All three of them continue to financially support their parents, and Mai sends her brother, who lives in Texas, one-third of her monthly salary. Both sets of parents are supportive of the pregnancy. However, neither mother can come and help with the care of the newborn, a traditional role of Vietnamese grand-mothers.

The Vuong family is a warm, hos-pitable Catholic family, with a secure sense of family loyalty, closeness, and strength. Traditional Vietnamese fami-lies have a patriarchal structure in which the eldest man is the head of the household and the woman is dutiful and respectful toward her husband. In the Vuong family, Tran is the head of the family, as is evident in the way he speaks for his wife and appears to be her caretaker. Mai is dutiful to her hus-band in the way she respects his opin-ion and serves him and their guest first. However, these roles are also flexible: all three members of this family share the domestic duties of their small two-room flat. They are also emotionally supportive and mutually respectful of each other as is evident in the gentle-ness Tran and Li showed toward Mai when she has difficulty understanding the questions of the English-speaking interviewer.

The Vuongs live among and work predominantly with Vietnamese immi-grants and refugees. This may signal social exclusivity within their ethnic community, because they have few non-Vietnamese friends. Consequently, this results in their being limited in their awareness of community services, such as childbirth preparation classes. This also decreases their opportunities to assimilate into their new culture and improve their English language skills. All three state that they do not know what to expect with pregnancy and child-birth, and they show concern regarding their lack of knowledge. They are presently receiving their knowledge from friends and neighbors, because they have no family in the immediate area. This could potentially lead to con-fusion, fear, and unrealistic expectations

of the course of the pregnancy and labor and delivery. Tran and Li seem to have formed an alliance in which they bond to support Mai and relate to her gently. Although culturally understand-able, this could foster her dependence on her family to meet her needs of effective communication.

The family anticipates the new baby with pleasure. Having been raised in traditional Vietnamese families, they respect their cultural heritage and believe the family to be important. When asked about raising their child in the American culture, Tran responded, "I think my baby was, born, okay I have to teach her. Sometimes we have to keep the Vietnamese idea in my family. I want to say no anything Vietnamese ideas excellent, but I think American idea something excellent. So we have to keep two of them in my family." Mai echoed, "Together."

In anticipating becoming parents, Tran and Mai seem aware that their child will be raised in a different culture and have some understanding of the challenge before them. Another strength of the potential parent-child system is Tran's involvement in the pregnancy. He speaks about needing to move to a larger home and shopping for the baby's bed. Having no role mod-els regarding pregnancy, childbirth, or the care of the newborn, the Vuong family has a knowledge deficit regard-ing the role changes and task realign-ment a new family member will bring into their home.

In traditional Vietnamese culture, the fathers are not expected to participate in childbirth; childbirth is regarded as a thing among women. Tran expresses feeling uncomfortable with entering the labor and delivery room. This may cause a conflict with the American expectation that fathers be involved in coaching the woman through labor and delivery. Because of a knowledge deficit regarding pregnancy, childbirth, and child care, Mai is at risk for difficulty in making the role transition to mother. Mai is reluctant to use her English language skills and has limited comprehension of the English language. This fosters dependency on her family and other members of her ethnic group to communicate for her.

The family members are interested in seeking knowledge in the areas that they feel are lacking and are interested in the child preparation classes offered by the clinic. Because extended family is so important in the Vietnamese culture, having no grandmother in the same geographic location may make the transition of having a newborn more difficult for this family.

RECOMMENDATIONS
1. The family needs to be encouraged to participate in childbirth preparation classes. This will provide anticipatory guidance in relationship to the labor and delivery process. Li or another woman needs to accompany Mai to the classes even if Tran feels that he wants to be involved in the coaching of Mai's labor and delivery.
2. The family needs to find a trusted friend who might give them reliable information regarding what is normal in pregnancy, labor, delivery, and newborn care. They also need to ask questions of their physician and the clinic nurses.
3. The health providers of this family need to be made aware of the family's cultural differences and work with them within their cultural context. An example of this would be not to pressure Tran to be Mai's labor coach but rather allow a woman to be with her.

4. Mai needs to be encouraged to continue English classes and to use her language skills to decrease her dependency on others to communicate. The clinic should not rely on written learning materials to provide instructions to Mai.

OUTCOMES
As an outcome of this family assessment, Mai and Li participate in the clinic's childbirth classes. They are also given needed attention when Mai came for her prenatal visits because the clinic staff members were aware of her needs and appreciated cultural norms of the Vietnamese family. Written teaching materials are used selectively because of Mai's limited ability to read and understand English.

SUMMARY

Matching learning objectives to appropriate learning methods and media is important to achieve positive results in patient education. Several examples were offered in this chapter to illustrate the design of interventions based on diagnoses, learning needs, goals, and patient learning objectives. Case studies illustrated interventions for individual patients, including tips for using home health care services to bridge the gap between hospital and home, and using an individualized care plan to accompany group teaching for a Vietnamese patient. Valuable tools for evaluating patient education materials and videos are also provided in this chapter. One teaching tool mentioned this chapter is presented in detail in Chapter 10.

STRATEGIES FOR CRITICAL ANALYSIS AND APPLICATION

1. Using the case study of Mrs. Fox, describe which instructional format and methods

you would choose for discharge teaching. Base the teaching on the patient's length of stay and priorities for patient learning. How would you coordinate your teaching with the physical therapist? Who else besides the patient should be included in teaching?

2. Select a sample patient education handout and a sample video addressing a topic of your choice. Evaluate them using the Suitability Assessment of Materials (SAM) criteria (Box 9.3). How would you improve them?

3. If you were asked to teach a 1-hour class to fellow nursing students about the need for their own adequate nutrition and exercise, how could you use the Health Belief Model as a guide to prepare the class?

4. Identify resources in your community that could be used to support the learning of non-English-speaking patients. Where can interpreter services be found? Where can health care providers obtain teaching materials written in other languages? What resources are available for patients to learn how to read and understand the English language?

To find the latest information

Key search terms
support groups, self-help groups, care maps, patient education AND video, PowerPoint, functional health literacy, low-level readers

Websites

- National Guideline Clearinghouse (Agency for Healthcare Research and Quality [AHRQ]): http://www.guideline.gov/; www.ahcpr.gov
- Evidence-Based Practice (Agency for Healthcare Research and Quality [AHRQ]): www.ahcpr.gov
- Evidence-Based Clinical Prevention (Canadian Task Force on Preventive Health Care [CTFPHC]): http://www.ctfphc.org/

- Research Related to Self-Help Support Groups (American Self-Help Clearinghouse): http://www.mentalhelp.net/selfhelp/
- Stanford Patient Education Research Center: http://patienteducation.stanford.edu/

REFERENCES

Agency for Healthcare Research and Quality (AHRQ). (2003, 6/30/2003). *National guideline clearinghouse*. Retrieved March 18, 2003, from http://www.guideline.gov/; www.ahcpr.gov

Agency for Healthcare Research and Quality (AHRQ). (2000). *Now you have a diagnosis: What's next? Using health care information to help make treatment decisions*. Retrieved March 12, 2003, from http://www.ahcpr.gov/consumer/diaginfo.pdf

Bodenheimer, T., Lorig, K., Holman, H., & Grumbach, K. (2002). Patient self-management of chronic disease in primary care. *JAMA, 288*(19), 2469–2475.

Boggs, P. P., & Rosenthal, M. B. (2000). Helping women help themselves: Developing a menopause discussion group. *Clinical Obstetrics and Gynecology, 43*(1), 207–212.

Bui, L. L., Last, L., Bradley, H., Law, C. H. L., Maier, B. A., & Smith, A. J. (2002). Interest and participation in support group programs among patients with colorectal cancer. *Cancer Nursing, 25*(2), 150–157.

Cantillon, P. (2003). Teaching large groups. *BMJ, 326*, 437–440.

Clark, M. C., & Lester, J. (2000). The effect of video-based interventions on self-care. *Western Journal of Nursing Research, 22*(8), 895–911.

Concordia University. (2003). *Microsoft PowerPoint 2000*. Retrieved July 14, 2003, from http://www.cuaa.edu/computing/softrain/powerpoint/index.shtml

Doak, C. C., Doak, L. G., & Root, J. H. (1996). *Teaching patients with low literacy skills* (2nd ed.). Philadelphia: J. B. Lippincott.

Engelke, Z. (1999). Take-out education extends teaching. *Patient Education Management 6*(7), 78.

Freda, M. C. (2002). *Perinatal patient education: A practical guide with education handouts for patients*. Philadelphia: Lippincott Williams & Wilkins.

Gaba, D. M. (2002). Two examples of how to evaluate the impact of new approaches to teaching. *Anesthesiology, 96*(1), 1–2.

Gorski, L. A. (2002). Effective teaching of home IV therapy. *Home Healthcare Nurse, 20*(10), 666–674.

Humphreys, K., & Moos, R. (2001). Can encouraging substance abuse patients to participate in self-help groups reduce demand for health care? A quasi-experimental study. *Alcoholism: Clinical and Experimental Research, 25*(5), 711–716.

Jaques, D. (2003). Teaching small groups. *BMJ, 326,* 492–494.

Johnson, J. (2000). An overview of psychosocial support services: resources for healing. *Cancer Nursing, 23*(4), 310–313.

Katz, D., Koppie, T. M., Wu, D., Meng, M. V., Grossfeld, G. D., Sadesky, N., et al. (2002). Sociodemographic characteristics and health related quality of life in men attending prostate cancer support groups. *The Journal of Urology, 168,* 2092–2096.

Kessels, R. P. C. (2003). Patients' memory for medical information. *Journal of the Royal Society of Medicine, 96,* 219–222.

Lamberg, L. (2003). Online empathy for mood disorders: Patients turn to Internet support groups. *JAMA, 289*(23), 3073–3077.

London, F. (1999). *No time to teach.* Philadelphia: Lippincott Williams & Wilkins.

Lorig, K. (2001). Self-management in chronic illness. In S. G. Funk (Ed.), *Key aspects of preventing and managing chronic illness.* New York: Springer.

Lorig, K. R., Laurent, D. D., Deyo, R. A., Marnell, M. E., Minor, M. A., & Ritter, P. (2002). Can a back pain e-mail discussion group improve health status and lower health care costs? A randomized study. *Archives of Internal Medicine, 162,* 792–796.

Lorig, K. R., Ritter, P., Stewart, A. L., Sobel, D. S., Brown, W. B., Bandura, A., et al. (2001). Chronic disease self-management program: 2-year health status and health care utilization outcomes. *Medical Care, 39*(11), 1217–1223.

Maloni, J. A., & Kutil, R. M. (2000). Antepartum support group for women hospitalized on bed rest. *MCN, American Journal of Maternal Child Nursing, 25*(4), 204–210.

Moore, L., Campbell, R., Whelan, A., Mills, N., Lupton, P., Misselbrook, E., et al. (2002). Self help smoking cessation in pregnancy: Cluster randomised controlled trial. *BMJ, 325,* 1383–1389.

Schultz, M. (2002). Low literacy skills needn't hinder care. *RN, 65*(4), 45–48.

Webber, D., Higgins, L., & Baker, V. (2001). Enhancing recall of information from a patient education booklet: A trial using cardiomyopathy patients. *Patient Education and Counseling, 44*(3), 263–270.

White, B. J., & Madara, E. J. (2004, February). *Self-help group sourcebook online.* Retrieved July 18, 2004, from http://www.mentalhelp.net/selfhelp/selfhelpgroups.org for American Self-Help Group Clearinghouse

Williams, M. V., Davis, T., Parker, R. M., & Weiss, B. D. (2002). The role of health literacy in patient-physician communications. *Family Medicine, 34*(5), 383–389.

Winzelberg, A. J., Classen, C., Alpers, G. W., Roberts, H., Koopman, C., Adams, R. E., et al. (2003). Evaluation of an Internet support group for women with primary breast cancer. *Cancer, 97,* 1164–1173.

Patient Education Resources on the Internet

Karen S. Zeliff

LEARNING OBJECTIVES

After reading this chapter, the student should be able to:

1. Describe the three components of a successful Internet search.

2. Describe e-mail, mail lists, newsgroups, chat rooms, and video conferencing, and their potential use in patient education.

3. Describe the information resources available on the Internet (such as search and metasearch engines, subject and review subject directories, databases) and the types of questions these resources can answer.

4. Apply a 10-step search planning and implementation process to locate educational and self-help resources for alternative therapies.

5. Identify six criteria for evaluating the quality of Internet information.

INTRODUCTION

Created in the late 1960s by the Department of Defense (Howe, 2001), the Internet has evolved from a tool designed to safeguard American intelligence secrets into a tool that has ushered in an information age. The Internet has grown into a vast publishing tool, offering access to information in multiple formats, from multiple resources, from multiple locations. Its customizable and non-linear construction provides the user with both novel opportunities and challenges for information retrieval. Although the structure of Internet publishing sometimes makes it difficult to retrieve selective and relevant information, continued efforts by librarians, archivists, commercial vendors, and government agencies to organize and classify Internet resources help this medium realize its potential as a unique educational tool. The Internet can be used independently or in tandem with other teaching tools. It offers resources and opportunities for personal interaction. The strategies for locating quality health and medical information on the Internet outlined in this chapter, although primarily directed at the patient educator, can be applied to self-directed learning by the patient, or by any person involved at any level in the delivery of health care.

Website addresses (URLs) change rapidly. If an address provided in this text does not take you to the site you are looking for, the title can be typed the into a search engine (eg, Google), to determine if it is still available.

The Internet: A Tool for Patient Education

Managed care is shifting the focus of health care toward chronic disease management and prevention. Consequently, there has been a shift toward personal responsibility for health outcomes. The Internet facilitates this by providing access to many resources that help people take an active role in maintaining physical well-being. By providing access to medical information, medical advice, support groups, and computer-based home monitoring systems, the Internet makes it possible for patients to assume much more responsibility for their own health care. In doing so, these health care consumers may challenge the traditional role of physicians providing care (Anderson, 2001). Informed health consumers no longer look solely to their physicians for health advice, passively following instructions with little information, and even less questioning. Instead, they expect to be active partners in resolving their health care problems, and believe that their personal health outcomes are improved by shared decision-making. They consult experienced health consumers and professionals from different clinical disciplines and backgrounds. Frequently, these active health consumers bring information derived from these resources to their health care providers, asking that the information be integrated into their treatment.

Of the 113 million Americans who have gone online, 64% have searched for health or medical information. Every day, about 6 million Americans go online for medical information, which is more on any given day than visits to health professionals (Nicoll, 2002). Many health care professionals think the rapid growth and lack of quality control of Internet information will lead to the spread of misinformation, with potential negative effects (Redwood, 2002). This view has not been supported by research. Although coverage of key information is poor and inconsistent, and reading levels are high, the accuracy of information provided on the Internet is generally good (Berland et al., 2001). Scant clinical evidence exists to indicate that the Internet has had a serious negative impact on public health outcomes. Health care providers are now being urged to collaborate with Internet-using patients, to improve the quality of their care and better disseminate new knowledge about illnesses and treatments (Tokarski, 2002).

Health care providers can integrate into their practices this new role as intermediary between patients and Internet information.

They can point patients to reliable information, ask professional organizations to endorse specific sites, and teach patients how to evaluate what they find. To be an effective Internet intermediary and prevent the proliferation of misinformation, health care providers must become discriminating information searchers. They must know how to find authoritative information on the Internet, understand which of these resources are appropriate for use under which circumstances, and accurately evaluate the quality of information published. This will help them not only to guide patients to information that will enhance their health and well-being but also to use the vast potential of the Internet for professional development and lifelong learning. Skills are needed to retrieve information, and it is recognized that these skills will need to be continuously modified in response to the rapidly changing context of the Internet.

The Information Retrieval Process

Although information needs vary widely from person to person, nearly everyone is adept to some degree at meeting his or her primary information needs. The Internet is just one tool that can be used to access information. Regardless of the source of information, there are three steps in the information retrieval process: definition, searching, and evaluation.

Definition

What do I need to know, and where is the best place to find the answer?

The person defines an information need, generally in the form of a question that needs to be answered. The person then determines, based on personal experience, the most likely resource that will answer the question. Having defined the need and selected the most likely resource for answering that need, the person proceeds to the second step of information retrieval, searching.

Searching

How do I use the resource I have selected to find the information I need?

Each person determines the best way to use the selected resource to answer the question. If retrieved answers do not satisfy their information need, searching strategies may be adjusted. If the selected resource does not provide the answer to the question, the searcher may investigate another source of information, or change the search strategy. Once information is retrieved, the searcher proceeds to step three, evaluation.

Evaluation

Does this information adequately answer my information need?

The information seeker reviews the information, and judges it for quality by applying criteria based upon satisfaction rates that are predetermined, often implicitly, by the searcher. If, however, the results of the information retrieval process are unsatisfactory, the searcher may go back to a previous step in the process, redefining the information need, looking for a new resource, attempting a new search strategy, or even determining that the need for information is not worth additional effort and simply discontinuing the quest.

APPLYING THE INFORMATION RETRIEVAL PROCESS TO THE INTERNET

This information retrieval process can be applied to locate information on the Internet. Once the question is identified, the best place to find the answer can be defined. The second step is to develop a strategy to retrieve applicable information quickly and efficiently. The third step, evaluation, is completed by establishing criteria that can be used to judge the quality of information retrieved from sites and documents on the Internet.

Defining Internet Resources: Knowing Where to Look for Patient Education Information

Internet health and medical resources come in two forms: tools that are primarily used for communication, and tools that are primarily used for data storage and retrieval. Communication tools consist of e-mail, mailing lists, newsgroups, and chat rooms. The two major information tools for retrieving data indexed by keyword are subject directories and search engines. A portal site is comprised of a customizable combination of both search engines and directories. Information is also available through proprietary data bases that do not index websites, but index other selective resources, such as peer-reviewed journals, and provide access to these data bases through a web interface. Each of these tools is distinguishable not only by its operational structure, but by its types of information and how it can be used as a patient education tool.

Communication Tools

Internet communication tools come in two formats: asynchronous and synchronous. People who communicate asynchronously with one another by e-mail, mail lists, and newsgroups do so during separate times. Synchronous or real-time communication occurs over the Internet by using chat or web conferencing.

ELECTRONIC MAIL (E-MAIL)
E-mail is one of the oldest Internet communication tools and is often the first exposure most people have to the Internet. Many users begin communicating with family, friends, and coworkers through e-mail, then begin to branch out to communication with strangers with common interests. Interestingly, only 38% of physicians in one study contact their patients through e-mail (Healthcare Information and Management Systems Society, 2002). While patients want to correspond with their doctors via e-mail, physicians are hesitant to use e-mail for physician-patient communication. Their reported concerns include:

- Legal concerns
- Lack of reimbursement
- Privacy concerns
- Limited time
- Interference with practice workflow
- Lack of e-mail use among the patients themselves

As more guidelines are set and adopted to govern questions of e-mail legitimacy and liability, access to providers and other clinical staff by e-mail will eventually evolve into a consumer demand that will drive the market. The ability for physicians, nurse practitioners, and patients to use e-mail may soon be seen as an enhancement to practice, by adding electronic communication with their patients directly into the medical record, making some office visits obsolete, and generally improving the provider-patient relationship.

MAIL LISTS AND LISTSERVES
Mail lists and listserves are e-mail exchanges among many people with a common interest. Mail lists are available for almost every health and medicine related subject or specialty. For example, PatEdNet, is a restricted mail list for professional patient educators. To subscribe, send a blank e-mail to join-patednet@lyris.med.utah.edu.

Mail lists foster a sense of community and broaden networks for self-help and support. The conversations that occur on mail lists provide a wide spectrum of perspectives and information on topics that relate to a particular health care issue or interest. Patients can use mail lists to ask questions, share confidences, or solicit and receive caring support in a way that may not always be available from family, friends, or their personal health providers. Mail lists represent dialogue that is frequently intimate, but not personal, since the response is broadcast to everyone on the list. Joining a mail list may provide dozens to hundreds of incoming e-mails to your box every week.

These lists encourage the breakdown of barriers between patients and health providers. Physicians who would not respond to their own patients via e-mail will advise in a consulting capacity to a group of subscribers on a listserve. Likewise, informed patients, who feel intimidated sharing concerns and doubts about treatment with their personal physicians, will not hesitate to engage a physician online with direct and pointed questions. This community of patients and clinicians, bonded together by shared experiences, provides unique opportunities for sharing specific and personal information. Also, this community is an outlet for expressions of grief, suffering, concern, and compassion. To find a mail list on a topic of your choice, use the search engines at Tile Net (http://www.tile.net) and Email Universe (http://EmailUniverse.com/).

NEWSGROUPS

In a newsgroup messages are not automatically sent to individual members' e-mail addresses daily. The broader range of input from a more diverse population is possible in a newsgroup, which, unlike listserves, does not require subscription before posting. To find a newsgroup on a topic of your choice, use the search engine at Google (http://groups.google.com/). Newsgroups lack some of the intimacy of mail lists because of their broader distribution. However, they provide a forum for grassroots opinions. For example, a newsgroup could offer a general discussion by well-informed consumers on the merits of a particular breakthrough in medical research, or a recent health care bill in Congress.

CHAT OR CHAT ROOMS (INTERNET RELAY CHAT)

One of the most popular forms of Internet synchronous communication is chat or chat rooms, technically known as Internet Relay Chat (IRC). Live conversations enable dialogue with other users, promoting intimacy and anonymity. Open channels may be open to a casual lurker, or chats may be scheduled, where a group of people gathers at a specific time to simultaneously discuss a particular issue.

Chat can be used as an adjunct to other types of educational formats for teachers, presenters, or authors to lead or facilitate groups in discussions. However, if discussions are not monitored, conversations can veer off-topic, or become monopolized.

WEB VIDEOCONFERENCING

In web videoconferencing, special cameras and software allow a user on one computer to receive a live sound and video broadcast from another computer, in real time. Online whiteboards allow the users to share documents and collaborate directly on materials while maintaining the online connection. Videoconferencing applications hold the potential for tele-education over distance between patient and educator, and for tele-health between provider and patient.

Information Tools

Hypertext markup language (HTML), with its hypertext links to additional information, provides a mixed blessing for information searchers. Because publication to the web is both easy and fast, the amount of information is increasing by thousands of web pages daily, creating potentially better access for patients to more current and in-depth information. Simultaneously, this proliferation of information on the Internet can be difficult for searchers who must filter and evaluate more material in the quest for accurate and relevant information on a specific topic.

There are two primary types of organizational tools:

1. **Subject directories.** These directories may be referred to as indexes or libraries, and may be reviewed or rated.
2. **Search engines and metasearch engines**

The primary difference between subject directories and search engines is recall and relevancy. Recall is the process of gathering the total number of documents on a particular topic. Relevancy is the process of gathering relevant documents on a particular topic. The index of a search engine is created mechanically, and tends to provide more recall than relevancy. Subject directory indexes are created by humans, and tend to provide more relevancy in their retrieval than do search engines. It used to be easier to identify whether a tool was a search engine or a subject directory. Now, most indexing sites have both. Still, it is useful to know the difference to assess and evaluate the results of search retrieval (Figure 10.1).

SEARCH ENGINES

Search engines use mechanical software programs that visit web pages routinely. These programs collect data for each page in a huge data base, break down the content into an index organized by keywords, move on to follow links attached to the page, and then initiate the process again.

The success of a search depends on three factors: creating exact matches between terms searched and terms used in the documents you want to find; the size and contents of the data base; and its features for searching its contents successfully.

A complex search, with highly specific terms and multiple concepts, requires a search engine. Determining which search engine to use varies according to the nature of the question and the specific features needed to refine or focus your search. Every search engine is different and varies according to size of the data base, currency of data base, search features, and indexing components. To ensure a greater degree of reliability in search results, it is recommended that users become familiar with at least three general search engines with varying capacities and features, and replicate their searches in each of them. Examples of search engines are www.google.com, www.altavista.com, and search.msn.com. To learn more about search engines, go to Search Engine Watch at http://www.searchenginewatch.com/.

METASEARCH ENGINES

Metasearch engines send a search to several search engine databases simultaneously, retrieving a listing of top-ranked listings from each source. Because metasearch engines search multiple databases, they give a quick overview, and work best with simple, straightforward searches. They are most useful for finding needles in haystacks, or information that can be described by a distinctive word or name, but is also unlikely to be found in many resources. Examples are offered in Table 10.1.

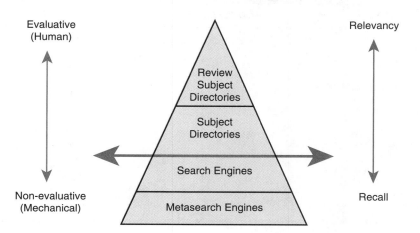

FIGURE 10.1 The search tool structure for the World Wide Web.

TABLE 10.1 Metasearch Engines

NAME	ADDRESS (URL)
Vivisimo	www.vivisimo.com/
EZ2WWW	www.ez2www.com/
Kartoo	www.kartoo.com/
Dogpile	www.dogpile.com
Mamma	www.mama.com
Fazzle	www.fazzle.com/
Ask Jeeves	www.ask.com
Metacrawler	www.metacrawler.com

For an updated list and detailed descriptions, go to Search Engine Watch at http://www.searchenginewatch.com/ and type "metasearch" into the search box.

SUBJECT DIRECTORIES

People organize websites into categories by subject content posted in subject directories, indexes, or electronic libraries. Although subject directories may begin with mechanical retrieval from a web search engine, they usually require some further filtering according to specific indexing schemes.

Subject directories can provide quick and easy access to primary, well-known sites on a particular topic. Subject directories give fewer results than search engines, often eliminating sites that refer to the subject in only a limited way.

Many health and medical related subject directories provide general overviews of health information and are good starting points to look for in-depth information. Many of these sites list links to medical information or handouts that are geared to patients and consumers.

REVIEW SUBJECT DIRECTORIES

A review subject directory further filters and refines a subject directory. Not only are listings on these websites indexed and displayed by subject, but they are frequently evaluated by specific criteria. For example, a review subject directory may rank sites according to the criteria of clinical applicability or appropriateness for use by a particular population of health providers or patients.

To obtain the best information on a topic, use a review subject directory of sites selected by a recognized authority on the given topic. Direct patients to a medical review subject directory because they are the most reliable method of assuring quality Internet information content on a general topic. The reviewers of these sites pay particular attention to identifying and verifying the accuracy of these sources of information. Table 10.2 presents examples of health and medical subject and review directories.

TABLE 10.2 Health and Medical Subject and Review Directories

NAME	ADDRESS (URL)	DESCRIPTION
Harden Meta Directory	www.lib.uiowa.edu/hardin/md	*Large listing of health sites selected for consistent connectivity.*
Health A–Z	www.healthAtoZ.com	*Consumer health site maintained by health professionals.*
HealthFinder	www.healthfinder.gov	*Produced by U.S. government—organized using lay language.*
Medhunt	www.hon.ch	*Sponsored by Health on the Net Foundation; targets information for patients, professionals, and physicians.*
MedicineNet	www.medicinenet.com	*Doctor-produced consumer health information.*
Omni	www.omni.ac.uk/	*Highly edited resources indexing medical information from the United Kingdom.*
Oncolink	www.oncolink.com	*Produced by the University of Pennsylvania Cancer Center; comprehensive listing of resources on cancer.*
Yahoo Health	www.dir.yahoo.com/health	*Popular listing of sites, plus chats and "ask an expert."*

PORTAL SITES OR PORTALS

Portal sites are a marriage of subject directory, search engine, newsreader, bulletin board, chat room, and even e-mail. Some of the best know portal sites are Yahoo's My Yahoo and Netscape's My Netscape. My Health-AtoZ is a recently developed health care–based portal site.

PROPRIETARY HEALTH INFORMATION DATA BASES

Many resources provide access to proprietary content information, or data bases. Although not technically part of the Internet or the web, they are accessible from a web browser and server. These data bases have a customer-friendly web browser interface, but their information is self-contained and is accessible only by use of an internal searching program or mechanism. These data bases are not accessible by general web search engines, and they use retrieval programs specific to their data base. These data bases are generally restricted for use by authorized subscribers who may or may not pay a fee for access. Examples include OVID and EBSCO.

Because each searching tool retrieves and displays data in a different way, each tool is useful for locating different types of information. The type of question should determine the type of site selected for finding information. The Noodle Tools website provides guidelines to help you choose the best search for your infor-

mation needs: http://www.noodletools.com/debbie/literacies/information/5locate/adviceengine.html

You may also refer to Table 10.3 for types of information needs that can best be met by a particular resource.

Searching for Internet Information Resources: Knowing How to Retrieve Information

The second step in the information retrieval process is to use the selected search tool effectively, by identifying the nature and scope of the information question, and specific techniques for retrieving information from each of the tools.

The searcher should start with an understanding of the types of information resources available on the Internet, and a general knowledge of which search tool can be used with each type of resource; then, plan a searching strategy. He should then think about the specific information needs and the most appropriate method to pursue answers.

When looking for information to give to a patient, consider the assessment of the learner's needs and abilities. This will help determine the type and format of information needed, and help to plan and develop a strategy for searching.

TABLE 10.3 Guide to Selecting Search Tools

INFORMATION NEED	INFORMATION TOOL
I want a broad overview of a topic.	Subject directory
I don't know where to begin to look for an obscure topic.	Metasearch engine
I have a complex search question that requires linking a number of concepts.	WWW search engines that permit Boolean searching
I want to meet/talk with people online.	Internet relay chat
I want to read discussions on current events.	News reader
I want a few relevant resources from sources I can trust.	Review subject directory
I want to find the e-mail address of a friend.	Database of people
I want to find information that occurred on a specific date.	WWW search engine that limits by date
I want to discuss professional issues with a small group of people in my field.	Monitored listserve
I want to locate information in another language.	WWW search engine that limits by language

The best way to get good results in an efficient way is to use a 10-step information retrieval process (Figure 10.2). Although this process is applicable to most queries on an Internet-based searching tool, it is easiest to understand this process in relation to searches conducted on a general web search engine. For that reason, the 10-step process is presented as it applies to a general purpose search engine, such as google.com. The clinical scenarios at the end of the chapter illustrate a sample search.

Step 1—Define the Problem Statement

The information retrieval process always begins with an information need, in response to an information problem, which is stated in the form of a single question. Although this may state the obvious, few people consciously and specifically define what it is they hope to find. Many people begin a search without realizing they are looking for answers to many interrelated questions. Some are better answered by one source than another. Some

have answers that build upon or redirect other questions. For example, a patient may ask a nurse for information that would help him or her understand a diabetes diagnosis better. Rather than searching on the single word diabetes, ask the patient about his or her information needs and add more details to the search statement based on the need to know about treatment, prognosis, genetic origins, or factors related to the patient's age, gender, or race.

Developing a good searching statement that translates into an effective machine-readable query involves defining these generalized information needs into a series of single, clear, and unambiguous statements.

Step 2—Identify Search Concepts

Once a single problem statement has been defined, it should be refined into discrete concepts. The user should clarify any ambiguity that may exist in each concept. For example, if seeking information on AIDS (acquired immunodeficiency syndrome), it should be determined if additional words or concepts in

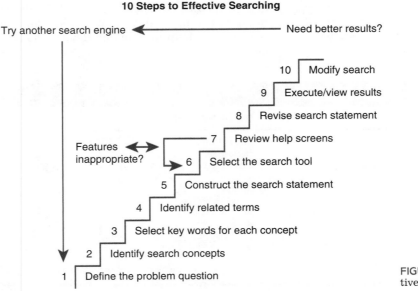

10 Steps to Effective Searching

Try another search engine ← ——————— Need better results?

10 | Modify search

9 | Execute/view results

8 | Revise search statement

7 | Review help screens

Features inappropriate? ↔

6 | Select the search tool

5 | Construct the search statement

4 | Identify related terms

3 | Select key words for each concept

2 | Identify search concepts

1 | Define the problem question

FIGURE 10.2 Ten steps to effective searching on the Internet.

a problem statement would help distinguish between the effects of human immunodeficiency virus (HIV), teaching aids, hearing aids, or nursing aids. Or, the user should ascertain: Is it more effective to use the term "drug therapy," or combine two separate concepts, "drug" and "therapy?" Word order may be significant in the interpretation of concepts. Concepts should be listed in order of their importance when defining the overall search statement.

Step 3 — Select Key Words for Each Concept

After determining the concepts that define the search statement, and placing them in order of importance, you should identify specific key words or phrases for each concept. A key word is a term that would most likely be used to name a particular concept in an index. When trying to identify a site that would discuss "childhood diseases" that occur "between birth and 6 years" should we select the key word child? Children? What about infant? Baby? Newborn? Preschooler? What about pediatric or pediatrics? Some health and medical sites will provide a browsable cross-referenced thesaurus of index terms (such as National Library of Medicine Medical Subject Headings). When in doubt about which key words to use, repeated efforts may be needed to locate the search terms most likely to return relevant results. To select alternative words, the fourth step in this process should be completed.

Step 4 — Identify Related Terms

After selecting the best key words, determine if synonyms or related terms exist that may be used by some search tools to define the concept. If initial attempts to apply the primary key words do not render quality results, substituting one or more synonyms or related terms into their search string may give better results. Many search tools allow truncation or wildcard symbols (see Step 7) to be used to retrieve words with a common root stem or words for which spelling is uncertain.

Step 5 — Construct the Search Statement

Once key words and related words have been selected, a search statement may be constructed that can be placed in a search window as a search string. Constructing the search statement consists of:

1. Selecting the key words (such as: diabetes, adolescence, drug therapy)
2. Ranking the key words according to priority and degree of relevance (such as: 1. diabetes, 2. drug therapy, 3. adolescence)
3. Grouping the key words systematically according to that search engine's principles of the logic (for example, using Boolean logic: diabetes AND drug therapy AND adolescence)

The traditional information retrieval algorithm used by search engines has been Boolean logic. Boolean logic uses the operators AND, OR, and NOT to combine terms and establish a relationship between terms. This system functions effectively in a database (such as Medline) when it is used within a limited data set that is indexed using a controlled vocabulary. One of the difficulties of understanding Boolean operators is that they are counterintuitive to the manner in which we usually use these terms. In general usage, the word OR is an excluder and the word AND is an includer (Figure 10.3).

Step 6 — Select the Search Tool

If a search statement has been defined carefully, it is relatively easy to decide what type of Internet tool should be queried to get the information you are looking for. If the statement is simple and comprised of one or two general key words, a subject directory is the best place to begin a search (see Table 10.2). Many of these subject listings also have search engines, which retrieve sites collected on the site directory based on key word

Boolean Operators

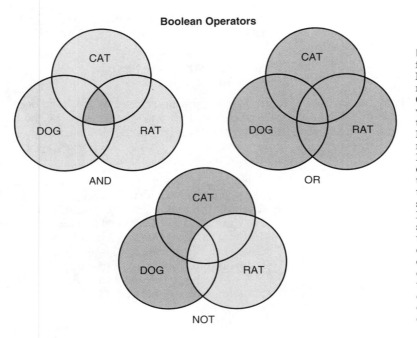

FIGURE 10.3 Boolean logic used for Internet search strings. The Boolean *OR* means one wants to retrieve *anything* on *either* cats OR dogs OR rats. In other words, a retrieval of *all* sites that contain *any* of those words. Boolean *AND* is not, as in natural language, an inclusive term. In Boolean logic the *AND* is an excluder. It requires that *only* those sites, that contain *all* of the terms (cats, dogs, and rats) should be in the retrieval. The Boolean operator *NOT* is a more selective excluder. It means those sites that include the specific search term should be eliminated from the retrieval. In other words, retrieval would be the set of all sites that include discussions of both cats and dogs, but not sites that also discussed rats.

searching. If a search is complex, requiring linking of multiple synonyms or concepts, a search engine would be required, such as Google.com.

Step 7—Review the Help or Tips Screen

A common mistake of novice searchers is to immediately apply the search statement they have created in Step 4 to the search engine they selected in Step 5 without reviewing the Help or Tips screen. Even the experienced searcher should review the Help screens frequently, because data base search tools evolve rapidly. Help screens give tips and strategies, accompanied by examples that reveal searching characteristics or capabilities that are unique to the specific search tool. Although subject directories and proprietary data bases generally have their own unique searching syntax, some elements are common to most of the primary web search engines (Box 10.1).

Step 8—Revise the Search Statement

Effective searching applies and executes the features and syntax rules that are specific to the individual search engine design. Having reviewed the help screens of the search tool selected for your query, and having noted particular features it uses to retrieve data sets, the searcher should return to the search statement created in Step 4 and revise it appropriately. It may even be appropriate, based on the nature of the search and the features provided by the search engine help screens, to return to Step 5 and select a different search engine.

Step 9—Execute Search and Review Results

Once the search has been executed, the results can be reviewed. Some worthwhile hits should occur within the first 10 sites listed in the retrieval. If this is not the case, the searcher should return to Step 6, review the

BOX 10.1 Common Search Engine Syntax Strategies

Use quotation marks around phrases or proper names of more than one word. Many search engines default to a Boolean OR. That means that if you type in "breast cancer," the search engine will interpret the statement as breast OR cancer, retrieving all of the sites that contain the word breast and include them with all the sites that contain the word cancer—regardless of what type or in what context. Placing quotation marks around the terms cues the search engine to search just for the occurrence of "breast cancer" as a phrase, with the terms taken together as a single concept.

Select search terms carefully and use the most uncommon and specific terms that will describe your topic. Common words produce many results. For example, if you were looking for information on how to prevent heart disease, instead of searching on the terms heart and disease and prevention, searching with the phrase "low-cholesterol diets" would retrieve more specific results. The more terms you can combine to describe the topic, the more restricted the search results will be.

Many search engines use characters as substitutes for the Boolean operators. Substitute a plus sign (+) for the Boolean operator AND. Substitute a minus sign (-) for the Boolean AND NOT.

Use nesting when using multiple Boolean operators. Search engines that permit long Boolean strings sometimes permit the use of ( ) parentheses to indicate "nesting," which instructs the search engine to conduct certain Boolean operations before others.

Use capitalization if words normally are capitalized in texts.

Truncation and Wildcards. Most search engines allow the use of a special character (usually an asterisk *) to search for words that have the same prefix. For example, by typing in "inform*" you can retrieve websites containing the word "informatics," "information," and others. Questions about correct spellings of words can sometimes be resolved by placing wildcard characters (such as a # or ? sign) in the center of word to retrieve all possible spellings. For example, searching for a proper name G###er would retrieve Gunter, Garner, Grover, and others.

searching tips again, revise the search statement, and execute the search again. If the search fails again to retrieve the desired results, return to Step 5 and follow the process through the remaining steps with another search engine.

Step 10—Modify Search or Execute Search in Another Database

No two search engines will ever retrieve identical data sets because they differ in search mechanics, which sites they have indexed, and the currency of the indexing. If first efforts do not provide the desired answer, or more good hits are needed, the searcher may return to

Step 5 and replicate the search in another search engine. The searcher should learn the features and syntax commands of three search engines well, and use these first for a search. Examples include www.google.com, www.hotbot.com, and www.altavista.com. The searcher may expand to other search engines after becoming familiar with, and monitoring, the changes of the original three.

Evaluating Internet Resources: Knowing What Information Is Appropriate

A listing of Internet resources that may answer a specific query has now been generated. Many of these resources are reliable and authoritative. Others are biased, inaccurate, and may even be deliberately misleading. This bias could provide the opportunity for misinformation, potentially causing harm to those who are using the Internet to locate health and medical information. All Internet users must become adept at critically evaluating the quality of information retrieved. How can a discriminating information searcher identify good content?

Many groups are committed to help both health care providers and consumers determine the quality of Internet information (Risk & Dzenowagis, 2001). These include:

eHealth Code of Ethics:
    www.ihealthcoalition.org/ethics/ethics.html
HON Code: www.hon.ch
American Medical Association (AMA):
    http://www.medem.com
The Health Summit Working Group:
    http://hitiweb.mitretek.org/iq/default.asp

Criteria for Evaluation

CREDIBILITY

Because websites are not filtered before they are published, the most important factor in evaluating the quality of the information on the Internet is determining the credibility of sources of medical information. Who publishes this site? What are the credentials for publishing the information? Are medically trained and qualified professionals writing or reviewing the content? Or is it written by a non-medically qualified individual or organization? Are they providing information or advice that is beyond the scope of their expertise? Who sponsors the information? Who reviews the content? Are clear references to source data provided, with specific HTML links to that data? Is the date of last modification posted?

A quality website displays the name and biographical information of all authors. It also includes the names and qualifications of the sponsoring organization and criteria for publication. The relationship of the author(s) to the sponsoring organization should be clear, to help the user determine motivation of sponsors and potential conflicts of interest.

When was the information originally published? When was it last updated? How relevant is the currency of the material to the topic being discussed? Due to rapid advancements, drug information should be current. Currency is less important for enduring content, such as anatomy information.

CONTENT

How accurate is the information on the site? Is it replicated in other resources in other media? Can the facts be checked for accuracy? Does the site provide links or references for these resources? Are clear distinctions made between clinical or scientific evidence and conjecture or personal testimonials? How well is the topic covered? Does the site claim to provide comprehensive coverage of a subject, but then fail to do so? Who is the intended audience of the site? Is the content clearly written? Does the site provide a disclaimer that describes the limitations of information on the site? All quality medical sites should provide a disclaimer that the material provided is for general information only, and that advice of a physician should be sought for authoritative information that relates to their specific issue.

DISCLOSURE

Is the mission and purpose of the site clearly stated? Is the material free from bias? Does it promote a particular position that casts doubt on the objectivity of the material? Does the site disclose identities of commercial and noncommercial organizations that have contributed funding, services, or material? If advertising is a source of funding it will be clearly stated, and the advertising policy will be displayed on the site. Can you clearly tell the difference between the informational material and advertising and other promotional material? If a site requires registration or other forms of collecting personal data about the site visitor, are the purposes for that information disclosed? Do statements attest to the confidentiality of information gathered in this fashion or does the site designate the manner in which the data will be used?

LINKS

Links are extensions of the original site, and therefore should be analyzed for their value in supporting the viewpoint demonstrated on the original sites. Do the links relate to the purpose and content of the site? Are criteria for links established and clear, supporting the content of the site? Are links described or annotated so viewers will have some idea of the nature of the linked site before following the link? Is it easy to navigate back and forth between links? Are site links maintained without a lot of dead links or links to outdated resources? Is the person or persons responsible for link selection identified and are methods of contacting them provided?

DESIGN

The ability to access information from a website is tightly tied to the arrangement of information. Design and layout of the site do not determine the quality of the content, but they affect the ability to access the content. Does the design facilitate the delivery of content and not distract from it? Is it easy to navigate? Does the overall design contribute to the purpose of the site in terms of balance in graphics, text, and multimedia elements? Do all pages within the site refer to the primary pages so users can clearly identify the source of information? Is the site organized effectively and does it reflect a logical structure? Does the page load quickly? Does the site meet the technical and equipment needs of most intended users? Is there an internal search engine to help users locate specific information without browsing through many pages? Is there a site map? Are links off the page described or annotated?

INTERACTIVITY

Is contact information provided for visitors who seek further information or support? Is the webmaster's e-mail address posted? This contributes to the site's authority, accessibility, and scope. Can users customize the content or features they view? If so, are methods used to profile the person clearly delineated? Are there options for use by people with hearing or seeing disabilities, viewers with low literacy levels, or foreign language users? Does the site provide a mechanism for an exchange of information between site viewers, such as discussion groups, forums, or chat rooms?

Evaluation at a Glance

A quick review of three components of every web page—the header, body, and footer—can help the user evaluate the quality of the site. The header usually provides the logo or link to the institution creating the information and to any sponsoring organization. Opportunities for interactivity also should be clearly visible somewhere near the top of the document, such as a search engine, e-mail, chat, or discussion links. The footer of the document generally provides information on the content author, the contact person for questions, the website designer, and date of creation or revision of the document, and any disclaimer for the scope of the material. A cursory review of the body of the document should clearly identify its intended audience and the purpose of the site, and testify to the balance and appeal of its layout, organizational quality, and navigability.

A structured way to check for quality is to use the IQ: the Health Information Quality Assessment Tool (http://hitiweb.mitretek.org/iq/begguide.asp). This interactive tool, developed by the Health Summit Working Group, helps you assess a website you choose.

Evaluating Materials for Patients

Clearly, information health care providers give to patients needs to be accurate and current, and produced by a reputable resource. The next step is to return to the assessment of the learner's needs and abilities. What does the learner need to know?

What does the learner want to know? Does this material contain that content? Can this learner understand this material, and apply it? Apply the Suitability Assessment of Materials (SAM) tool to evaluate the material (see Chapter 9).

One advantage of content downloaded from the Internet is the size of the type can be adjusted to the needs of the reader. A patient with visual impairment may need information to be presented in a 16-point typeface or larger. Information can be made larger on screen with a zoom in feature, available on toolbars of either web browsers or PDF readers.

Some learners may need an illustration to best understand a concept. One way to find this is to go to Google.com and, above the box for your search term, click on "Images" instead of "Web." For example, enter the word "swallowing" to get a number of anatomical illustrations.

Some learners may need audio or video clips to better understand the content. One way to search for audio or video clips is to enter into the search engine your search term with "AND audio" or AND video." For example, go to Google.com and enter "colonoscopy AND video." See Table 10.4 for more sites of interest.

TABLE 10.4. Sites for Patient Education Information

NAME	ADDRESS (URL)	DESCRIPTION
AAFP—Health information for patients	www.familydoctor.org	Includes self-care flowcharts, and education resources by topic.
Drug reference center	www.nursespdr.com/	Complete monographs on drugs.
Health A–Z	www.healthAtoZ.com	Consumer health site maintained by health professionals.
HealthFinder	www.healthfinder.gov	Produced by U.S. government, provides fact sheets.
HealthTouch	www.healthtouch.com	Single-page patient education documents from professional organizations.
HealthWeb	www.healthweb.org	Strong emphasis on full text educational materials.
Intelihealth	www.intelihealth.com/IH/	Topical information by experts at Harvard.
Kid's Health	www.kidshealth.org	
Lab Tests Online	www.labtestsonline.org	
Mayo Clinic Health Watch	www.mayoclinic.com	Topical new items, experts.
MedicineNet	www.medicinenet.com	Doctor-produced consumer health information.
Medline Plus	www.medlineplus.gov/	Health information from the National Library of Medicine. Links to medical dictionaries.
Merck manual online	www.merck.com/pubs/	Full-text of the 1992 manual online.
Netwellness	www.netwellness.com	Links to clinical trials, physician referrals, and online textbooks.
NIDDK Digestive and diabetes disease briefs	www.niddk.nih.gov/health/health.htm	High quality fact sheets produced by National Institutes of Health.
NOAH	www.noah-health.org	Material in Spanish. Strong mental health focus.
OSU patient education materials	http://medicalcenter.osu.edu/referringphysicians/patienteducation.cfm	Well-formatted teaching guides.
RxList	rxlist.com	Searchable database of drug information.
Virtual Hospital	http://www.vh.org/	Produced by the University of Iowa, containing textbooks and booklets for health care providers and patients.
WebMD	my.webmd.com/webmd_today/home/default	Physicians and journalists provide health information.

USING THE INFORMATION RETRIEVAL PROCESS TO MEET PATIENT NEEDS

To most effectively and efficiently use the Internet for teaching patients:

1. Develop a general road map of the Internet so learners can locate resources on a specific topic.
2. Use the 10-step searching plan and techniques for narrowing down resources to specific, relevant educational materials.
3. Review and evaluate materials review to assess the quality of the resource in terms that are specific to the patient's educational need.

Health care providers can use the Internet and the information retrieval process to

- expand their knowledge about a specific condition or treatment
- retrieve materials to integrate into teaching, or
- help the patient use the Internet to self-educate.

So far this chapter has focused on finding quality information. The Internet can also be used to direct patient education. For learners who are physically and mentally able to use computers, the Internet can enhance motivation and provide a participative learning environment. For example, a patient may need some additional information, facts, or concepts that can broaden an understanding of his or her health situation and contribute to a change in behavior. Many Internet sites contain brief, easy to read or print, factual information that describes, in language appropriate to the patient, particular concepts related to symptoms, disorder, or treatment.

The Internet can be a source of fact sheets, articles, illustrations, animations, video demonstrations, discussion groups, and interactive activities for health promotion. Through these, it can be a tool to increase knowledge, reinforce skills, change attitudes, and support healthy practices.

Although skills are learned through doing, the Internet can reinforce teaching of home care skills. A website may offer step-by-step directions, perhaps with illustrations, audio, or video to further describe a specific activity. The learner can use materials from the Internet as often as needed.

The Internet can help patients shape healthy attitudes toward their illness or treatment through Internet discussions or chat groups with persons who have similar health problems. These resources can help patients and their families cope with the changes brought on by illness and reinforce desired belief systems.

Three factors determine how the Internet is used in patient education, and how much it is used:

1. **Technological access factors.** These include features and location of the computer, the quality and stability of the Internet connection, and the amount of time the instructor or patient can use the equipment.
2. **Technological competency factors.** These include the computer and Internet literacy level of the instructor and learner, and the comfort level each has using them in the education process.
3. **Physical and emotional factors.** These include physical limitations (such as pain and fatigue; visual, audio, neurological, and motion deficiencies) and emotional limitations (such as depression, anxiety).

Many of the technological barriers to Internet use can be overcome with a little effort and perseverance, and competency can be improved with practice, and by using tutorials. It takes little dexterity (and only a little practice) to move a mouse or to type on a keyboard, and with time and patience, most patients can achieve these skills.

Many of the physical problems associated with computer use can be overcome with simple adjustments. Computers can be an especially appropriate medium for patients who have difficulty seeing or hearing other mediums of instruction. Text on computers can be configured to up to 72-point typeface to allow for reading by people with vision problems. Headphones can be attached and audio files can be made loud enough to be understood by patients with hearing problems. Special software can read the text aloud. A computer with an Internet connection may be the tool that pulls a depressed or anxious patient out of self-involvement, encouraging interaction and providing distraction, a sense of competency, and hope.

When a patient cannot access the Internet directly, the health care provider can print appropriate information and provide it to the patient. Caution should be exercised when downloading or printing information off the Internet to comply with copyright restrictions. Many sites specify restrictions, such as giving permission to print one copy to give a patient. For additional information on electronic copyright, see the Library of Congress Copyright Office site at http://www.loc.gov/copyright/.

The Internet can be used many ways in the patient education process. The following three case studies suggest ways to apply the information retrieval process to clinical practice.

CASE STUDY 10.1

SELF-DIRECTED LEARNING

A 45-year-old woman has been taking Prozac for 6 months to alleviate the symptoms of depression. She has experienced some mild side effects from the drug. Friends have told her that St. John's Wort is an effective, natural alternative treatment for mild depression. After the patient consults her physician, she asks the nurse educator for help to learn more about St. John's Wort. The patient says she wants to (1) talk to other people who used the product and see what kind of reaction they have had, (2) determine if any studies (preferably clinical trials) have been conducted on St. John's Wort, and (3) determine if any information on the Internet compares the effectiveness of Prozac and St. John's Wort.

STRATEGIES
What can the nurse do?

Strategy 1. The nurse determines that the information for query 1 is most likely in discussion groups, listserves, and newsgroups. A search of St. John's Wort in the Google Groups search engine (http://groups.google.com/) reveals at least 10 groups, including alt.support.depression.manic.moderated, sci.psychology.psychotherapy, and alt.support.depression. The nurse suggests to the patient she can read some of the discussions on those newsgroups, and post her questions on one. The nurse also suggests the patient can use that site to make connections with others who currently use St. John's Wort.

Strategy 2. The nurse determines that the information for query 2 is most likely in an authoritative proprietary data base of peer-reviewed medical journals, such as Medline. The nurse has two medical sites already bookmarked, Ovid and PubMed. The nurse goes to the PubMed site (http://www.ncbi.nih.gov/entrez/query.fcgi) and reads instructions about using search terms. (PubMed basic search uses natural language queries.) The nurse types in "St. John's Wort clinical trials" and retrieves references to 124 articles that match this topic. The nurse browses several abstracts and finds a recently published article on a double-blind, placebo-controlled trial to test the efficacy of St. John's Wort for depression, and a review of the evidence-based literature on St. John's Wort. She asks her hospital's medical librarian to order both articles.

Strategy 3. The nurse uses the 10-step plan to search the Internet for information that compares the effectiveness of Prozac and St. John's Wort for depression.

Step 1. Are there any studies that compare the effectiveness of St. John's Wort and Prozac as a treatment for depression?

Step 2. Depression, St. John's Wort, Prozac. Comparison, effectiveness, treatment.

Step 3. Because the words comparison and effectiveness are likely to generate many irrelevant hits, it would be better to restrict the keywords to depression, St. John's Wort, Prozac and treatment and add the other terms only if needed and only if conducting the search in a database that uses subsearching.

Step 4. Begin by asking if there are generic words for Prozac or medical terms for St. John's Wort? If not, are there additional terms that could be used for depression (such as major depression, depressive disorder, bipolar)? Would it be better to search for the concept "drug therapy" rather than treatment? Do you need to account for possible alternative spellings, such as Saint for St.? Should you use a truncation symbol on the term treatment (ie, treatmen*) to retrieve the singular and plural forms of the word?

Step 5. Because many concepts will require combining, it might be useful to use a complex Boolean operation algorithm to ensure the proper relationship of terms. For example, a search statement that captures most of the elements in Step 5 may look like:

Depression AND Prozac AND ("St. John's Wort" OR "Saint John's Wort") AND ("drug therapy" OR treatmen*)

Step 6. Because this is a complex Boolean search, her first attempt in the search was in AltaVista Advanced Search (www.altavista.com). AltaVista also allows you to limit the search by a date range; given that St. John's Wort has received a lot of news coverage recently, this could be a helpful feature. AltaVista also provides ranking of results by selected keywords; the nurse may want to select the term Prozac as the most unique identifier and have those results ranked first.

Step 7. After reading the advanced tips screen on the AltaVista page, the nurse notes that all of the parameters used in the search, Boolean operators, phrase searching, and nesting are available, although you see no mention of truncation. The Help screens also tell you how to enter the date range.

Step 8. The search appears to be formulated correctly according to the help screens, so we need not reuse the search strategy for this example.

Step 9. The nurse executes the search and gets no results, and AltaVista suggests:

- Check your spelling.
- Try different or fewer keywords.
- Remove quotation marks or plus signs.

The nurse builds the query without Boolean operators, in the Advanced Web Search section:

all of these words: depression Prozac
this exact phrase: John's Wort
any of these words: drug therapy treatment
and gets 4,913 results.

Step 10. The nurse knows HotBot uses
Boolean operators, and tries her original search at www.hotbot.com. She
gets 198 hits.

CASE STUDY 10.2

WORKING WITH CHILDREN AND ADOLESCENTS

A nurse is working with a 12-year-old
boy who has recently been diagnosed
with insulin-dependent diabetes. He is
active in sports and is the captain of his
soccer team. He generally feels good,
so it is difficult for him to take his illness seriously. He admits to skipping his
medication sometimes, and not being
careful about his diet. The nurse and
the patient's mother would like the boy
to take more interest and responsibility
for monitoring his illness. The nurse
knows the family has a computer in
their living room, which he uses to play
games and to chat with a group of his
close friends.

STRATEGIES
What can the nurse do?
The Internet is an especially valuable
tool for educating children and adolescents because of its multimedia components and interactivity. By making
learning fun and interesting, educators
can frequently get children and adolescents to overcome anxieties about a
health issue and participate more fully
in their own health care. The nurse can:

1. Develop an Internet searching strategy to retrieve information on children and diabetes.
2. Discover a site titled "Children with
Diabetes" and begin to explore related links.
3. By clicking on a hypertext link titled
food links on the main page, discover an animated food pyramid that
can help the patient learn more
about the kinds and amounts of
food he should eat. He can even
download a full-color food pyramid
that he can hang on his wall to help
him remember food groups.
4. Explore some links to software,
read the reviews, and determine if
any free shareware computer programs can help with tracking medication and food. The patient finds
one he can download and install. He
is excited at the thought of using
software to monitor the changes in
his glucose level and is eager to try
it.
5. Explore additional links and learn
about many diabetes summer camps
where he can go to learn more about
his illness. The patient seems both
surprised and eager to ask his parents if he could go to a camp outside his home state.
6. Discover an online chat room. The
nurse and patient find that enter-
tainer Alan Thicke, father of a child
with diabetes, is currently online discussing diabetes.
7. Discover a link to the American
Association of Diabetic Educators.
The nurse finds some interesting
audiovisual materials to order that
will help the patient and other young
patients with diabetes take more
control of their illness.

CASE STUDY 10.3

WORKING WITH FAMILIES

A nurse enters the room of a young woman who has recently undergone a radical mastectomy for breast cancer. The woman is single, and her closest relative and primary caretaker is her younger sister. Although the patient is sleeping comfortably, the nurse finds the sister crying by the patient's bedside. The nurse asks if she can help, and the sister seems eager to talk. The sister confesses that although she feels comfortable about the clinical decisions and quality of care her sister is getting, she is worried about her own ability to adequately care for the patient during her illness. The patient will be living with the sister during chemotherapy, and the sister is not sure how to respond to the needs of the patient or how to help her own family (she has two young children) understand what is happening to their aunt. The sister also expresses some concern about her own potential risk of developing breast cancer.

STRATEGIES

What can the nurse do?

1. The nurse has a list of resources on major medical topics. This list has been reviewed and evaluated according to the seven criteria of quality. The nurse opens her bookmark listings under cancer and clicks on Oncolink (http://www.oncolink.upenn.edu/). Oncolink is a major resource for cancer topics, has been a long-standing site of good reputation, and is sponsored by the University of Pennsylvania Cancer Center.
2. The nurse notices immediately a hypertext link titled "Coping With Cancer," which leads to another page of resources titled "Caregivers."
3. The nurse clicks on a link that enables the patient's sister to join a caregiver listserv.
4. Also, a link to a "Hospice/Homecare Family Caregiver Cancer Education Program," with fourteen modules of step-by-step instructions related to caring for a cancer patient. The nurse prints out the first page, with the link (http://www.oncolink.upenn.edu/books/books.cfm?b=22) so the sister can access it from home, and read sections as she needs the information.

The nurse checks another bookmarked link, the National Cancer Institute (http://www.nci.nih.gov/). She finds information that delineates the risk factors and screening procedures for estimating the likelihood of breast cancer. She also finds, on this site, an interactive Breast Cancer Risk Assessment Tool, which can help the patient's sister understand her risk for breast cancer.

SUMMARY

The Internet is a vast publishing medium that provides a unique opportunity for communication, information dispersal, and education. Its continued global growth both in total numbers of users and frequency of use has ensured continued commercial development for some time to come. As technologies develop that enable computer equipment to increase in performance and decrease in cost, accessibility to much relevant and customized information will increase. A primary target for Internet development is the professional health provider and the consumer health markets. As security systems are enhanced and computerized patient records become more commonplace, data and order entry will increasingly be delivered electronically at the point of care. Patient records will be integrated with links to the medical literature, pharmaceutical information, clinical decision-making tools, patient education handouts, and brief continuing education opportunities for a provider who needs to be updated to the most recent information related to his or her patient's disease, treatment, or procedure.

Patient information will increase both in quantity and formats, with an emphasis on multimedia delivery. It will become easier to customize information and accommodate the learning styles and educational assessment profile of each person. New hardware and software development will enhance and increase the opportunities for self-directed learning by both provider and patient, ultimately resulting in improved health outcomes. To prepare for the acceleration of technology-based and Internet-accessible learning, health care providers must develop skills that integrate information technology into daily practice routines. They must adopt an attitude toward computerized educational technology that is open, flexible, and adaptable. Health care providers must become discriminating information searchers, qualified information intermediaries, committed to lifelong learning.

The ability of computers to store and organize large quantities of information makes them a very useful tool for identifying the impact of specific interventions. This leads us to the next chapter, evaluating patient education outcomes.

STRATEGIES FOR CRITICAL ANALYSIS AND APPLICATION

1. Discuss when the Internet is an appropriate vehicle for answering health-related questions, and when it is not.
2. Develop an Internet searching strategy for locating and compiling a reference list of evidence-based complementary and alternative medicine therapies.
3. Outline and develop a plan for using the Internet and an interpreter to help a mother who speaks only French understand the health issues of her child who has been diagnosed with sickle cell anemia, and how she can be involved with the child's care.
4. A young patient suffering from partial paralysis from stroke is confined to a wheelchair. The patient has sufficient dexterity to manage a computer keyboard and wants to communicate with other patients who have had strokes. Develop a plan for helping him or her access support groups, listserves, and Usenet resources.
5. Apply the 10-step search planning and implementation process to locate educational and self-help resources for non-English-speaking patients.

To find the latest information

Key search terms

listserve, listserv, search engines, metasearch engines, patient education resources, health education

Websites

- Patient Education Network (PatEdNet): http://www.med.utah.edu/pated/patednet/
- Web Searching Tips: http://www.searchenginewatch.com/facts/index.php

REFERENCES

Anderson, J. G. (2001). *How the Internet is transforming the physician–patient relationship.* Retrieved July 18, 2004, from www.medscape.com/viewarticle/415047_print

Berland, G. K., Elliott, M. N., Morales, L. S., Algazy, J. I., Kravitz, R. L., Broder, M. S., et al. (2001). Health information on the Internet: Accessibility, quality, and readability in English and Spanish. *JAMA, 285*(20), 2612–2621, 2655–2616.

Healthcare Information and Management Systems Society. (2002). *2002 HIMSS/AstraZeneca Clinician Survey.* Retrieved July 18, 2004, from www.himss.org/

Howe, W. (2001). *A brief history of the Internet*. Retrieved July 20, 2003, from http://www.walthowe.com/navnet/history.html

Nicoll, L. H. (2002). Patient education in the Internet era. *CIN: Computers, Informatics, Nursing, 20*(6), 215–216.

Redwood, H. (2002). *Patient education: The end of one-way traffic*. Retrieved April 21, 2003, from http://www.healthandage.com/PHome?gm=2&gid2=1992&fa=1&path=null&x=72&y=2

Risk, A., & Dzenowagis, J. (2001). Review of Internet health information quality initiatives. *Journal of Medical Internet Research, 3*(4), e28.

Tokarski, C. (2002). *Physicians urged to collaborate with patients who use Internet for health information*. Retrieved February 28, 2003, from www.medscape.com/viewarticle/446272_print

Evaluating Patient Education Outcomes

LEARNING OBJECTIVES

After reading this chapter, the student should be able to:

1. Describe how evaluation and documentation of learning can be integrated into patient care.

2. Identify four levels of evaluation, and provide examples of patient learning outcomes that can be identified in each level.

3. Discuss how the problem-oriented record (POR) can be used to encourage interdisciplinary collaboration.

4. List 10 patient education mistakes that can have a negative impact on outcomes, and how they can be avoided.

INTRODUCTION: ASSESSING OUTCOMES

It is clear from practice that the instructed patient fares better than the uninstructed one. However, health care providers do not consistently evaluate patient education outcomes. Although evaluation is an essential component of the patient education process, it is often misunderstood and neglected. Why do health care providers so often neglect evaluating patient education and sharing their progress through documentation?

To evaluate means to determine the "significance of" or "worth of" by careful appraisal or study. Both health care providers and patients may feel threatened by the thought of evaluation. Some may worry about being personally devalued or judged unworthy. Some may recall the humiliation of failing a test, and may not want to feel that way again. Some may fear that if they fail to achieve what others expect of them, they will lose love, support, assistance, esteem, and credibility.

The purpose of evaluation is to measure the results of care, to define specific outcomes, and to redirect patient care. It is not intended to place a value or a worth on patients or health care providers. Outcomes must be measured to assess the cost, quality, and effectiveness of care and organizational performance.

Patient education can be evaluated at many levels and many stages. The degree of success of patient education with a specific patient and family can be measured at four different stages in the process:

1. during the intervention
2. performance after learning
3. performance at home
4. overall self-care and maintenance

The degree of success of patient education can also be measured at the program level, at each of these four stages. Strategies for evaluating organizational and community programs are discussed in Chapters 12 and 13.

Before teaching begins, the goals and measurable objectives of teaching are defined. At evaluation, the health care provider determines if these measurable objectives have been met. In doing so, the health care team can determine if the patient has the self-care skills and appropriate resources for continuing care to be safely discharged.

The patient education process is a continuous loop of assessment, goal setting, intervention, and evaluation (Figure 11.1). As learning needs change, so do goals and interventions. Evaluation links to assessment, and the process continues. Evaluation is not an end point; it measures progress. If the patient did not meet the goal, it is important to determine why not, to decide how to better individualize the intervention.

This chapter defines evaluation, addresses methods of data collection, and discusses how to use the information from the evaluation process to reinforce learning and to plan future learning opportunities for individual patients and their families. This chapter also addresses documentation because the patient's record should reflect what the patient knows, understands, or performs.

SCOPE OF EVALUATION

Evaluation is closely related to assessment. Both involve formulating criteria or questions, gathering and categorizing data, and writing a summary statement. These findings are used in patient care planning. Assessment usually refers to building a data base that includes nursing diagnoses and outlines the patient's needs or problems. Evaluation is essentially the follow-up assessment that is continuously conducted as nursing interventions are performed. Therefore, evaluation occurs throughout the learning activities and is used to assess the patient's progress toward meeting learning objectives.

When learning goals are not constructed through collaboration, but imposed on the learner by the health care team, they are often not met. For example, a staff nurse from an outpatient clinic in the Boston area shared this experience:

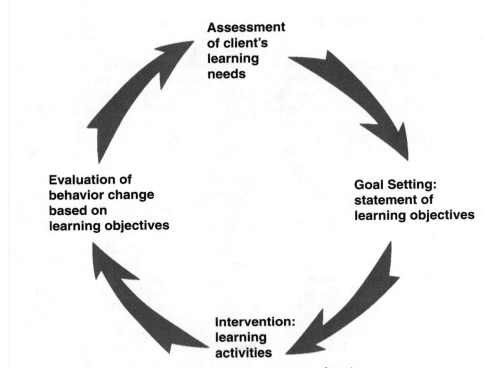

Assessment of client's learning needs

Goal Setting: statement of learning objectives

Intervention: learning activities

Evaluation of behavior change based on learning objectives

FIGURE 11.1 Evaluation is part of a continuous process in patient education.

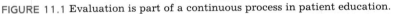

There are numerous barriers when educating a patient with HIV/AIDS. One of the more pronounced barriers I have encountered in my career is when the nurse recognizes the need for a patient to change behaviors, but the patient does not agree to this goal. A person with HIV/AIDS has a great responsibility to society to slow the rate of transmission of this virus. We can facilitate education, provide information, and make recommendations for a healthy lifestyle, but the ultimate responsibility is the patient's. The educator is further challenged when the patient is an active injection drug user, or when the patient has expressed a loss of hope for the future. Instilling that hope and setting individualized goals with patients is the first step in overcoming barriers to patient education and ultimately changing behaviors.

Evaluation is conducted using the behavioral objectives discussed in Chapter 8. Behaviorally defined objectives clearly describe what to evaluate and how to evaluate it. The active participation starts when the patient and family collaborate to identify the learning objectives. They define what is expected, participate in learning activities, and seek feedback to direct performance. Now they are active participants in evaluating learning.

The adult learner needs to be involved in the process, from deciding the goals, defining the desired outcomes, and learning the skills to reach those outcomes. Confidence alone is not enough to change behaviors. Providing information alone does not change behaviors, either. But when combined, when the learner has self-efficacy, knowledge, and skills, behaviors can change to improve health outcomes.

The process of self-evaluation can increase the learner's recognition of progress and accomplishments. Positive feedback and support from others reinforces this sense of success.

Evaluation is also a learning opportunity for the teacher. The progress or lack of progress made tells the teacher if the approach needs to be modified, or if other teaching strategies should be used. Were the objectives clear? Were important factors missed in the assessment? Were the teaching methods appropriate? Was more review needed?

Both the learner and teacher benefit from feedback that reinforces success and identifies problems. At times evaluation is conducted in a formal manner, using oral feedback and documenting outcomes in writing. This may be done when other information is updated in the chart, after classes or skills training, and before a patient's discharge from the hospital or outpatient office. Just as the assessment process involves asking questions to gather specific information, so does the evaluation process. The evaluation process should include:

- Measuring how well the patient met the learning objectives.
- Indicating needs to clarify, correct, or review information.
- Noting learning objectives that are unclear to the patient, family, or health care providers.
- Pointing out shortcomings in the teaching interventions, specifically addressing content, format, activities, and media.
- Identifying how teaching could have been better individualized to improve outcomes.

It is the patient educator's responsibility to:

- initiate the evaluation
- summarize the findings
- communicate findings to the rest of the health care team through documentation in the patient record
- give constructive feedback to the patient and family

- plan future experiences to reinforce learning
- design learning opportunities to foster behaviors that were not initially accomplished

The teacher must understand each component of the patient education process, and know what questions to ask. Evaluation is the time to measure behavior, look critically at patient care, and identify problems that have prevented learning.

THE FOUR LEVELS OF PATIENT LEARNING OUTCOMES

The guidelines of the Joint Commission on the Accreditation of Healthcare Organizations emphasize the need for evidence of patient learning outcomes (Joint Commission on Accreditation of Healthcare Organizations, 2003). The standards support setting realistic goals that are appropriate to length of stay. They do, however, expect teaching to be individualized to each learner's needs.

Measuring learning outcomes can be accomplished in any setting, even if the patient is there only a matter of minutes. Learning can be evaluated at four different levels, with each successive level representing a more precise measure of the effectiveness of teaching (Winfrey, 2003). Evaluation at each level is provided with the response to a single question. The four questions are: "Did they like it? Did they learn it? Did they use it? Was teaching worth it in the long run?" Box 11.1 provides a summary of these four levels of evaluation.

Level A: Patient and Family Involvement During Interventions

As the teaching intervention is implemented, the teacher evaluates the involvement of the learners. Are the learners willing to

BOX 11.1 The Four Levels of Evaluation

Level A: Patient and family involvement during interventions
Question: Did they like it?
When: Immediate, at the time of the intervention
What it measures: reactions, feelings, perceptions, satisfaction
About: content, teaching tools, environment, teaching style

Level B: Patient performance immediately after learning experience
Question: Did they learn it?
When: Right after learning
What it measures: skills, knowledge, attitudes
About: progress made toward meeting learning objectives

Level C: Patient performance at home
Question: Did they use it?
When: At home, away from the health care setting

What it measures: remembering and applying knowledge in home setting
About: Changes in behaviors, whether new knowledge and skills are applied, whether opinions and attitudes are changed

Level D: Patient's overall self-care and health management
Question: Was teaching worth it in the long run?
When: Over 1 year later
What it measures: impact, improvement in health care outcomes
About: improved quality of self-care, maintaining health

Resources: Winfrey, E. C. (2003). Kirkpatrick's Four Levels of Evaluation. Retrieved July 27, 2003, from http://coe.sdsu.edu/eet/Articles/k4levels/index.htm and Clementz, A. R. (July 22, 2002). Program Level Evaluation: Using Kirkpatrick's Four Levels of Evaluation to Conduct Systemic Evaluation of Undergraduate College Programs. Retrieved July 27, 2003, from web.bryant.edu/~facdev/Program%20Level%20Evaluation.doc

assume responsibility for learning? Do the learners seem alert and interested? Did the learners know what they were expected to do, and why? Do the learners understand instructions? Do they ask questions? Are learning experiences relevant to the patient's unique situation? Is teaching individualized to account for the culture and beliefs of the learners? Do the learners participate in discussion, demonstrations, and problem solving? Were concepts too basic? Or did the learner feel overloaded and overwhelmed by the amount of instruction and information? What are their reactions, feelings, perceptions, and satisfaction with the process? Do they like it? How did the family participate?

Level A measures the teacher's ability to individualize teaching to the learner's needs and readiness to learn. It is a great challenge

to counsel patients during the initial shock of an illness or disability, help them accept it, and encourage them to focus on how they will live their lives in the future. It is important to share with the health care team interventions and evaluation of the patient's responses related to this counseling. The level of involvement of the learners at this stage determines, to a great degree, the potential for success at subsequent levels of evaluation.

Level B: Patient Performance Immediately After Learning Experience

Immediately after teaching, the following questions should be asked: Did they learn it? Did the learners acquire the skills, knowledge, attitudes identified in the objectives? To what extent did the learners meet objectives?

It is more relevant to document the learner's performance, rather than what was taught. Outcomes should reflect knowledge and ability to participate in self-care. You do not know if learning took place until you evaluate learner comprehension and recall. Overlooking this step is a missed opportunity that may have important clinical implications (Schillinger et al., 2003). The evaluation at this level determines the effectiveness of an intervention, and what and how to teach next. This is especially important in situations vulnerable to miscommunication, as when the learner has poor health literacy skills, or speaks a language different from the teacher (Dreger & Tremback, 2002). Return demonstration and teaching back are essential evaluation methods that should be used after every teaching session. Chapter 3 discusses how to optimize use of an interpreter to ensure learning took place.

Level C: Patient Performance at Home

This third level of evaluation of learning occurs after the learners leave the health care setting. Did the learners remember and apply knowledge in the home? Did they use it? Did behaviors change? Were new knowledge and skills applied? Did opinions and attitudes change as a result of the teaching? Did the learners get written discharge instructions they could understand? To what extent did they follow the plan? If they had difficulty, was this a result of not remembering, inability to perform the skill, or misunderstanding instructions? Did they change their minds about willingness to perform the behaviors? Did physical limitations or financial barriers prevent them from self-care? Was a continuing care provider identified and told where teaching left off, to promote continuity of care?

Research shows families may misinterpret or not recall information given to them before discharge, even when it is offered clearly and with sensitivity. For some learners, the need for information is greatest after discharge,

when situations are encountered that require specific information (Paterson, Kieloch, & Gmiterek, 2001).

Level D: Patient's Overall Self-Care and Health Management

This level of evaluation answers the questions: Was teaching worth it in the long run? What was the impact of teaching? Did health care outcomes improve? Was the quality of self-care improved, and did it stay improved over time? Was health regained or retained? This evaluates learning one year or more after the initiation of teaching. Was the patient readmitted for the same medical problem, when it could have been prevented? Was overall management successful in preventing or controlling health problems? Did physiologic data, such as blood pressure and blood glucose level, handling emergencies, and readmission rates reflect successful self-care? Often, success at this level depends on the ongoing evaluation and reinforcement of teaching by the continuing care providers.

Which Level of Evaluation Is Best?

Comparing the Four Levels of Evaluation

It is best to collect and summarize data from a combination of evaluation sources. When summarizing results, ask: To what extent were the learning objectives accomplished? The answer to this initial question leads to more questions including:

- If the behavior was successfully performed, how can it be reinforced?
- If the behavioral objective was not met, was the learner able to perform the behavior in the past?
- If the learner could perform it in the past, why has he failed to perform it now?

Evaluation does not end the patient education process. Instead, it becomes another starting point. Data is gathered, feedback is offered about the learning experience from the patient, the family, the health care providers, and the institution. Health care providers look for feedback about the quality of their interventions. When feedback is used positively, it can be a powerful learning tool that guides behavior.

Carefully consider the conclusions drawn from evaluation. Often data are limited or absent at one level of evaluation. If so, conclusions at a higher level may be inaccurate.

For example, if information is collected at level D (overall self-care) to reflect that blood pressure has not come under better control, you need to conduct evaluation at all levels before you assume the patient did not know how to follow the regimen (level B) or that he or she did not follow the treatment plan at home (level C). Ideally, evaluation occurs at each level and modifications are made to the teaching plan to build success at each level.

Evidence of patient learning in each evaluation level can be assessed by anyone on the health care team, anywhere along the continuum of care. All levels of evaluation provide important evidence. For example, you discover a patient does not perform a skill at home, such as insulin administration or blood glucose testing. Was that patient ever instructed in that skill? Until that information is gathered it is not clear what intervention is needed to correct the situation. If the status of patient education has not been documented along the line, valuable time may be lost recreating the assessment of learning needs and abilities.

The authors frequently hear health care providers say, "I'd love to do patient education, but I don't have the time to teach and document it, with all the paperwork and other demands." Opportunities for patient education are lost during the typical day in every setting. For example, bath time can be used for teaching the patient with diabetes about good skin and foot care, the surgical patient about dressing or cast care, the patient with chronic obstructive lung disease about breathing exercises. Medication time can be used to teach the patient with congestive heart failure how to take his or her pulse before self-administering medication, or to teach the patient with rheumatoid arthritis to safely taper off steroids. Every patient encounter is an opportunity for patient teaching. The astute health care provider who capitalizes on these moments should always document the evaluation of teaching in the patient's chart.

EVALUATING PATIENT EDUCATION INTERVENTIONS

This step in evaluation considers the performance of both the teacher and the learner. Was the teaching environment set so the health care provider was a consultant, and the patient a colleague? Did the patient and family collaborate in establishing learning goals and objectives? Was the educational process interesting, clear, and stimulating to the learner? The answers should guide modification of the process in future encounters. Box 11.2 offers some questions to guide evaluation of the patient education process.

It is also important to evaluate the teaching interventions used.

Evaluating format and content. Was the patient taught by self-study, individual instruction, or group instruction? Was the format compatible with the learning objectives and with the patient's condition and learning style? Was the format effective in giving the patient the necessary facts and training to learn the desired behaviors?

Evaluating teaching activities and media. Was the patient given an opportunity to actively participate, ask questions, and practice? Were the patient's past experiences used as resources for learning? Were the patient's social roles and developmental tasks acknowledged? Was learning practical and problem centered? Was there an opportunity for immediate application by the learner? Were the learning methods and media appro-

BOX 11.2 Evaluation Checklist for Patient Education

Was the original assessment complete?
- Did the patient participate in goal setting?
- Did the patient perceive the identified problem as important? Did the patient want to change?
- Did the objectives clearly state observable patient behaviors?
- Were the objectives realistic for the patient?
- Were the interventions tailored to meet the objectives?
- Did new problems pose obstacles to behavioral change?
- Was behavioral change measured and documented accurately?
- Is there a skill deficiency? Should there be changes in the teaching interventions?

priate for the types of learning objectives? Did the media deliver the message in a manner that the patient and family could understand?

Evaluating patient and family satisfaction. Do the patient and the family have suggestions for improving the patient education experience? Which activities did they find most helpful and which did they find least helpful? Did they feel supported in the learning environment? Were their concerns addressed? Did they feel confident with the staff's preparation to teach? Was the content understandable and practical?

Evaluating the resources and staff recommendations. Were staff and facility resources adequate for teaching? If not, which unmet staff needs posed barriers to patient learning? Do health care team members have suggestions? How do they assess the quality of the patient learning experience? Was teaching the

patient and family coordinated between members of the health care team? Did they feel prepared to teach? If not, what training should be offered to the staff? (Refer to Chapter 5.)

Evaluating Patient and Family Performance

Learning objectives measure the patient's ability to assume self-care. Learning objectives are the behaviors the patient will perform to show that he or she has mastered knowledge, attitudes, and skills. They are tailored to the patient's individual goals.

Chapter 8 described the three components of a learning objective: performance, conditions, and criteria. To evaluate patient education, the teacher uses performance, conditions, and criteria to measure the patient's progress. Qualitative and quantitative data must be collected accurately to measure these components.

For example, the following is an example of a learning objective: The patient will draw up and administer 22 units of insulin using sterile technique at 7:00 AM on 3 consecutive days. Qualitative data might include the following statement: "The patient could perform sterile technique in preparing the injection but could not accurately measure the units of insulin." Quantitative data might include this statement: "The patient could perform sterile technique correctly only once. In the other two efforts, he or she contaminated the needle by placing it on the table uncapped." Specific data help to acknowledge progress that is made toward meeting the objective, and help focus education on problem areas.

Evaluating Performance in the Home

Evaluating performance in the home is often difficult because continuing care is not always possible from the hospital, clinic, or school setting. Outpatient follow-up may be difficult because the patient is discharged to a different city, follow-up appointments are infrequent, home health services may not be available, or there is little communication about patient teaching between agencies.

The health care team needs to know how the patient is doing at home. Does the patient feel competent to manage self-care? Does the home environment present any barriers to self-care? Is the regimen flexible enough? Can the patient handle problems or temporary relapses constructively? If emergencies have occurred, did the patient or family respond appropriately? Does the patient still assume responsibility for self-care?

Unfortunately, health care providers often do not learn about patient difficulties until a crisis, such as a visit to the emergency department or a hospital readmission. A number of interventions can improve evaluation of home performance, such as telephone follow-up, postcards, e-mails, home visits by students, and better communication between the health care providers along the continuum of care.

Home health care is growing, particularly for geriatric care. The older patients' ability to care for themselves is dependent upon a good assessment, and adapting what needs to be taught to the learner's competence levels. Effective communication and teaching skills are essential to management of the older patient's condition and may ensure, or at least extend, the time that patient can remain living at home (Barry, 2000).

Evaluating Self-Care and Health Maintenance

This level of evaluation takes a broad look at the patient's course of care before and after the learning of new behaviors. Information is collected about absences from work or school, hospitalizations, episodes of acute complications, and daily management. Research data are usually gathered to measure the long-term value of patient education interventions. In addition, the data may be used to substantiate requests for third-party reimbursement of patient teaching and negotiated managed-care contracts.

Treatment goals, such as medication, nutrition, and exercise outcomes, are continually evaluated. Clinical and financial outcomes include decreased drug spending, decreased hospitalization, decreased emergency department visits, and decreased outpatient visits for acute episodes.

Methods of Measurement

There are several ways to gather information to evaluate learning. Evaluation becomes part of the learning experience when it is an exercise shared with the learner. Feedback reinforces positive behaviors, and guides the correction of misunderstandings and performance problems. By presenting the learner with problems to solve, the learner practices applying the information while the teacher evaluates how well the new information has been integrated.

There are seven methods commonly used to evaluate patient education: direct observation, patient records, reports, tests, interviews, critical incidents, and length of stay.

Direct Observation

Watching the patient perform a skill or having him or her role-play a situation offers two valuable opportunities. First, accurate, descriptive data can be collected. Second, the learner receives immediate feedback and guidance. Direct observation should be used whenever possible, rather than relying on reports and assumptions. Patients should be encouraged to demonstrate self-care activities, and give professional guidance to reinforce learning. Examples of opportunities for direct observation are when the patient changes dressings, administers medication, performs breast self-examination, or selects foods according to a prescribed diet.

Preventive education for children also can be evaluated through return demonstration. Age-specific teaching for burn prevention by a pediatric nurse practitioner helps young children create an escape plan and has them demonstrate "stop, drop, and roll." Second and third graders crawl through a simulated smoke tunnel, and older children learn about burn staging and skin grafting through simulations (Gregory, 2000).

Patient Records

Although health care professionals begin teaching, much of the actual learning occurs in the home when the patient and family assume total responsibility. Reinforcement of positive behavior is essential, but it is not easily provided when opportunities for observation are lacking.

The patient should be asked to keep specific records and to present them to the health care team at a later time. This reinforces the patient's responsibility, reinforces positive behaviors, helps the patient evaluate his own progress, and provides the team with data for evaluation. This method has worked well in evaluating compliance with medical regimens, diet modification, stress management, and treatments carried out at home. Patients may keep records of data such as blood sugars, blood pressures, or weights. When possible, objectivity should be increased by supplementing the patient records with direct observation.

Reports

Patient and family reports are used as sources of data, although their objectivity is often questioned. Measurements, such as pill counts, weight, and blood tests, can accompany reports.

Health care providers should carefully construct questions to elicit reports from the patient and family. For example, they might ask, "What medicine did you take today and at what times did you take them?" rather than, "Are you taking your medication as you were instructed?" More specific and descriptive data may be obtained in this manner. Patients can be taught to be good reporters if they are given specific directions about collecting and recording significant information, and if they are told how they are expected to contribute to the evaluation process.

Tests

Tests reveal current cognitive knowledge, but they may not be the best evaluation tools because patients may become anxious about testing. Before you present a test, assess the learner to make sure this test would be appropriate for this person at this time. Introduce tests in a nonthreatening way, as questioning, and use the results to reinforce progress toward meeting cognitive objectives.

Tests are most appropriately used with adult learners as a presentation of problems, as in "what would you do if . . ." They help guide patients and give feedback, and can be used before learning activities and repeated at intervals following instruction. When evaluating knowledge, present problems in a sequence from simple to complex, appropriate for the level of the patient's health literacy skills, making success possible. Tests can measure the patient's progress, and they offer objective data about learning retention. Tests can be used in the process of evaluating daily management decisions made by patients and their families dealing with chronic illness.

Interviews and Questionnaires

PATIENTS AND FAMILY

Patients and their families may be interviewed or given written questionnaires to assess their expectations, opinions, degree of confidence in new knowledge, and self-efficacy. In these interviews and questionnaires, patients may evaluate their own progress, define their learning needs, and offer suggestions for future training.

The authors have used questionnaires to evaluate prenatal classes, newborn care instruction, and stress management classes. The questions should be phrased so that the learner can understand them. Specific questions that do not require long, general responses should be asked. Questionnaires are inappropriate for patients and family members with poor literacy skills. The evaluator might ask a patient to write a letter describing the birth experience or a surgical experience, and explain how prepared he or she felt for it. The patient can offer suggestions for how to best prepare others based on his or her experience.

STAFF

Everyone on the health care team, of every discipline, collects information evaluating the knowledge and skills of a patient and family, intentionally or incidentally. An evaluator should review the patient's chart to learn what the health care team members have documented. If it is found that professionals who work closely with the patient and family have not been documenting their evaluations of teaching, they should be asked to do so, focusing on specific, measurable behaviors. Teaching will be much more efficient and effective if team members collaborate.

Critical Incidents

The patient's chart should be reviewed for critical incidents, such as readmission and complications. Emergency room visits may reflect patient learning needs.

Length of Stay

Patient education can reduce length of stay by enabling the patient to better participate in recovery and prepare for discharge. Teaching goals should be set realistically, based on the estimated length of stay associated with the diagnosis-related group (DRG) or the case type.

Identifying Needs and Performance Problems

The behavioral objectives in the learning process (see Figure 8.1) guide the nurse in the evaluation process. If the desired behavior is accomplished, opportunities should be pro-

vided for reinforcing the positive behavior. Clinic visits, home visits, telephone calls, and community resources offer such opportunities. The patient and the family can demonstrate the knowledge and skills they have retained and ask for the review or guidance they need. The health care team should encourage patients to take advantage of these learning resources.

When new behaviors are not learned, or only partially learned, barriers to behavior change should be reassessed and readdressed. Pipe and Mager (1997) provide a model for problem solving to determine patient learning needs (Figure 11.2). If a skill deficiency is present, the evaluator should reconsider whether the particular behavior is important and necessary. Is it a survival skill? If so, and the patient has never been able to perform the skill, additional training should be provided. If the skill will be used infrequently, feedback and practice should be arranged. For example, insulin injection is often learned with some initial difficulty, but the skill is used so often that it is retained and reinforced. Breast self-examination is performed less often, so this technique and the importance of its performance may need more reinforcement.

If the patient has demonstrated the ability to perform the skill but has not continued to perform it, four additional questions direct the teacher's problem solving. Mager and Pipe suggest that if performing the skill somehow "punishes" the patient, the nurse must identify the source of punishment and remove it.

1. Why does the patient feel punished? For example, patients who are on special diets often complain that they cannot follow their diet while socializing with friends. Locating other sources of support, such as support groups of dieters, may remove the feeling of being different or punished.
2. Does the patient see the performance as unrewarding? If so, arrange positive consequences by offering additional support and more frequent follow-up visits and

---

WHEN CLIENTS FAIL TO MEET LEARNING OBJECTIVES: IS THERE A SKILL DEFICIENCY?

Yes	No
1. Has the client ever demonstrated the ability to perform the skill? If not, *formal training* is required.	1. Is the performance of the skill punishing? If so, *remove punishment.*
2. Is the skill used often? If not, *arrange practice.* If so, *arrange feedback.*	2. Is nonperformance rewarding? If so, *arrange a positive consequence.*
	3. Does the client feel that it doesn't matter if he performs the behavior? If so, *arrange a consequence.*
	4. Are there obstacles to performing the behavior? If so, *remove obstacles.*

FIGURE 11.2 *Note.* Pipe, P. & Mager, R. F. (1997). *Analyzing performance problems: Or you really oughta wanna* (3rd ed.). Atlanta: Center for Effective Performance. Adapted with permission.

reporting mechanisms, so the patient will see his improvement more clearly.

3. Does the patient think that it doesn't matter whether he or she performs the behavior? If this is the case, as with patients with hypertension who fail to take their medications regularly, more frequent blood pressure checks can reinforce the patient's awareness of the seriousness of omitting the medication.

4. Do obstacles prevent the patient from performing the behavior? If so, review these obstacles and help the patient deal with them. For example, the snack machine at work, which contains only candy and chips, may be less of a temptation if the patient brings a nutritious snack. If a mill worker feels self-conscious about wearing a protective mask on the job, because "nobody else wears one," the company manager and employee health nurse may insist all employees wear the recommended masks.

Become a detective to help patients overcome stumbling blocks in the learning process. This requires the skills of making astute observations, using active listening, and approaching individual situations creatively.

The continuous cycle of teaching and learning brings us back to formulating objectives. The health care provider, the patient, and the patient's family must once again discuss their mutual goals: What does the patient want? What can the health care team do to assist him or her in carrying out new behaviors? Negotiation and the learning contract are as important in evaluation as they were in planning. The original learning contract should be modified, as necessary.

Feedback

Feedback is a communication process that involves sharing perceptions. Constructive feedback supports and guides the patient and family in learning. Health care institutions ask for feedback from the public about how they are meeting community health care needs. Nurses often comment that they wish patients, families, and staff would give them more positive feedback about the care they provide.

There are two types of feedback: positive and negative. Positive feedback compliments a person's behavior. Negative feedback communicates displeasure or disappointment with a person's behavior. Most people describe positive feedback as being of great importance to them. It means more when it comes from someone we respect, from someone who values us, and from someone who understands our situation. In patient learning, patients and their family members expect to receive feedback from nurses and other team members.

The best feedback, whether positive or negative, is constructive and helpful. For example, getting negative feedback about something you cannot change is not helpful at all. Box 11.3 describes the characteristics of constructive feedback and includes tips for giving feedback to the patient and family in ways they can understand and use.

DOCUMENTATION OF PATIENT EDUCATION

Written documentation of all aspects of patient care, including patient education, is essential. Documentation is critical for communication among team members, to provide a legal record, to support quality assurance efforts, to meet JCAHO standards, to promote continuity of care, and to facilitate reimbursement. Documentation should reflect the following elements of patient care and patient education:

- Initial assessments and reassessments
- Nursing diagnoses, patient learning needs, priorities
- Interventions planned
- Interventions provided
- Patient's response, outcomes of care
- Ability of the patient and family to manage needs after discharge

---

BOX 11.3 Guidelines for Obtaining and Giving Constructive Feedback

Characteristics of Constructive Feedback
- Descriptive rather than judgmental, it offers objective data and suggestions for improvement.
- Specific rather than general, it does not include absolute words such as *always* or *never*. It is concerned with the here and now.
- Focused on the person's *behavior* rather than on the person.
- Given at the earliest opportunity after the behavior is performed; it is timely.
- Considers the needs of the learner. It is given to help, not to hurt.
- Directed toward a behavior about which the learner can do something. The person will only become frustrated and discouraged when he or she is unable to control a situation.
- Involves sharing information and offering guided choices rather than giving advice such as "You should...."

- Considers the amount of information that the learner can handle. It does not overload the person.

Tips for Giving and Soliciting Feedback
- Ask whether feedback is wanted. It is most useful when it is solicited rather than imposed.
- Be prepared to listen.
- Give positive feedback first. Reinforce positive behaviors, then discuss weaknesses.
- Don't argue or push. Present alternatives.
- Ensure that your feedback is interpreted correctly.
- When requesting feedback from others, tell them what kinds of specific information you want. Offer them structured questions, but encourage them to use open-ended responses.
- When you want feedback from others, be open to it. Observe patients' expressions or comments. Listen for the intended message.

Documentation takes time, especially in light of increasing patient acuity, complex care, and expanding clinical responsibilities. However, timely, accurate documentation shows the basis of clinical judgments and evidence of care provided to the patient.

Documentation is most efficient when all components are designed to fit together. Documentation should be streamlined to avoid duplication of charting and to accurately reflect care, problems resolved, and problems referred. To demonstrate quality care, all clinical data and the contributions of all health care team members need to be integrated into a single patient-centered chart or data base. The method does not matter.

Documentation may be computerized, with data entry at a bedside terminal. Research on the use of bedside computers (Nahm & Poston, 2000) shows a statistically significant increase in the quality of nursing documentation, as well as a decrease in variability in charting. This study demonstrated that documenting with a point-of-care, integrated computer system can increase compliance to JCAHO standards without negatively affecting patient satisfaction.

A documentation system should be concise, organized, and focused on patient outcomes. A glance at the chart should clearly show what the patient knows, can do, and still needs to learn. Statements such as "patient teaching done" are meaningless, because they describe the caregiver's behavior but give no information about the status of the learner's self-care skills.

There is no special form or format for documenting patient education. A better checklist or flow sheet may help, but only if the documentation form is the problem. More often, poor documentation is the result of inadequate assessment and evaluation skills, or not holding health care providers responsible for documentation. Creating new forms often leads to fragmented communication, the perception that patient education is separate from routine care, and the belief that patient teaching requires an unrealistic amount of extra work. If a new form is creat-

ed, the staff should be involved in its design, and it should eliminate one or more existing forms. The question should be: "Where is patient education currently documented and is it working? Is the charting of everyone on the health care team integrated, so the chart is an effective communication tool?"

Critical pathways (Chapter 12), which identify key learning outcomes and related variances, should be a focus of interdisciplinary teaching. Chart audit results can be used to direct quality improvement initiatives, including staff development toward improved patient education skills. Documentation of patient education should be incorporated into employee appraisals.

A review of the common components of a documentation system illustrates how documentation of patient education can be integrated into the patient record. The components are:

Admission assessment (data base)
Problem list
Care plan or critical path
Flow sheets (optional)
Progress notes
Discharge summary

Admission Assessment

Patient profile and history are completed by the health care team on admission. Functional assessment is highlighted to aid the formulation of nursing diagnoses. Patient assessment forms vary according to setting and patient needs. Assessment is described in Chapter 7 and emphasizes the identification of ways to individualize teaching, such as readiness, language, and physical problems. Assessment forms may be designed to red flag high-risk patients, to pinpoint potential problems that identify specific learning needs.

Problem List

The front of the chart has a list of actual and potential health problems identified by health care providers, individually or collaboratively. Medical and nursing diagnoses are included in this list. A date is entered next to each problem as it is identified, and another date is recorded to reflect when the problem is resolved. Standardized care plans may be generated based on DRGs and nursing diagnoses.

Care Plan or Critical Pathway

An individualized care plan for each patient includes medical and nursing diagnoses, patient goals (including learning goals), interventions (including patient education and discharge planning), and actual outcomes.

Flow Sheets

Routine or repetitious actions can be systematically documented on flow sheets. Flow sheets, either on paper or computer, can be kept at the bedside to record data such as vital signs, medication, and positioning. Flow sheets list observations in a clear, concise check-off format to encourage rapid and immediate documentation. Findings or patient responses outside of normal limits must be recorded in the chart notes. This method of charting assumes that all abnormal findings, or variances, are charted; this is referred to as "charting by exception." If flow sheets are used to record patient education, the data entered should be the documentation of evaluation of understanding, not what was taught.

Progress Notes

Narrative notes show the patient's progress as viewed by all health care professionals involved in the patient's care. Evaluation of the patient's responses to nursing interventions should be evident. Each problem may be referenced with a number corresponding to the problem list.

Patient education can be effectively documented in the progress notes section of the medical record. Because patient education is a problem-solving process, documentation includes a clear statement of needs or problems, significant data, and the plan for care. It is essential to document the outcomes of care. Narrative notes also encourage the charting of the patient's own words to illustrate outcomes of patient education and evidence of individualized care.

POR and SOAP

Dr. Lawrence Weed (1971) developed the problem-oriented record (POR), a systematic tool for communication and problem solving. All team members (physicians, nurses, physical therapists, dietitians, pharmacists, and social workers) contribute to the one problem list that focuses on patient problems rather than on provider problems. Team members write narrative and discharge notes using the SOAP format to document subjective and objective data, assessment (or identification) of problems and the planned course of intervention. The SOAP note was later modified to include intervention, evaluation, and revision, and referred to as SOAPIER. This method increases awareness of the contributions of others and encourages the members to function as a team. There are no divisions of notes by discipline. All health care professionals document information on the patient's progress notes. The patient is clearly the center of the team and the focus of care.

We recommend this method, and in our own experiences in patient education, it has increased communication and collaboration. It helps team members to know what has been taught by others and facilitates reinforcement of learned behaviors.

The POR highlights the use of the patient education process, which is based on problem solving. Narrative notes begin by naming the problem, and they then offer subjective and objective data, the assessment, and the plan, as detailed in Box 11.4

Many formats exist for progress notes that can promote interdisciplinary coordination, a focus on the patient's functional health problems, and a record of the patient's learning outcomes as an integral part of documenting care. Regardless of the type of progress note, the focus should be on the patient, and the

BOX 11.4 The SOAP Format for Notes in Problem-Oriented Records

Problem: refer to the number of the problem on the problem list

S: Subjective data—what the patient reports

O: Objective data—what is observed through the senses and diagnostic tests

A: Assessment—patient responses to health problems

P: Plan—includes diagnostic, therapeutic, and patient education interventions and reflects immediate and future actions and the evaluation of these actions

For a SOAPIER note, add:

I: Intervention

E: Evaluation

R: Revision

patient's response to treatments, eg, How does this diagnosis affect this patient?

Discharge Summary

Summaries or reports written at the time of discharge or transfer communicate to other health care providers the patient's needs for reinforcement and continued learning. This documentation is important because learning does not end at the door. It often begins in the hospital, but it continues in the clinic or home. Notes and telephone consultations can be used to communicate assessments and ongoing learning needs to continuing care providers.

A significant amount of patient learning occurs after patients leave the sheltered hospital environment, and most need continuous teaching to responsibly and capably manage their daily care. Suggestions for patient-centered discharge instructions are offered in Chapter 9. Many agencies require that dis-

charge instructions be developed in triplicate; the patient and family sign a copy for the patient's record indicating instructions were received, a copy is given to the patient, and a copy is provided to the individual or agency responsible for continuing care. Patient contracts may also be entered as a permanent part of the patient record (see Chapter 9).

CLINICAL APPLICATION OF EVALUATING PATIENT EDUCATION OUTCOMES: CASE STUDIES

The case of Mrs. Dawe, who is struggling with her daily management of diabetes and hypertension, continues.

CASE STUDY 11.1

EVALUATION OF MRS. DAWE'S BEHAVIORAL CHANGE

After the home visit for Mrs. Dawe, the nursing students offered a summary of patient learning outcomes. Reassessment of patient needs and modifications to the teaching plan are also noted.

Problem 3: Altered Nutrition. Mrs. Dawe correctly outlined food exchanges for breakfast, lunch, and dinner using her American Diabetes Association meal plan. She wrote three sample menus for each meal. She included one-half cup of ice cream in one of these meals and substituted accurately. She returns to the clinic for her first weekly visit with 2 days of food intake recorded in her notebook. She followed her diet plan on both days. She reports that on the last 5 days she "cheated" on her diet and ate several desserts, failing to record what she ate. She states that she feels guilty not following the diet and explains that she knows weight control is important for her diabetes management.

Her weight at the clinic visit is unchanged from her last clinic visit. The nurses review her goals and learning objectives. Mrs. Dawe states that she is still interested in following her diet and wants a nurse's help in doing so.

The nurses reinforce Mrs. Dawe's knowledge about her diet and her understanding of the importance of weight control for her condition. The nurses stress she must take responsibility for changing her habits. They offer to help her come up with strategies to confront problems. She states she would like to resume her diet plan today and come back to the clinic next week. The nurses agree, and remind her she had 2 days of success with her plan, and is able to do it.

Problem 4: Altered Tissue Perfusion. Mrs. Dawe reported that she took her medicine and showed the nurses the record of medication in her notebook. She reports that she omitted salt in cooking during the week and that she did not use any canned foods except for water-packed fruits. When asked to list ten high-sodium foods, she does.

Her blood pressure at the clinic visit is 188/96 mmHg.

Mrs. Dawe reports that it was less difficult than she thought to avoid high-sodium foods, and that Mr. Dawe had encouraged her to do so. In fact, when she was about to use canned tomato sauce in cooking, Mr. Dawe reminded her of its high sodium content. The nurses commend the Dawes on their positive behaviors and show them how the blood pressure measurement highlights their success.

Boxes 11.5 and 11.6 illustrate SOAP notes written by the nursing student to document Mrs. Dawe's care.

BOX 11.5 March 31 Home Visit of Mrs. Dawe

Nursing Note

Altered Nutrition

S: "I want help with my weight problem. I know I'm too heavy and it's making my diabetes difficult to manage. My diet is too limited. I just can't follow it."

O: 5'3" tall, weight 170 lb. at last visit, 45 lb. above prescribed weight. Unable to follow American Diabetes Association meal plan. Gets little exercise except for housework.

P: Negotiate weight loss goals. Change diet to updated ADA low-fat meal planning. Outline menus with Mrs. Dawe and make referral to the dietitian to build variety into her meal plan. Discuss importance of weight loss in management of diabetes. Refer to diabetic luncheon.

Schedule clinic visit for 1 week from now.

Altered Tissue Perfusion

S: "I know I need to cut down on salt and lose weight to get my pressure down."

O: Blood pressure 220/190 today. Reports taking medication.

A: Blood pressure poorly controlled. Food intake recall reveals salt used in cooking and at the table, with canned foods frequently included.

P: Continue medication as ordered. Patient to keep written records. Follow weight-reduction diet as ordered. Omit salt in cooking and avoid canned foods. Mrs. Dawe agrees with the plan. We discussed high-sodium foods to be avoided. Return to clinic in 1 week for blood pressure check.

BOX 11.6 April 7 Clinic Visit of Mrs. Dawe

Nursing Note
Altered Nutrition

S: "I followed my meal plan the first 2 days, but cheated after that. I just couldn't pass up desserts when I thought about having them. I didn't write down what I ate, because I was embarrassed. I really do want to lose weight and wish you would help me to do it."

O: Weight 170 lb. (unchanged from last visit). The 2 days of recorded meals indicated Mrs. Dawe followed diet plan.

A: Having trouble following with meal plan. Understands meal spacing and can select menus. Understands importance of weight control but does not per-

form necessary behavior modifications.

P: Review goals. Stress Mrs. Dawe's responsibility. Offer assistance for problem-solving and role-playing. Reinforce 2 days of positive behavior. Return visit in 1 week.

Altered Tissue Perfusion

S: Reports taking medication. Reports omitting salt in cooking.

O: Blood pressure 188/96 today.

A: Blood pressure lower. Good cooperation with reducing sodium intake. Knows name and dosage of medication. Identifies high-sodium foods to avoid.

P: Reinforce progress. Continue weekly blood pressure checks.

CASE STUDY 11.2

MR. STRAMINSKY'S AMBULATORY SURGERY

Mr. Straminsky is 73 years old. His wife, Alice, is 70 years old. They live in the suburbs, 30 miles from a large teaching hospital where Mr. Straminsky is to have a bladder biopsy in ambulatory surgery. He was a patient in the same hospital 3 years before when he had a coronary artery bypass graft.

Nurses in the ambulatory surgery unit recognize all patients have some degree of anxiety before the procedure. During the preoperative assessment, the nurses ask about concerns the patient and family have. Patients usually come to the ambulatory surgery center 2 days to 4 days before surgery. Before

beginning teaching, the nurse assesses the following factors:

The patient's knowledge about the expected surgery or procedure
The patient's previous surgical experiences or hospitalizations
Other illnesses the patient may have
The patient's support systems
The patient's concerns about his or her occupational or related issues (such as when activity or work can be resumed)
Effective ways of coping with pain

Unfortunately, nurses at the center find that they usually have about 15 minutes to complete the assessment, and often patients do not share their concerns in depth with the nurse. This is particularly true of older patients.

Patient teaching preoperatively for Mr. Straminsky addressed what to expect in the surgical procedure and instructions for discharge. The patient and his wife said they understood; however, Mrs. Straminsky made a comment about how they had seen so many doctors, specialists, residents, and medical students, and they were overwhelmed with instructions. They were given a pamphlet explaining the ambulatory surgery unit and told the logistics of arriving the next morning for the surgical procedure.

The nursing diagnoses identified for most patients in this unit are appropriate for Mr. Straminsky:

1. Knowledge deficit related to the ambulatory surgery unit and the surgical procedure
2. Anxiety related to surgical procedure and discharge from unit

The short teaching session with the Straminskys seems to go well. The Straminskys ask questions about the procedure and repeat what they should do after discharge. They seem interested and capable.

When they return for the husband's bladder biopsy, the admissions nurse greets them. They were asked to report at 6:30 AM, and they arrive early, at about 6:00 AM. Mr. Straminsky is assigned a bed and his wife waits for a few minutes before joining him. Throughout the morning, Mrs. Straminsky seems anxious. Despite the procedure, which according to the health care team goes well, Mrs. Straminsky seems distracted and unsettled. She tells the nurse assigned to recovery that she was not well prepared for this "ordeal."

The nurse recognizes patients and families have many concerns and worries that they do not share with health care providers (Barry, et al., 2000). She gives Mrs. Straminsky a blank piece of paper and asks her to write her concerns, reviewing her experience. This evaluation method helps the patient (or in this case the spouse) verbalize her feelings, and it can also be used to better teach other patients. Mrs. Straminsky agrees and begins making notes. Three days later, her "surgical experience" is delivered by mail to the nurse.

MY HUSBAND'S BLADDER BIOPSY

The various physicians who have sent my husband and me for the many outpatient procedures are intelligent, caring, and extremely busy people. They certainly never indicated that they were sending us to the Ritz, but neither did they prepare us specifically for conditions in a large suburban outpatient facility.

In the first visit, more discussion, or a videocassette, would all have been helpful. Some of these things could certainly be the responsibility of the hospital.

The first shock to me was the size of the tiny cubicles to which a patient is assigned. The only similar situation I have seen was an emergency room 25 years earlier. My sister had been taken there after an accident. I accepted the lack of privacy because of the need for immediate attention in that case.

This time we were scheduled and asked to report at the usual crack of dawn. One lonely nurse was on duty and she got my husband into bed. I was allowed to sit in a straight chair by his side as many other patients joined us, each in his curtained rectangle, each giving his history, giving blood, giving urine, and surrendering all thought that some items might be personal and private. There was no way to avoid hearing the details of others' dilemmas.

When my husband was finally wheeled away to surgery, it was a relief for both of us. I escaped first to the cafeteria, then to a waiting room near surgery. After the surgeon spoke to me about my husband, I was allowed into a recovery room where he was blessedly alone with a nurse in attendance.

"Good," I thought, "He'll be here in peace and quiet for a while."

It was a short time. Groggy, he was wheeled back to the outpatient area, now a bustling place. We were informed that as soon as he could urinate on his own, my husband would be discharged. There were many disappointing trips to the lavatory, and often other patients were waiting to use the facility. We waited about 8 hours before he was discharged. I believe it was that time that I asked if it would have been better if he were admitted to the hospital. We were advised that neither Medicare nor our insurance would cover the cost, and the nurse advised against it. Evidently patients do best spending as little time as possible in hospitals!

"You don't want him to be in the hospital; terrible things happen in hospitals," were the exact words from the spouse of another patient. At least in the outpatient facility I could sit with my husband and watch for those terrible things.

The nursing staff was wonderful. Competent, professional nurses stayed aware of all that was going on. I imagine that they too wish for a better environment for themselves and their patients.

This experience (which bothered me much more than it did my husband) could have been alleviated by some preparation such as the ones suggested at the beginning of this account. In addition, a waiting area adjacent to the patient holding area could have a video or slides to help explain what is happening.

After reading Mrs. Straminsky's letter, the nurse realizes that more explanation of the physical layout of the unit is needed in the preadmission program. She also knew that patients and families experience more anxiety than they expect to feel because of the loss of control on the morning of surgery. The nurse decides to convene a group of patients and family members who had surgical procedures on the unit and ask them to share questions or concerns that they each had before, during, or after the procedure.

The staff created a 15-minute videotape to add to the preadmission program, showing what the facilities looked like and following-up on a patient through the surgical procedure. It could also be shown the morning of surgery. The videotape features a spouse who described how she handled such things as waiting, getting information about her husband's status, and so forth. This videotape is shown to groups of patients the day before the surgery, and a nurse is available to answer questions after the film. She finds that patients and family members learn from each other and also get support from each other, which may continue through the surgical experience on the unit.

COMMENTARY ON THE STRAMINSKY CASE

Research indicates that preoperative information alleviates anxiety and aids in postoperative recuperation (Walker, 2002). However, preoperative instruction for the family has been largely overlooked. When a family member's fear and anxiety is alleviated, he or she can be a better source of support for the patient. Fear and anxiety have different characteristics and are subjective experiences. We know through the case study of the Straminskys that sensory experiences of the spouse can be a source of anxiety caused by lack of preparation. Particularly with older patients, preparation can decrease anxiety related to the ambulatory surgery environment. Continuously evaluate the patient and family's perceptions of the adequacy of preoperative instruction.

age aspects of his own care. Mr. Horton's anxiety decreases when measured 24 hours after contracting with his primary nurse. When teaching attempts are hampered by the patient's anxiety and depression, CCU nurses can use patient contracting as a powerful intervention that gets results.

CASE STUDY 11.3

MR. HORTON IN THE CORONARY CARE UNIT

Mr. Horton is the 67-year-old owner of a large retail store. He is admitted to the coronary care unit (CCU) with symptoms of coronary artery disease. Like most patients in this situation, he is anxious, depressed, and angry.

The nurses in the CCU use patient-nurse contracts to help physiologically stable patients regain a feeling of control. The nurses recognize the routines and sensory experiences of the CCU are depersonalizing and that unit procedures and policies (such as restricting visitors, telephones, and newspapers) make matters worse. They also know research indicates that stress reduction measures to counteract environmental stressors positively affect patient attitudes and the return of functioning.

COMMENTARY ON THE HORTON CASE
Mr. Horton was oriented by audiotape to patient-nurse contracting, and then a nurse worked with him to offer choices about visiting privileges, hygiene time, room arrangements, teaching preferences, activity, and other areas of patient concern. The contract was shared with the nursing staff, who honored the terms of the contract whenever possible. Through this process, he was taught about how and why to man-

SUMMARY

Evaluation occurs at different points of the teaching and learning process and uses different methods to gather the types of information needed. Evaluation measures the degree to which patient learning goals have been met and uses findings to improve or redirect patient care. Documentation of patient education focuses on patient outcomes: knowledge, skill, and health behaviors. Good documentation facilitates communication between health care providers, improves continuity of care, satisfies legal responsibilities for charting patient care, and provides evidence that standards for accreditation are met. Understanding patient expectations and improving patient satisfaction are key to providing patient- and family-centered care. Through evaluation we learn valuable lessons from our patients and their families about teaching priorities, who needs to be taught, how to share responsibility for learning with the patient and family, and how difficult long-term change can be.

Despite good intentions, new knowledge, skills, and behavior modification strategies, patients may only partially achieve their health outcomes goals. Obstacles to change are often less tangible than, for example, exposure to party foods or pressure from family and peers. Obstacles may include poor self-efficacy, low self-esteem, and the patient's view of himself as a whole person. The feedback and counseling offered to patients in the health care setting may help them place greater value on themselves and their health. This often takes time, and many patients have difficulty accepting their own responsibilities in daily health management. Some choose the comfort of old habits over the challenges of change. The provider–patient relationship offers an opportunity to help the patient assume his or her role as a member of the health care team. It is important to communicate confidence in the patient's ability to choose responsibly. It is also important to offer encouragement and guidance for change. Evaluation of patient education can strengthen the provider-patient relationship and continue patient-centered care. Documentation of evaluation of patient learning provides critical evidence of such patient-centered care.

In addition to meeting agency mandates for evaluating and documenting the outcomes of patient education, health care providers gain important personal and professional rewards by engaging in the process. In acute care settings, teaching can make the critical difference in helping a patient survive through an illness or injury. This chapter addressed evaluation with individual patients. Chapter 12 applies evaluation to groups of patients through case management, disease management, and research.

STRATEGIES FOR CRITICAL ANALYSIS AND APPLICATION

1. Consider care provided in the following settings: preoperative visit in day surgery, prenatal outpatient visit, recovery room, medical-surgical orthopedic unit, pediatric office, home health, long-term care, elementary school, and occupational health. Identify what types of patient learning outcomes are realistic, in which level they belong (Level A, B, C, or D), and how you would document them in the patient record.
2. Describe two strategies health care providers can use to involve patients and families in evaluating patient education efforts, and offering suggestions for

improving patient education services.
3. Describe two ways members of the health care team could become more involved in evaluating patient education efforts, and offer suggestions for improving patient education services.
4. How would you assess whether a new form is needed for documenting patient education in your agency? How would you involve health care providers of all disciplines in this process? What are the pros and cons of creating a new form? Which existing form or forms could be eliminated?

To find the latest information

Key search terms
evaluation, teach back, health care outcomes, patient education outcomes

Websites
- Effective Communication in Health Care Setting Requires Active Participation of Both Patients and Physicians (DeWalt, D. A.): http://www.ama-assn.org/ama/pub/article/12208-7632.html
- Through the Patient's Eyes: Health Literacy: What Patients Know When They Leave Your Office or Clinic (Schwartzberg, J., & Lagay, F.): http://www.ama-assn.org/ama/pub/category/5154.html

REFERENCES

Barry, C. A., Bradley, C. P., Britten, N., Stevenson, F. A., & Barber, N. (2000). Patients' unvoiced agendas in general practice consultations: Qualitative study. *BMJ, 320,* 1246–1250.

Barry, C. B. (2000). Teaching the older patient in the home assessment and adaptation. *Home Healthcare Nurse, 18*(6), 374–387.

Clementz, A. R. (2002). *Program level evaluation: Using Kirkpatrick's Four Levels of Evaluation to conduct systemic evaluation of undergraduate college programs.* Retrieved July 18, 2004, from http://bryant2.bryant.edu/~assess/recources.htm

Dreger, V., & Tremback, T. (2002). Optimize patient health by treating literacy and language barriers. *AORN Journal, 75*(2), 278, 280–283, 285, 287, 289–293, 297–300, 303–304.

Gregory, C. (2000). Age-specific education targets burn prevention. *Patient Education Management, 7*(2 Supplement), 2.

Joint Commission on Accreditation of Healthcare Organizations (JCAHO). (2003). *2004 hospital accreditation program standards.* Retrieved 6/17/2003, 2003, from http://www.jcaho.org/accredited+organizations/2004+standards.htm

Nahm, R., & Poston, I. (2000). Measurement of the effects of an integrated, point-of-care computer system on quality of nursing documentation and patient satisfaction. *Computers in Nursing, 18*(5), 220–229.

Paterson, B., Kieloch, B., & Gmiterek, J. (2001). 'They never told us anything': Postdischarge instruction for families of persons with brain injuries. *ARN: Association of Rehabilitation Nurses, 26*(2), 48–53.

Pipe, P., & Mager, R. (1997). *Analyzing performance problems: Or you really oughta wanna* (3rd ed.). Atlanta: Center for Effective Performance.

Schillinger, D., Piette, J., Grumbach, K., Wang, F., Wilson, C., Daher, C., et al. (2003). Closing the loop: Physician communication with diabetic patients who have low literacy. *Archives of Internal Medicine, 163,* 83–90.

Walker, J. A. (2002). Emotional and psychological preoperative preparation in adults. *British Journal of Nursing, 11*(8), 567–575.

Weed, L. (1971). *Medical record, medical education, and patient care.* Cleveland: Press of Case Western University.

Winfrey, E. C. (2003). *Kirkpatrick's four levels of evaluation.* Retrieved July 27, 2003, from http://coe.sdsu.edu/eet/Articles/k4levels/index.htm

Case Management and Patient Education Programs

LEARNING OBJECTIVES

After reading this chapter, the student should be able to:

1. Explain why case management systems, with the goals of controlling health care costs and improving the quality of care, emphasize the need for patient and family education.

2. Describe how patient learning outcomes are integrated in critical pathways and patient care maps.

3. Describe two ways you can provide leadership in promoting patient education as an integral part of case management.

4. Identify the philosophical differences of traditional and progressive health care providers that can challenge unification of patient education efforts.

5. Discuss the types and sources of power that you can use to promote patient education and to secure needed resources.

6. Describe 3 ways to measure outcomes of patient education programs.

7. Write two specific aims for a proposed study to test the efficacy of patient education for patients older than 65 years of age with non-insulin-dependent diabetes.

INTRODUCTION

Case Management: Controlling Costs and Improving the Quality of Care

Case management has been used for more than 25 years to allocate health care resources across various settings to meet individual patient needs. The term case management originated in 1863, when it was applied to coordinate community services for the sick and poor. When reimbursement incentives for health care shifted in the 1980s, case management was adapted to inpatient, acute care settings and various outpatient settings (National Tuberculosis Center, 2000). Case management promotes team collaboration, includes the patient and family, and incorporates clinical and financial outcomes. Patient education is an integral part of case management because it enables patients and families to participate in care and to gain survival skills needed to promote decreased length of stay and safe discharge.

Integrating Patient Education into Case Management Models: Product and Process

Case managers, managed care coordinators, and clinical specialists often coordinate patient and family education rather than deliver it. They fulfill the roles of manager, consultant liaison, advocate, facilitator, gatekeeper, negotiator, educator, and researcher. If they do not directly deliver patient education, they are instrumental in coordinating case management system development. They also must promote innovative, interdisciplinary patient education interventions as part of patient care, design ways of evaluating complex patient needs and responses, and assess staff knowledge and skill to teach patients (Powell, 2000). These roles enhance the power to improve patient education, yet simultaneously challenge the case manager to appear neutral in the eyes of the interdisciplinary team and to gain the trust and respect of clinicians and administrators.

Process issues, including assessing and using power, dealing with politics in the organization, and promoting constructive change are key to successfully leading case management efforts (Lachman, 1999). The development process for case management plans (also called clinical pathways and critical pathways) is a 10-step process (Tahan, 2002). The first four steps are done by a steering committee, the last six steps are done by an interdisciplinary team.

1. Design the format of the pathway.
2. Select the target population.
3. Organize the interdisciplinary team (6–10 members).
4. Educate and train the team in the process.
5. Examine the current practice.
6. Review the literature for evidence-based practice.
7. Establish the length of the pathway (consider length of stay).
8. Write the content of the pathway.
9. Conduct a pilot study of the pathway.
10. Standardize and normalize the case management pathway.

These plans often come in paired formats: one for the health care providers and one for the consumers. The consumer format provides patients and families with information about the plan of care and the treatment options or expectations, and it enhances informed decision-making. A good plan can help health care providers link structure, processes, and outcomes to best identify where improvements can be made (Tahan, 2002).

The most challenging task throughout this process is gaining consensus. The authority of the steering committee, the structure and training they provide, the selection of team members, the commitment to evidence-based practice, and the use of a facilitator help the process move smoothly. Turf battles, arising from different points of view from various disciplines and individuals, must be recognized and addressed. These process issues and the use of power and politics are covered in the second section of this chapter.

PRODUCTS OF CASE MANAGEMENT

Key Elements of Case Management Models

Every organization tailors case management models to its own environment and organizational culture. However, they all include these key elements:

- Standardization of care through the use of clinical pathways or some form of prescribed clinical protocols
- Identification of factors that facilitate or hinder meeting goals of care promotes system improvements
- Comparison of expected and actual outcomes provides outcome evaluation
- Optimization of resource use
- Enhancement of continuity of care
- Support of collaborative team practice
- Facilitation of communication (Smith & Danforth, 2001)

Critical Pathways

Clinical guidelines can be translated into care plans that detail the expected progress of patients in terms of essential steps and time frames. They promote team collaboration, clinical consistency, and continuity of care. These interdisciplinary care plans come in many styles: critical pathways, clinical pathways, critical paths, clinical protocols, care maps, or care tracks. A systematic review of the literature suggests their use reduces the cost of care and length of hospital stays, increases quality of care and patient satisfaction, and improves continuity of information and patient education. Critical pathways should be evidence-based, and individualized to specific patient needs. Although some studies suggest critical pathways have no impact on outcomes, there is no evidence they have any negative impacts (Renholm, Leino-Kilpi, & Souminen, 2002).

Critical pathways are developed collaboratively by all of the health care professionals involved in patient care. The goal is to incorporate an interdisciplinary perspective, identify expectations and events that are critical to achieving a desired length of stay, and implement strategies that improve the quality and cost-effectiveness of care. The critical pathway does not take the place of physician orders. Timing and content for effective patient teaching are emphasized in the pathway. Other activities addressed include consultation, diagnostic testing, discharge planning, activity, diet, and medication.

An example of a patient care map for open-heart surgery patients at High Point Regional Hospital in North Carolina is shown in Figures 12.1 and 12.2. It is designed for DRG #106 (coronary artery bypass graft with catheterization) based on a length of stay of 4 to 5 days. The cardiovascular clinical care coordinator incorporated patient focus groups in the design of the patient care map. Based on patient input, the care coordinator collaborates with physicians, home health, and cardiac rehabilitation to develop a second care map (patient plan), which addresses the patient's course during the first 2 weeks after discharge. The care map is designed as a picture plan to aid the teaching of patients with limited reading skills. It also explains in narrative the expected events during the patient's recovery.

Most hospitals have adopted some form of critical path and care map system for patient care. Similar efforts to coordinate and standardize clinical care may be referred to by different names, including clinical paths, practice guidelines, and coordinated care plans. Time lines for critical paths can occur by visit (home health), by month (extended care), by week (rehabilitation units), by day (medical-surgical unit), or by minute (emergency department).

Critical pathways have been successfully applied in a wide range of patient care situations, including burn wounds (Mamolen & Brenner, 2000), carotid endarterectomies (Kallenbach & Rosenblum, 2000), and endoscopies (Terry, 2001).

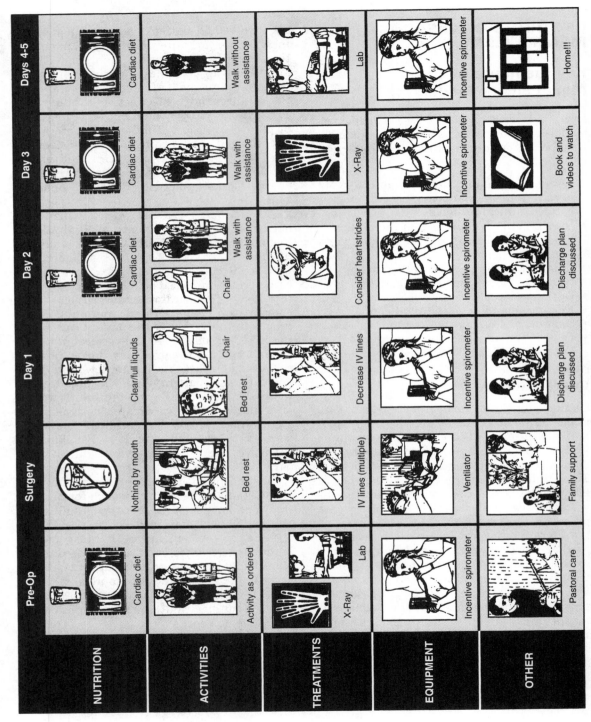

FIGURE 12.1 High Point Regional Hospital open heart surgery patient plan (picture path).

Open Heart Surgery Plan

Welcome to High Point Regional Hospital. This plan is to share with you and your family a picture of what to expect during your hospital stay, one day at a time. If you have questions or concerns, please ask your doctor, nurse, or members of our health care team.

Before Surgery: This is a busy day for you, but you can still enjoy your cardiac diet/food until midnight. You can also do the same activities the doctor has ordered for you until surgery. You will have a chest x-ray and blood and urine tests done. Teaching by your health care team members will also be done today. This will include: coughing, breathing exercises, ankle exercises, the equipment used to watch you during and after surgery, and about the surgery itself. A visit from Pastoral Care is also available.

Surgery: The events of the day of surgery begin at an early hour. Medicine will be given to you that makes you sleepy and relaxed. Your only activity will be bed rest. Before surgery, please do not get up after taking your medicine. After surgery, you will wake up in the Surgical Intensive Care Unit (SICU) with a breathing tube in your mouth, which is connected to a ventilator (breathing machine). You will not be able to talk until the tube is taken out, but the nurses will ask you yes/no questions so you can let the nurses know what you need. The nurse will explain things to you. Your family may visit you in the SICU at pre-set times, since it is a good idea for them to get some rest, like you, after you return from surgery. The doctors and nurses will also explain to them what is happening and why.

Day One After Surgery: By morning, the breathing tube is usually removed and you can talk again and start taking sips of clear liquid (apple juice, jello). You will wear an oxygen mask and will work on your deep breathing and coughing. An IV will be kept in place, but all the other equipment will be removed, if not needed. Usually you will be transferred to the Cardiac Telemetry Unit (CTU) where you continue your progress towards going home. Your activity will gradually increase during the day and you may get up in the chair. Your emphasis is to stay comfortable and rest.

Day Two After Surgery: Your diet will return to a cardiac diet. Your activity will increase and you will get in the chair several times. Teaching for going home will be continued.

Day Three After Surgery: You will continue with the cardiac diet throughout your stay. Your activities will increase each day. You will have an x-ray. You might feel sore, so please take your pain medicine to keep you comfortable. The most important activities for you to do are coughing and deep breathing. You and your family or care person will watch videos and learn discharge activities daily to help get you ready to go home. Your discharge plans will be reviewed and finalized.

Day Four or Five After Surgery: You will be walking and doing your coughing and deep breathing exercises by yourself. You will have blood tests. You will be ready to go home.

Remember, each person is special and may progress at a different rate. The plan is adapted to meet the needs of all our patients. It will allow you to set goals for yourself and keep you on course to go home. All your needs are taken into consideration as we work with you to return home. For more information, please read your books: *Going for Heart Surgery, What You Need To Know,* and *Moving Right Along After Open Heart Surgery.*

FIGURE 12.2 High Point Regional Hospital open heart surgery plan (text).

Patient Case Management and Variances

The term patient case management describes the close tracking and specialized individual intervention along the continuum of care that are needed to manage high-risk, high-cost patient cases. Case management frequently targets patients vulnerable to readmissions and an unpredictable course of care, such as:

- Low-birth-weight infants
- Pediatric patients with special needs
- High-risk obstetric patients
- Patients with terminal illness
- Patients with multiple trauma
- Patients with human immunodeficiency virus (HIV) or acquired immunodeficiency syndrome (AIDS)
- Patients with radical surgeries (such as amputation)
- Patients on long-term ventilation

Variances, or deviations from the projected critical path that prevent the patient from staying on the expected course, are identified. For example, when a new diagnosis is identified, the plan of care is revised. Variances are tracked to improve quality of care. When patient outcomes vary from those expected, the variance and its reason are documented. Common reasons for variances are detailed in Box 12.1.

Although exceptions are expected as plans are individualized, the targeted length of inpatient stay remains unless it can be justified by the variance. Variances may extend the length of stay, or shorten the length of stay when patients progress more quickly than expected. All variances are noted, with efforts to resolve negative variances and to examine positive variances that may lead to decreasing lengths of stay.

Disease Management Programs

Critical pathways apply to episodes in care, such as a procedure or hospitalization. Disease management programs provide population-based health care to patients with

---

BOX 12.1 Common Reasons for Variance

- Patient condition, complication
- Patient pain, fatigue
- Patient decision
- Patient's limited mental status
- Medication or treatment not administered
- Additional tests needed
- Care map modified because of admitting diagnosis or pre-existing condition
- Family decision or unavailability
- Equipment, medication, referral, transfer bed not available

---

chronic illness. The goal of disease management is to provide optimum, cost-effective care to individual patients across their lives. These interdisciplinary programs use evidence-based clinical guidelines and critical pathways to guide practice. In addition, they use integrated data management systems to track patient progress across care settings, which facilitates continuous improvement of treatment algorithms. Activities of case managers in disease management programs include:

- baseline assessment
- educational interventions
- evaluating patient outcomes
- evaluating program outcomes (Huston, 2002)

Documentation of Case Management

Documentation that supports case management continues to evolve. The trend toward computerized systems, often called decision support systems, integrates many facets of tracking, communication, and quality improvement. Software programs are capable of developing reports for physicians, nurses, and other staff, which reflect actual length of stay, patient and procedure variances (including those related to patient education outcomes), and actual outcomes of care. A charting-by-exception format is commonly used with bedside computer terminals.

Discharge Creep and Issues of Timing Implications for Patient Education

Patient education is a key component of case management. Critical pathways help the health care team keep the big picture in mind, and focus on the goals of care. Consequently, discharge teaching begins at admission and is integrated into every interaction with the patient and family. As length of stay decreases, critical paths must be redrawn to reflect a new time line for the delivery of procedures, tests, treatments, and patient teaching. For example, a 7-day patient education program cannot be condensed into 4 days, and keep the same learning goals. In addition, all days are not equal. When allocating teaching responsibilities to the path, consider the patient's physical and psychological ability and the need for reinforcement of learning. Given shorter stays, if patient safety and self-care goals are to be met, patient education must be coordinated across the continuum of care.

Patient education programs may be evaluated by averaging the lengths of stay for a patient population that has participated in a patient education intervention (usually for the purpose of making a case for the program's impact). Consider the following advice:

The median is the same as the 50th percentile rank, the score in a distribution of scores above and below which one-half of the scores fall. It is the middle score, if all scores are laid out in numerical order. The median is less sensitive to outlier scores than is the arithmetic mean (the average of all scores). Therefore, the median is a better statistic to use when evaluating impact on length of stay, particularly when outliers can reduce the appearance of a program's success for most patients.

Individualization of Case Management Care

Case management and critical pathways facilitate application of evidence-based, standardized care. They provide a consistent structure that frees up health care providers to attend to individual differences in patients and families. This structure promotes patient-centered care by assuming collaboration between the patient, family, and interdisciplinary health care providers.

Reaching outcome goals is dependent upon this collaboration. Health care providers do not make patients well. When patients and families are part of the goal-setting process, they are most likely to change behaviors to reach those mutually determined goals. Adherence to these new behaviors:

- is highly personal because illness has personal meaning to each patient
- requires readiness and stamina
- takes time
- involves perceived gains and losses, and benefits must outweigh the costs

Adherence requires a positive relationship between the patient and interdisciplinary health care providers aimed at the patient's highest level of comfort, health, and self-sufficiency. Individualization of patient education involves assessment of the learner, and using the right teaching intervention at the right time (Henry & Zander, 2001).

PROCESS ISSUES IN CASE MANAGEMENT

Philosophical and Power Issues: Implications for Case Management and Patient Education

When care coordinators, case managers, nurse managers, and staff nurses involved in creating critical paths are interviewed, they invariably mention philosophical issues and power or political issues. Confronting these issues is essential to successfully streamline and integrate patient education into innovative case management efforts, including the development of critical paths and expert patient teachers (Benner, Tanner, & Chelsa, 1996; Powell, 2000).

Despite evidence indicating that patient education improves the quality of care and reduces costs, patient education efforts must compete for budgets and organizational influence. With the focus of patient education on interdisciplinary planning and coordination involving many providers, and frequently crossing divisional lines in the institution, a political coalition is necessary to support patient education services. Building these coalitions involves several philosophical and political issues.

Philosophical issues concern one's approach to patients and basic beliefs about how patient education should be implemented. These issues tend to vary with educational background; health care professionals tend to practice patient education in a manner consistent with their own educational preparation. Power and political issues usually concern control—who teaches what, to whom, and when.

This chapter explores the impacts that different professional roles and institutions exert on the delivery of patient education, and presents skills that will enhance the effectiveness of confronting philosophical, power, and political issues in promoting patient education. These skills will also help prepare the health care professional become an agent for change.

Traditional Versus Progressive Health Professionals

Through years of nursing practice, we have noticed that, in general, two types of health care professionals exist: traditional or progressive. Although we speak of health care professionals as all professional disciplines on the health care team, the following discussion focuses on physicians and nurses.

The traditional health care professional is accustomed to a hierarchical approach to medical care, in which the physician is the dominant decision-maker and the focus of patient care activities. Those who subscribe to this model view the physician as totally responsible for all aspects of the patient's care and tend to regard the patient as belonging to the physician. The physician operates from a position of centralized power. This model assumes the physician always knows what is best for the patient and the patient concurs with this attitude. The patient exhibits this concurrence by responding without question to the medical regimen.

Physicians practicing in medical and surgery specialties often apply this traditional approach to patient education. They are among those with a high risk of medical malpractice suits. This risk may account for this group's less than enthusiastic acceptance of patient education done by other members of the health care team. This group of physicians must be persuaded that patient education can actually reduce litigation. Accurate and concise documentation will establish a channel of communication, keeping the physician aware of all information given to his or her patients.

A traditional nursing orientation to patient education is associated with nursing education prior to 1970, when nurses were taught in a medical model, often with physician instructors. The current approach to nursing education in both degree programs and continuing education has resulted in a more eclectic, holistic appreciation of humankind that does not depend on one particular approach or model.

The progressive health care professional may be younger, more accustomed to patient-centered care provided by an interdisciplinary team, and less likely to view the physician as the dominant or sole decision-maker. The progressive health care professional eschews centralized power in favor of decentralization, so that all team members have authority in their specialty areas.

Both traditional and progressive approaches are appropriate; the traditional approach may be better suited to some situations than the progressive approach. However, as readers can probably tell, our bias is in favor of the progressive health care professional.

Philosophical Issues

SELF-CARE APPROACH

Self-care is Dorothea Orem's conceptual basis for nursing practice. Self-care is defined as the voluntary regulation of one's own function and development to maintain life, health, and well-being (Orem, 2001). The nurse's function is to help the patient achieve a level of wellness consistent with the patient's own lifestyle and value system, but not necessarily with the value system maintained by the health care providers. In self-care, the patient controls his or her medical regimen and makes choices regarding medical management.

In the United States, traditional health care by physicians emphasizes acute management, which leaves little opportunity to assist the patient in mastering self-care activities and skills. On the other hand, nursing promotes self-care, health promotion, and prevention of illness, encouraging greater independence from the traditional health care system. Patient education is an integral part of self-care practice, because knowledge and skills are needed to promote health and to manage problems related to disease. Ideally, patient education reduces a patient's dependency on the health care system, or does not increase the need for services.

Consumer desires and pressures are influencing professional attitudes toward self-care. The philosophy of many nursing and medical schools now includes patient-centered care. In addition, the standards of the Joint Commission on the Accreditation of Healthcare Organizations (JCAHO) support the promotion of self-care and wellness skills.

PATIENT EDUCATION MODEL

Progressive and traditional health care professionals adhere to different models of patient education. In our experience, traditional health care professionals tend to approach patient education from the medical model perspective of content: diagnosis, prognosis, and therapy. Although most medical students receive this type of education, nursing students, especially recent graduates, usually receive instruction in teaching and learning theories, which assert that although information is imparted, there is no guarantee it is learned.

Nursing students are required to put teaching and learning theories into practice, and almost all recent nursing graduates can remember being evaluated on a patient education project. But as these theories assert, all students do not learn and practice the precepts as comprehensively as they should. A recently evaluated baccalaureate nursing student said to a patient, "Because you've had a heart attack before, I know you understand what it's all about. I'll leave you a handout that will give you more information." The student made no effort to assess the patient's level of understanding, or possible misconceptions about the previous myocardial infarction. This student wrongly assumed that delivering information constituted patient education. (For more information on assessment in patient education settings, see Chapter 7.)

The traditional health care professional frequently views patient education as the imparting of information, whereas the progressive views patient education as an interactive collaboration. Consequently, progressive health care professionals also understand the value of tailoring teaching to individual patient needs and beliefs.

INFORMATION SHARING

Progressive health care providers are generally more willing to share information with patients. One nurse related an incident that occurred in a hospital where she worked, in which several physicians did not want their patients told about the potential side effects of a particular medication. In another example, a nursing student was forbidden to make home visits to an oncology patient because the physician did not want the student to tell the patient the possible side effects of chemotherapeutic agents. When a physician forbids a nurse to give information to a patient, issues of power and control are definitely at stake (Benner, Tanner & Chelsa, 1996).

Obviously, instances occur when nurses impart incorrect information or choose the wrong time to attempt patient teaching. A nurse may completely overwhelm a presurgical coronary bypass patient with teaching, so the patient approaches surgery with an unhealthy level of anxiety. It is the nurse's responsibility to ensure that his or her information is correct and that he or she properly assessed the patient's ability to learn. It is the physician's responsibility, in keeping with the patient's right to know, to impart all pertinent information to the patient in such a manner that the patient can understand.

One of the best ways to get physicians to support patient education is to show how it benefits them. Find out what patients repeatedly phone the physician about during or after office hours, such as pain or constipation. Find out what physicians find themselves repeating to patients over and over again. Provide a handout to remind patients of what they were taught. An orthopedic surgeon may sit down with a patient and review exercises that the patient is to perform after surgery. Create a teaching sheet to reinforce the instruction and use it for follow-up. It can also include information on how to deal with pain. When patients remember and follow instructions better, resistant physicians learn to appreciate the contributions of patient education.

HOLISM

Holistic medicine is the art and science of healing that addresses the whole person, including body, mind, and spirit (Ivker, 2003). It views the person as a total, nonfragmented human being, who is a sum of all his or her parts.

When we assume the holistic approach, we are interested in the total person, not just his or her diseased or dysfunctional part. The medical model separates mind from body from spirit, applying a nonholistic approach. One looks at the child's broken leg, diagnoses it through the use of x-ray films, casts it, and prescribes an analgesic. According to the medical model, the fractured femur is the dysfunctional part, the part that is treated. A holistic approach expands the focus on the child with the broken bone to include assessing the parents' need to be taught childhood safety. When the holistic approach is applied to patient education, it becomes clear that teaching includes more than just information about a single dysfunction or problem.

Another example of holism and its effect on patient teaching involves a 44-year-old man with gastric carcinoma. A nursing student who had cared for the patient in the hospital made a home visit to evaluate his status and teach, as needed. She found the patient's family had learned the necessary skills of dressing changes and tube feedings and they were doing much better with the physical care than had been expected. However, she noted that the teenage son exhibited inappropriate behavior by ignoring his father. During discussions with the mother and son she learned that the son feared a bloody, gruesome death scene. The nursing student could clarify the misconceptions and alleviate a great deal of the adolescent's anxiety. Her holistic approach also included a referral to a local hospice group.

In the past, most nursing education paralleled medical education, and nurses were instructed according to the medical model. Some nurses still subscribe to the medical model but, as nursing education has progressed, many nurses abandoned the old model in favor of a view of the patient as a unified whole. There is also a growing trend among physicians to subscribe to a holistic concept, and it is not unrealistic to hope for a unified nursing-medical approach in the future.

EDUCATION FOR THE CHRONICALLY ILL

Viewpoints about educating chronically ill patients differ between traditional and progressive health care professionals. Most progressive professionals believe that patients with chronic illnesses need more in-depth education than is ordinarily offered by the medical regimen (that is, more information than listing when medications should be taken). Progressive health care professionals teach about chronic illness in an effort to help the patient attain the highest level of wellness possible.

Between 95 percent and 99 percent of chronic illness care is given by the person who has the illness. The patient is in charge of his or her own health, and the daily decisions patients make have a huge impact on outcomes and quality of life (Funnell, 2000).

Patients with chronic diseases need to understand:

- Their illness is serious. If they don't believe it is a problem, they will never make changes to improve their health.
- Their condition is essentially self-managed.
- They have options.
- They can change their behavior (Funnell, 2000).

For example, a nurse spent 3 hours with a 12-year-old girl who had insulin-dependent diabetes and her parents, educating them about the intricacies of diabetes management. This preadolescent girl and her family had to learn about insulin administration, diet, exercise, blood glucose monitoring, and the signs and symptoms of hypo- and hyperglycemia, and how to work this regimen into the lifestyle of a 12-year-old. The patient and her parents needed to set goals for her care. They had to weigh the option of less strict control against the possible dangers of later complications and even premature death.

When an adolescent is diagnosed with non-insulin-dependent diabetes, it is likely other family members are glucose impaired. Obesity; high-fat, low-fiber diets; and lack of physical exercise are also a common family pattern. It is helpful to review the entire family dynamic and help the family make healthy lifestyle choices. Long-term plans must be made and long-term goals defined by the patient, family, and the health care provider.

Power and Political Issues

COMPLIANCE

It has been said that health care professionals take credit for their patients' successes and blame patients for their own failures. In reality, the responsibility is shared in both cases, but ultimately the patient has more control of the outcome than we do (Funnell, 2000).

Traditional health care professionals often claim that the goal of patient education is compliance, and view patient education as worthless if it cannot be proven to increase compliance. They may also view patient education as a form of coercion or a violation of free choice (Bastable, 2003). However, progressive thinking sees compliance with a medical regimen as an important, but not sole, goal of patient education. A significant process occurs between education and compliance, in which the goals are mutually established, the patient internalizes the teaching, and then makes informed choices about applying the teaching to his or her life. It is the coercive aspect of compliance that relates this issue to power and control. Who has power in a patient education situation, the health care provider or the patient? Obviously, the patient should have the control, but too often patient educators try to control the situation for the patient, subtly threatening removal of support or services if instructions are not followed.

Health care providers, especially physicians, have usually been viewed as authority figures who must be obeyed. As consumers demand greater accountability of health care professionals, many providers have dropped the traditional, paternalistic roles. The emerging role of the health care professional is to provide clinical expertise and information, collaborate with the patient to solve his or her problems, and support the patient throughout the process (Funnell, 2000).

RESPONSIBILITY FOR TEACHING

Traditional and progressive providers also frequently disagree on who should teach patients and families. Almost all health care providers have a legal responsibility to provide health teaching for their patients. Yet some physicians still believe they are the only providers who should teach. In some hospitals, physicians require that the rest of the health care team should wait for an order before their patients may be shown hospital-approved videos or literature. Although in some cases a physician's order is required to facilitate third-party payment for patient teaching, in many situations the requirement of a physician's order for patient education is an issue of power and control.

A physician's reluctance to let nurses perform patient education as an independent function may be related to previous experiences involving novice nurses who were clinically unprepared to teach (Benner, Tanner, & Chelsa, 1996). The educational programs for licensed practical nurses (LPNs) do not prepare them to assess and plan for patient education. This is not to say that few LPN patient educators carry out effective patient teaching, but it is unrealistic to expect all of them to be as well prepared, without staff development and continuing education. Granted, some professional registered nurses (RNs) are ineffective as patient teachers because of lack of preparation or personality factors. A few experiences with these nurses tend to dampen the enthusiasm of even the most strongly patient education–oriented physician. However, nurses who have been rebuffed in their patient education efforts by physicians are inclined to lose some of their enthusiasm. Patient education must be a team effort.

Most nurses are not interested in appropriating the physician's role in discussing the diagnosis, prognosis, and therapy with the patient. Instead, they interpret their role in patient education as that of making themselves available for clarification and discussion of daily management of the problem. If we accept the goal of nursing as the promotion and maintenance of health in individuals, families, groups, and the community, this role is appropriate for the nurse. Again, collaboration is a key to effective patient education. It is often necessary to spend time one-on-one with physicians to garner trust and to gain support for patient education.

PATIENT EDUCATION REFERRALS

The third political issue is the willingness to refer patients to other patient education resources, especially self-help groups. It is frequently appropriate to refer patients to community resources to receive ongoing support and ongoing teaching from like-affected people. Examples include patients with substance abuse problems, and families of patients with Alzheimer's disease.

Health care providers may not know about groups and online computer resources to which patients could be referred. Part of this lack of awareness represents a lack of concern regarding the development of patients' coping and adaptive resources.

A more disturbing attitude, however, is the paternalism found among traditional health care professionals who are reluctant to suggest community resources unless they can vouch for their value. The idea of ownership of patients is not congruent with the prevailing belief that adults are responsible, autonomous human beings who make their own choices about health care. If a health care provider refuses or neglects to give a patient information about self-help groups, he or she has single-handedly decided that the patient cannot judge whether such a self-help group might be useful. This attitude effectively places the power for decision-making in the health care provider's hands instead of in the patient's, where it rightfully belongs.

All health care providers should acquaint themselves with self-help and support groups that offer services for their patients. Consumers know what sort of support they need, and are becoming aware that the medical system does not have the resources or structure to provide complete support for the chronically ill, the handicapped, the needy, the deviant, and the socially isolated. It is not a question of giving our power away. Health care consumers already have the power to access community resources and take responsibility for self-care. Our only options are to stubbornly struggle to regain control, or collaborate to ensure quality care.

Power in the Patient Education Setting

Power is the ability to influence others. Health care providers have begun to recognize power as a legitimate function, and educators promote its use.

RECOGNIZING TYPES AND SOURCES OF POWER

Power is a quality that is developed over time with a great deal of hard work. The clues to recognizing power and influence in others are subtle. To implement patient education, first recognize where power resides by asking the questions in Box 12.2. Because power includes decision-making and control of resources, get the correct answers to these questions and approach the power source or sources.

Power emanates from various sources, which in turn strengthen or lessen the power. The following typology of power outlines its sources, starting with the most and ending with the least influential:

1. Expert power
2. Positional power
3. Personality, or charismatic, power
4. Social power

Expert power is the most effective type of power. The person with expert power knows what he or she is talking about, and people respect what he or she has to say. This person may or may not possess positional power. A nurse who attempts to coordinate or initiate a patient education program on pain management must have expert power to succeed, pro-

---

> **BOX 12.2** Questions to Determine Who Has the Power Regarding Patient Education in an Institution
>
> - Who decides if this patient is to receive teaching?
> - Who assesses the value of a teaching program and mandates its operation in the hospital?
> - Who approves necessary funding for audiovisual equipment to enhance patient education?
> - Who knows what is really going on in this institution?
> - Who seems to be "in control" at meetings on patient education?

---

viding pertinent information in a logical, concise manner, citing evidence-based guidelines for analgesics.

Expert power may be a type of formal power (as in a clinical nurse specialist) or it may be informal power (as in the staff nurse everyone turns to when a patient needs teaching). Formal education or on-the-job training can develop expert power, but expert knowledge makes this person credible. Being an expert on the costs and benefits of patient education, especially financial, is an important source of expert power.

Positional power is always formal power, because it is invested in the person by an institution or organization. Persons with positional power have the ability to hire and fire, to authorize pay increases, and to set limits of acceptable behavior. Positional power is an obvious asset to the nurse who tries to initiate a patient education program. Nurses who have assumed the roles of care coordinator or case manager can learn to use their position and administrative mandates as a source of power.

Personality, or charismatic, power is less effective than expert or positional power. All of us have known people with tremendous power because of a dynamism that sets them apart from others. Most people can name political or religious leaders with charismatic power. Likewise, most people know coworkers with power based on their personalities. We know a physician who began a successful in-house patient education program that was quickly adopted by the medical and nursing staff because of the power of his personality. Power by personality is more efficacious if it is combined with either expert or positional power. The support of a person with charismatic power can be a tremendous asset in beginning a patient education program.

Social power is the fourth and least effective type of power. Social power is the power that one has through social relationships and friendships. It is power given by a group to its informal leader. The aspects of social power that make it least useful are its dependence on relationships, its lack of substance, and the underlying premise that something is owed in return for the granting of social power.

Social power, like expert power and charismatic power, can be formal or informal. Educators and nurse managers frequently use social power to induce staff to accept changes. When launching a new patient teaching program, having a staff development session over lunch and sharing public acknowledgement with staff for their successful development efforts are helpful strategies that capitalize on social power. It is not unusual for chief nurse executives in large hospitals to use charismatic power to advocate for new programs; in fact, nurse executives are probably more productive if they can use these types of power in addition to the more formal kinds. A combination of power types is usually effective, but expert power is a necessity for anyone who wants to be recognized as an able leader for patient education.

DEVELOPING POWER

Once who has the power and the type of power have been identified, many directions can be taken to gain support for patient education efforts. An obvious response is to develop expert power. Because this usually takes some time to develop, it may be desirable to gain knowledge from the one with expert power. This is also the time to gather as much formal training and education as possible, through reading books and journal articles, and attending seminars and classes.

One nurse who was hired as coordinator for patient education in a community hospital spent the first 6 months in her new position identifying powerful figures among physicians, nurses, and other hospital personnel. She also improved her already formidable knowledge about patient education by attending conferences on patient education, by reading extensively, and by working closely with graduate students in health education to develop a needs assessment for the hospital. She researched innovative patient education models that had been shown to improve patient outcomes and decrease costs. After 6 months she solidified her power, which was previously positional, by displaying her knowledge of patient education needs in the hospital and by being recognized as an expert in her field. Positional power continued to support her authority, and expert power enhanced and strengthened her power in the hospital.

After assessment of the institutional power structure and establishment of a power base, change may be necessary.

Planned Change and Change-Agentry Skills

The nature and process of change is still not well understood, although many social scientists and some nursing leaders have developed theories and models to attempt to explain it (see Chapter 4). The skills involved in providing patient education also can be applied to change organizations: assessment, planning, implementation, and evaluation.

Seven skills listed below are especially useful:

- Coordinating
- Collaborating
- Consulting
- Negotiating and bargaining
- Confronting
- Reframing
- Coercing

Coordinating

Change agentry in patient education involves organizing and uniting various approaches and health care professionals in a way that ensures high-quality patient education is delivered. Coordination as a change-agentry skill recognizes the contributions and capabilities of others involved in patient education, and arranges programs to meet the needs of varied patient groups.

For example, an advanced practice nurse in a community hospital used coordination by facilitating decision-making by the patient education committee, rather than asserting her power or authority. She openly recognized the professionals on the patient education committee as the experts, and she assisted them in designing teaching protocols as part of the critical paths.

Collaborating

The process of working in a creative and egalitarian manner can further promote the welfare of the patient in the patient education setting. Health care professionals of all disciplines can appreciate the effectiveness of sharing of expertise through collaboration. Collaboration precludes the negative approaches of territoriality and ownership of patients.

In the above example of the patient education committee, collaboration was used creatively by the coordinator to set a tone of cooperation. She used validation as a strategy to prevent members of the task force from becoming entangled in the decision-making process. Validation consisted of documentation and carefully written minutes that were circulated before every meeting. By validating the process that was taking place, she could establish a spirit of mutual cooperation and appreciation of others' contributions.

Another way in which she used collaboration was through her obvious ability to work within the environment of the community hospital and to deal with the constraints imposed by the institution. Because she could work creatively with administrators and physicians, the nurse executive immeasurably improved her chances of successfully implementing a hospital-wide patient education program.

Consulting

The relationship between a patient education specialist and the consultee who seeks his or her skills is reciprocal. The consultant has effective communication skills and uses them to assist the consultee in developing patient education resources and programs. By providing consultation for difficult patient situations, case managers and clinical specialists can provide the mentoring and precepting other health care professionals need.

For example, the patient education coordinator assumed her role as consultant by first clarifying her own understanding of her role. She realized that she occupied a staff position and not a line position; thus, there were limits on her authority and ability to discipline, hire, fire, or set policy. Instead, she had been employed for her considerable managerial and organizational skills, to provide the impetus for the establishment of a patient education program.

She avoided a common consultant mistake by actually teaching patients, and did not interject herself into the work setting. When using consultation to effect change, it is inappropriate to assume the actual work of educating patients. It is more effective to teach the staff how to assess learning needs and evaluate understanding, the principles of teaching and learning theory, and other relevant information.

Furthermore, this coordinator assumed the role of consultee herself when she sought help from other departments. In addition to increasing her visibility in the hospital, she managed to secure some valuable contacts for later use. For example, the coordinator consulted the medical records department to determine the most frequent diagnoses on admission. Her ability to move from the consultee to the consultant role provided beneficial role modeling for the staff.

Negotiating and Bargaining

To promote and provide patient education, the health care provider must negotiate agreements. The agreements usually involve the procurement or delivery of education to a patient group with learning needs. Negotiating is a positive process through which both parties derive satisfaction. In the patient education setting, bargaining may also occur between a nurse and a patient, with both parties negotiating for mutually satisfactory and achievable goals.

Bargaining is a splendid change-agentry skill that many of us rarely use. However, it must be accomplished in a setting in which rationality and calmness prevail. A patient education coordinator can avoid emotional debates. If someone exhibits obnoxious, strident behavior during meetings, it should not be held against the person in future meetings.

One coordinator bargained effectively when the goals of certain patient education programs were questioned. Instead of compromising goals, however, she agreed to changes in content and strategy. When bargaining is used as a change-agentry skill, remember that negotiating a bargain is a give-and-take proposition, and some important ideas may have to be traded away.

A clinical nurse specialist who served as associate director of a diabetes teaching center negotiated to achieve her desired ends regarding establishment of outreach patient education centers for Chinese and Hispanic patients with diabetes. The med-ical director of the center was eager to have the center accredited by the American Diabetes Association, a long and tedious task that he was unwilling to do himself. The nurse informally bargained with the physician, using her willingness to oversee the accreditation process in exchange for the physician's willingness to approve the outreach programs.

Confronting

The various perceptions held by different people in a patient education setting must be clarified and compared. Confrontation involves a face-to-face encounter between health care providers, or between a health care provider and a patient or family member. Reserve confrontation for situations involving a lack of direct, open communication. Use confrontation only after other change-agentry skills have been exhausted.

When using confrontation as a change-agentry skill, be aware it usually evokes two levels of response: emotional and intellectual. Recognize and identify the emotional response, but do not respond to it. The intellectual response allows room for reasoning. Do not use confrontation in an attempt to impose beliefs on another, but to establish an environment that will encourage a new approach to the problem. For example, when a patient education coordinator realized that territoriality was becoming an issue, she turned the decision-making focus toward patient care and patients' rights.

The term confrontation often has negative overtones. Skillful use of confrontation minimizes its adversarial aspects. When involved with confrontation, consider the amount of authority and support held by the person being confronted. If the person is not powerful, the optimal method of confrontation may be to override him or her. If he or she does possess support and authority, summon the committee members to attempt to change his or her mind. These group members must have equal influence and power for this method of confrontation to work.

Reframing

When a situation is viewed in an entirely new light, old ideas and methods can be replaced with new approaches. This reframing is different from confronting in that the situation is reworked or restated. This frequently involves introducing an entirely different perspective into patient education. When old problems are broached in a different light, new directions can be taken.

This different perspective on patient education may be introduced by a patient, the administration, or a particular committee member. An example of reframing occurred when defining patient education to the medical staff of an outpatient center as not just an attempt to gain compliance, but a basic feature of the patient's right to know. One physician who pondered this idea said, "I see what you are saying; it's like informed consent."

Coercing

Legal authority can be used to gain an end that is not attainable in any other less forceful fashion. Coercion avoids emotional overtones, focusing instead on institutional and government regulations. Coercion is better applied to recalcitrant groups of health professionals who are unwilling to institute patient education than it is to individual patients.

Coercion is usually a last-resort change-agentry tool; apply it only when all else has failed. When a patient education coordinator was stymied by one "blocker" physician, she used coercion by having an administrator exert power from above, after showing him the blocker was obstructing the goals of the organization. This change-agentry skill makes many of us feel uncomfortable; it is not a skill we are taught or are encouraged to use in clinical practice. At times, however, it is the only effective way of achieving the desired goal.

The use of critical incidents, such as a high rate of diabetic readmissions or JCAHO probationary accreditation, can coerce reluctant people or institutions to affect change. When the staff of a community hospital was informed that they did not meet JCAHO criteria for acceptable patient education, they ceased arguing the merits of patient education and began planning better programs.

Other Strategies

Using open-ended questions to probe the attitudes of recalcitrant patient education task force members has led to greater understanding of some unspoken, underlying issues. When opposition is strong, retreating and compromising rather than continuing to wage war may be a good tactic. When using this strategy, however, it is unwise to go back to the beginning of the process because all gains would thus be nullified.

Another strategy is to reinforce the base of support for change and make the base stronger. A change agent should constantly reinforce his or her position through the help of others. It is also important to look inward if things are not going well. Perhaps the change agent has provoked an undesirable response. Increasing credibility is another strategy to effect change. Showing is better than talking, and it is imperative that other health professionals believe the change agent is an expert in his or her area. High visibility in an institution does not guarantee credibility.

EVALUATING PATIENT EDUCATION PROGRAMS

Credibility can be enhanced through evidence, and it is important to apply evidence-based practices. However, there are many aspects of patient education that have not yet been systematically studied and evaluated. It is important not just to evaluate the effectiveness of specific patient education programs, but also to share your findings through publication, so others may learn from your experiences and build on your successes.

One way to analyze the cost-benefit ratio of a patient education program is to systematically calculate its direct and indirect costs, and compare the totals to the benefits of the program. Welch, Fisher, and Dayhoff (2002) have created and validated a worksheet to facilitate this process.

HEALTH OUTCOMES RESEARCH AND PATIENT EDUCATION

Health outcomes research is a body of research that covers quality of care to outcomes for patients. Generally, outcomes research serves as a guide to policy rather than as solely a guide to practice, although outcomes research obviously influences practice. The methodological perspective of outcomes research typically uses populations rather than individuals for samples and generally employs correlational designs that allow for statistical inferences. However, as Figure 12.3 illustrates, it is possible to employ various levels of analysis to determine health outcomes.

In the past, quality of care has routinely been monitored in hospitals through outcomes such as mortality rates or infection rates. However, because of greater sophistication in statistical techniques and greater public interest, it has been found that quality of care and practice patterns vary from institution to institution, from provider to provider, and in different regions of the country. These variations are then reflected in the levels of analysis that must be considered when planning a study of quality of care.

Quality of care can be evaluated on the basis of structure, process data, or outcomes data. Structure refers to organizational components, such as staffing patterns, collaborative practices, and characteristics of hospitals. Process data include the components of the encounter between the health care provider and the patient (eg, for nurses involved in patient education, this includes knowledge levels of patients). Outcomes data refer to the patient's subsequent health sta-

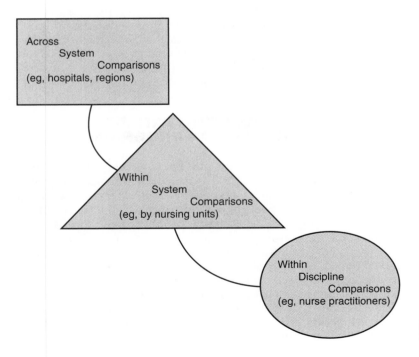

Across
   System
      Comparisons
(eg, hospitals, regions)

Within
   System
      Comparisons
(eg, by nursing units)

Within
   Discipline
      Comparisons
(eg, nurse practitioners)

FIGURE 12.3 Levels of analysis for measuring quality of care

tus, such as an ability to perform self-care related to diabetes or improved mobility. To have nurse-sensitive patient outcomes, it is important to measure outcomes that are amenable to nursing practice. Additionally, the outcomes should have reliable and valid measures. It is difficult to identify patient outcomes that are specific and sensitive to nursing intervention only (most outcomes are influenced by multiple care providers). Therefore, it is more logical to study the processes of care and, secondarily, to link processes to outcomes.

Patient education could bring about positive health outcomes in areas such as functional status, behavioral changes, knowledge, family coping, and symptom control through the process of patient education. Research that could be conducted to measure health outcomes includes a study designed to ascertain if all patients from three hospitals in one city who received discharge teaching post-myocardial infarction (MI) had the same functional health outcomes at one year post-MI. Such a study would demand an across-systems comparison of hospitals.

CASE STUDY 12.1

A YOUNG MAN WITH HIV DISEASE

Chris is a 24-year-old male intravenous drug abuser with a three-year history of HIV disease. He is seen in a large university practice in San Francisco. During the initial encounter with the NP, a large amount of data is collected, including history of present illness, review of symptoms, and previous medical history, childhood illness, medication history, history of STDs, habits, dietary habits, travel history, and pets.

The physical examination consisted of laboratory studies and a complete physical examination, including a general assessment, oral exam, fundoscopic exam, lymph node assessment, skin, neurologic exam, cardiovascular exam, and gastrointestinal and genitourinary exam.

The NP uses this encounter to establish a therapeutic relationship with the patient. She listens to his concerns about his lifestyle and its impact on his illness. He has a history of male prostitution to obtain money for drugs, and he did not always use condoms. The NP and patient contract that the patient will cease any high-risk behaviors and practice only safe sex. In consultation with the consulting attending physician, the NP determines the degree of immune suppression and stages the disease for this patient.

Chris has HIV RNA levels at 20,000 copies/mL of plasma and a CD4 count of less than 150 cells. This is within the guidelines for initiating antiviral therapy. The NP consults with Chris and determines if he is ready to commit to an antiviral therapy, stressing the need for adherence. Initially the decision is made to hold off on treatment until Chris can stabilize his drug habit and housing issues.

COURSE
The NP sees Chris every 2 weeks. The NP and Chris agree that the priority is to place Chris into a drug rehabilitation program. The NP is familiar with resources in the community and helps Chris contact the admissions counselor.

In addition, Chris is referred to a social worker to locate a drug-free housing referral when he completes his detoxification program.

The NP schedule of health care maintenance activities included regular screening exam and lab studies to monitor his illness and complications. In addition, as the therapeutic relationship develops, the patient seeks additional information about therapies and medications. When his detoxification is complete, he makes an informed decision about therapy and begins a multiple drug therapy. Also, the NP notices that, once detoxed, Chris displays symptoms of depression and refers him to a mental health provider for counseling and group therapy.

With time, the NP refers Chris to a network of services available through the HIV community in the Bay area. The NP meets regularly with other providers of care; she remains updated on intervention strategies and sources of services available in her area.

CASE COMMENTARY

Chris's case illustrates that patient education services are needed by patients with AIDS, especially during the period treatment decisions must be made. Now that the treatment armamentarium has been increased, a diagnosis of AIDS does not portend certain death, and patient education needs are similar to those for patients with all chronic illnesses. The gay community has successfully pushed the medical community to offer as many treatment options as possible and often informs health care providers of the treatment strategies. Thus, the nurse who attempts patient education with an informed person with AIDS should persevere in attempts to maintain the most up-to-date information about pharmacologic and nonpharmacologic interventions and be open to suggestions from patients.

Because many health care providers are unfamiliar with the lifeways of the gay community, the health care professional should admit this to the person with AIDS and maintain an open, caring, and professional relationship. Moral debates regarding sexual behavior and gay life choices have no place in the health care arena. If health care profes-

sionals cannot care for persons with AIDS in a nonjudgmental manner, then they should not work in this area of health care.

When caring for a gay man in the terminal stages of AIDS, health care providers appreciate that this person may be faced not only with mortality but also with the need to tell his family of impending death and his lifestyle choices. The informed health care provider can be exceptionally helpful to family members by giving them information, offering support, and allowing for privacy. The definition of family should be redefined to include the patient's partner and other gay friends who have become part of the family of the AIDS patient.

Intravenous drug abusers (IVDAs) are the fastest growing group of persons with AIDS in the United States. They may be of any gender, cultural, ethnic, or racial group. Sharing of syringes is responsible for a huge surge of cases in this population. The IVDAs are a challenging group with which to work. Because chemical dependency is often associated with denial, pharmacologic treatment may be more difficult to maintain. Patient education is difficult with this group until abstinence from alcohol and intravenous drugs has been achieved. Therefore, referral to Alcoholics Anonymous and Narcotics Anonymous support groups is essential. Self-destructive behavior is common and the health care provider should be alert to signs of impending suicide. The health care professional should be aware that this group of persons with AIDS is one of the most stigmatized groups in American society and is thus a vulnerable population. Patient education should always be accompanied by caring concern.

DEVELOPING RESEARCH PROPOSALS TO STUDY THE EFFICACY OF PATIENT EDUCATION

The next level of evaluation of patient education interventions or programs would be a formal research study. This chapter will now outline one way to produce a proposal that meets the guidelines of the various institutes of the National Institutes of Health (NIH), using the U.S. Department of Health and Human Services, Public Health Service (PHS) form 398. Examples are drawn from portions of an approved but unfunded proposal submitted by Dr. Rankin to the National Institute of Diabetes & Digestive & Kidney Diseases (NIDDK). This proposal was chosen because the research involved patient education. The PHS format was chosen because it is one of the most rigorous and can be modified for submission to foundations or other funding sources. Form 398 is revised frequently, but the same basic elements of the application are consistent.

Developing a research proposal is a precise and tedious process that involves following the grantor's guidelines and gathering necessary materials. The most difficult aspect of designing a research proposal is the conceptualization that must occur before writing the proposal. Answering the question "What do you want to know?" is the most difficult part of the proposal process. Once the investigators have determined what it is they want to know, research texts, methodologists, and statisticians can be consulted for aspects of design, sample specification, and data analysis.

The same type of proposal format is used regardless if the research is qualitative or quantitative. In general, qualitative research seeks to generate hypotheses and deals with data that cannot be structured in a numbers format, whereas quantitative research includes data that can be structured in a numbers format or can be transposed into a numbers format. Whether research is qualitative or quantitative depends on the question being asked and the type of data available.

The longest and most important section of the proposal is the research plan. The proposal has nine sections (six of which are covered here):

1. Specific aims
2. Background and significance
3. Preliminary studies
4. Research design and methods
5. Human subjects
6. Vertebrate animals
7. Literature cited
8. Consortium/contractual arrangements
9. Consultants/collaborators

These sections are found in almost all foundation and other agency proposal formats, although they may have different titles. Items 7, 8, and 9 are well outlined by the agency or foundation and, in the case of vertebrate animals, do not apply to patient education research. Many private foundations ask the investigator to summarize in lay terms how the findings will benefit the population studied. Many different approaches to writing a research proposal exist, and this discussion represents only one approach.

Specific Aims

The specific aims section of a proposal addresses the broad, long-term objectives of the proposed study. This section, which appears first, should be a concise and articulate attempt to grab the reader's interest. This section should be approximately one page; thus, the investigator must present a succinct, compelling argument for the study. Some investigators choose not to write their aims until they have developed the study in detail, so the aims reflect the study design and methods precisely. Specific aims should be translatable into research questions or hypotheses.

The specific aims that were derived for a study to improve health outcomes for ethnic minorities with diabetes mellitus were twofold:

The primary aim of the proposed study is to conduct a randomized clinical trial to test the effectiveness of educational interventions (1 day versus 4 days) and family member support (family member present or absent) on selected outcome measures (metabolic control, knowledge levels, family support, quality of life, depression, and family function) at four data collection points (before intervention, and 3, 12, and 24 months after the intervention). A secondary aim describes the incidence of cardiovascular and renal complications in a sample of immigrated Chinese people with diabetes because the data are not now available.

The specific aims section also referred to a previous study funded by NIDDK that was preliminary to the randomized clinical trial and included operational definitions of important variables.

Background and Significance

The purpose of the background and significance section is to critically review the literature and document areas of existing knowledge that may be inadequate and specifically identify the gaps that the study is expected to fill. The background and significance section may include a theoretical model that will be tested in the study. Theoretical links to extant theories should be documented, so that the findings can later be interpreted within a theoretical framework. Literature that is reviewed should include recent work in the field and classic studies. Again, this section must be strongly stated and must demonstrate why the proposal is sufficiently unique and deserves funding.

The background and significance section in Dr. Rankin's proposal set the stage for continued study of Chinese immigrants with type 2 diabetes mellitus. Leventhal's self-regulation model was the theoretical framework used (see Chapter 2). This section included the independent variables (the educational and family support interventions to enhance metabolic control) and the dependent variables (diabetes quality of life, depression, and

glycosylated hemoglobin levels). The background and significance section concluded with the following statements:

The importance of health education programs to teach self-care management skills to persons with diabetes has been highlighted by recent reports of the Diabetes Control and Complications Trial (DCCT) indicating that careful metabolic control in insulin dependent diabetes mellitus delays the onset of complications. Health education for people with chronic illnesses is also a national priority as described in the objectives of Healthy People 2010 (U.S. Department of Health and Human Services, 2000). It is a national goal to increase the proportion of people with chronic illnesses receiving formal patient education as part of illness management to 40%. Chinese Americans with non-insulin-dependent diabetes mellitus (NIDDM) living in the San Francisco Bay Area are a rapidly growing minority population that has not been sufficiently studied. Although educational and psychosocial interventions can enhance not only short-term control of NIDDM but also quality of life for patients and their families, failure to adequately address cultural factors in the designing, implementing, and testing of these interventions can reduce their effectiveness and perpetuate current disparities in health care for minorities.

The background and significance section of a proposal offers the investigator an opportunity to lay the groundwork for the study of an important phenomenon. Although the investigator may believe that her proposal offers a unique chance to study patient education, it should be recognized that many proposals to study the efficacy of patient education have been funded in the past; therefore, a proposal must be exceptional to garner funding.

Preliminary Studies

The preliminary studies section allows the investigator to report on his or her previous work in the same or similar areas. In this section, pilot work should be explained, so that the reviewers have an opportunity to review the investigator's expertise in the field. In nonfederal applications, this section may not be explicitly included. A summary of pilot work completed by the example study included the following statements:

This study allowed the Principal Investigator access to an important site for data collection from Chinese subjects with diabetes; critical contacts were made, and two data collection tools were translated into Chinese. This study also offered the opportunity to pilot a one-day course with the Chinese participants although there was no opportunity to compare a Chinese one-day to a four-day course during this study. Answers on the Diabetes Educational Profile (a questionnaire) indicated that diabetes mellitus was perceived as a stigmatizing illness over which this group had little control and about which they had little information. Other significant information related to the enthusiasm about doing self–blood glucose monitoring, which had not been in the repertoire of this group's behaviors before; with instruction in Chinese many of the subjects began self–blood glucose monitoring.

A second study, also of Chinese immigrants with type 2 diabetes mellitus, was also included in the preliminary studies section.

Research Design and Methods

The research design and methods section describes the design (eg, experimental versus quasiexperimental) and the procedures that will be used to achieve the specific aims of the study. This section also includes the methods by which data will be gathered, analyzed, and interpreted. Any statistical procedures to be used in data analysis must be described in detail. A power analysis to determine sample size should also be included. If the methods are comprised solely of qualitative methods, then, likewise, the procedures for analyzing qualitative data must be described. Some private foundations refer to this section simply as procedures; however, no matter how the section is titled, it should be sufficiently

detailed to allow the reviewers to understand how the study will be carried out and how the data will be analyzed. With increasing sophistication on the part of reviewers and less funding available, the investigator must be comprehensive and articulate in describing the research design and methods. The following portion of the proposal describes the proposed design:

A three-factor, randomized clinical trial with a longitudinal, repeated measures design to test selected dependent variables is planned. The two between-subjects factors are length of intervention (1 day versus 4 days) and family support (family present or absent) and the one within-subjects factor is time (before intervention, 3, 12, and 24 months after intervention). Dependent variables are biobehavioral and cognition based: metabolic control measured by glycosylated hemoglobin (HbA1c) tests, Michigan Diabetes Research and Training Center (MDRTC) diabetes knowledge levels, family support, and emotion based: psychosocial impact, quality of life, depression, and family function. Data are collected before the intervention begins, and at 3, 12, and 24 months after the intervention.

This section also included subsections on setting, recruitment strategies, sample criteria, sample size, descriptions of the teaching interventions, and descriptions of the various data collection instruments (questionnaires) and equipment (a piece of portable medical equipment that analyzed HbA1c), procedures and measurement, and data analysis. For example, the portion of the proposal that related to coding and missing data read:

Data will be entered on a personal computer using the SPSS-9 for Windows statistical package. After data reduction to the appropriate subscales, analysis will proceed using SPSS-9. Two-tailed levels of significance will be set at .05. Missing data will be handled as follows: When no more than 20% of the items from a scale or subscale are missing, the mean of the scale or subscale will be substituted for that person's missing values;

however, if more than 20% of the items are missing, the scale or subscale will be treated as missing for that person. Descriptive statistics will be computed on demographic and medical data including data pertaining to cardiovascular and renal complications. Additionally, the four groups will be compared on major covariates (eg, age, gender, education, income, and cardiovascular and renal complications) to determine that random assignment equally distributed the covariates.

The investigator should use precision and care for the research design and methods section. The authors recommend that a statistician be consulted to review this section of the proposal. Most institutions, whether hospitals or academic settings, have consulting statisticians available for this type of assistance.

Human Subjects

Human subjects is the last section in the PHS proposal format. Whether an agency requires this section in the formal proposal, the investigator must gain human subjects' clearance before commencing a study. In addition to describing the procedures that will be used with subjects or study participants, the principal investigator must also include the plans for the recruitment of subjects, the consent process, the nature of the information to be provided to prospective participants, and the method of documenting consent. Issues regarding consent are covered in Chapter 6 of this book. The human subjects section of the proposal must include any potential risks to study participants and procedures for protecting subjects against potential risks. The purpose of obtaining human subjects' clearance through an institutional review board is to protect study participants to as great an extent as possible from any physical, psychological, social, legal, or other risks. This step of the grantsmanship process is of extreme importance and must never be neglected.

Concluding Remarks on Writing a Proposal

Conceptualizing, designing, and writing a research proposal is a creative endeavor that takes approximately 3 months to 6 months, depending on the resources needed. We have found that proposals that are reviewed by a group of one's peers before submission to the funding agency have a much better chance of receiving favorable reviews and funding. Colleague input may save valuable time and prevent having to rewrite proposals that are not favorably reviewed. Other means of learning the ropes of writing a proposal include mentorship by senior nurse scientists and proposal writing workshops. Many proposals are not funded during the first submission, but are patiently reworked and resubmitted for second or even third considerations. Although the process is time consuming, it is invaluable in terms of garnering funding and gaining clarity about one's own research directions.

SUMMARY

This chapter addressed the innovation necessary to strengthen patient education programs. It is necessary to visibly incorporate patient teaching in the process of critical pathway design and implementation. Patient education should be realistic, based on length of stay as reflected by care maps; variances for patient teaching should be tracked with those for other interventions. Thus, patient education becomes part of total quality programs in the organization and outcomes can be evaluated. Positive outcomes, such as safer discharges and cost savings, can provide needed support to justify staff time and resources for patient education programs. Patients and families should also be involved in planning care so that designs are patient centered.

Every health care professional can provide needed leadership for patient education innovations. Direct care providers who know about critical paths, are skilled at teaching, and are enthusiastic about teamwork with other disciplines can help to make high-quality, low-cost care a reality. Case managers, care coordinators, or patient education coordinators advocate for both the patient and the staff nurse not only through their clinical expertise but also by developing consensus and gaining needed political support. Specifically, they advocate for two of the most needed resources to deliver quality patient education: allocating the time of direct care providers to teach and providing staff development to promote expertise in the practice of patient education for all professional staff.

This chapter has reviewed evaluation of patient education programs, and presented an approach to writing a research proposal using actual examples from a proposal. Research on patient education has become increasingly sophisticated, a fact that has helped the health care provider who needs to convince the skeptic of its efficacy. As the potential of patient education is increasingly appreciated, the research will continue to reflect the positive outcomes engendered by effective patient education. The next chapter moves beyond acute care settings, to address community-based patient education programs.

STRATEGIES FOR CRITICAL ANALYSIS AND APPLICATION

1. Consider the various settings in which care is provided for the patient before, during, and after total hip replacement. Describe how the use of patient focus groups could help nurses identify learning priorities and redesign patient education for the inpatient period.
2. Describe how community-based nursing case management might improve patient education efforts for early discharge postpartum patients and their families.
3. Propose a strategy you could use to gain political support for an innovative new program you developed to replace an existing program that is outdated because of decreased length of stay in your practice setting.
4. If you had to convince the board of trustees in your local hospital to fund an office of patient education, which arguments based on research would you use?
5. What is the purpose of the background and significance section of a research proposal? What important points should be covered in this section if your proposal deals with prevention and detection of tuberculosis in the homeless community?

To find the latest information

Key search terms
case management, critical pathway, care plan, outcome measurement, research proposal, grant writing

Websites
- American Holistic Health Association: http://ahha.org/
- The Change Agent Tool Box Series (National Technical Assistance Center for State Mental Health Planning): http://www.nasmhpd.org/ntac/toolbox/

REFERENCES

Bastable, S. (2003). *Nurse as educator: Principles of teaching and learning for nursing practice* (2nd ed.). Sudbury, MA: Jones and Bartlett Publishers.

Benner, C., Tanner, C., & Chelsa, C. (1996). *Expertise in nursing practice: Caring, clinical judgment, and ethics*. New York: Springer Publishing Company.

Funnell, M. M. (2000). Helping patients take charge of their chronic illness. *Family Practice Management, 7*(3), 47.

Henry, S., & Zander, K. (2001). Improving patient adherence: Case managers can assist patients in adhering to their treatment plans by focusing on education and individualization. *CareManagement, 7*(4), 13–18.

Huston, C. J. (2002). The role of the case manager in a disease management program. *Lippincott's Case Management, 7*(6), 221–227.

Ivker, R. S. *Comparing holistic and conventional medicine*. Retrieved August 10, 2003, from http://ahha.org/articles/ivker.htm

Kallenbach, A. M., & Rosenblum, J. (2000). Carotid endarterectomy: Creating the pathway to 1-day stay. *Critical Care Nurse, 20*(4), 23–26, 28–29, 31–36.

Lachman, V. (1999). Breaking the quality barrier: Critical thinking and conflict resolution. *Nursing Case Management 4*(5), 224–227.

Mamolen, N. L., & Brenner, P. S. (2000). The impact of a burn wound education program and implementation of a clinical pathway on patient outcomes. *Journal of Burn Care & Rehabilitation, 21*(5), 440–445; discussion, 439.

National Tuberculosis Center. (2000). *Fundamentals of tuberculosis case management: Self-study module number 2*. Retrieved August 6, 2003, from http://www.umdnj.edu/ntbcweb/casemgmt.html; http://www.umdnj.edu/~ntbcweb/tbcmfn00.htm

Orem, D. E. (2001). *Nursing: Concepts of practice* (6th ed.). St. Louis: Mosby.

Powell, S. (2000). *Case management: A practical guide to success in managed care*. Philadelphia: Lippincott Williams & Wilkins.

Renholm, M., Leino-Kilpi, H., & Souminen, T. (2002). Critical pathways. A systemic review. *Journal of Nursing Administration, 32*(4), 196–202.

Smith, G. B., & Danforth, D. A. (2001). *Hospital-based case management: Part I*. Retrieved August 7, 2003, from http://nsweb.nursingspectrum.com/ce/ce74.htm

Tahan, H. A. (2002). A ten-step process to develop case management plans. *Lippincott's Case Management, 7*(6), 231–242.

Terry, L. (2001). Educational care path for the endoscopic patient. *Gastroenterology Nursing, 24*(1), 34–37.

U.S. Department of Health and Human Services. (2000). *Healthy People 2010: Understanding and Improving Health*. Retrieved July 10, 2004, from http://www.health.gov/healthy people; http://www.healthypeople.gov/

Welch, J. L., Fisher, M. L., & Dayhoff, N. E. (2002). A cost-effectiveness worksheet for patient-education programs. *Clinical Nurse Specialist, 16*(4), 187–182.

Community-Based
Patient Education Programs

Marilyn P. Verhey

LEARNING OBJECTIVES

After reading this chapter, the student should be able to:

1. Describe the purpose of a community needs assessment.

2. Develop a plan for a community-based health education program.

3. Identify settings for community-based health education programs.

4. Implement and evaluate a community-based health education program.

INTRODUCTION

Educating communities or groups of people can be difficult because the boundaries of communities are not always clearly defined. Rissel and Bracht (1999) identify two general categories of communities: geographical communities and communities of interest. Geographical communities include neighborhoods, towns, and cities. Communities of interest consist of aggregates of people who are linked through a common interest or characteristics (such as breast cancer survivors, people committed to preventing domestic violence, or families of the chronically mentally ill). When a needs assessment indicates that community-based education is desirable, the implementation process must proceed in a careful and organized fashion. The program design must consider economic realities and include evaluation methods.

This chapter describes concepts relevant to tailoring patient education programs to meet the needs of communities. It presents two examples of community-based programs: a health promotion and education program for adolescents in a school-based health center, and a peer advisor program for older patients who are recovering at home after a myocardial infarction.

COMMUNITY-BASED HEALTH EDUCATION PROGRAMS

Community Needs Assessment

Patients are assessed in the context of family, socioeconomic, educational, and cultural influences. Likewise, communities are assessed in relation to their interfacing systems. Communities do not exist in a vacuum; social, economic, organizational, and environmental influences must be considered. Within this context, people may join to identify issues that matter to them, such as drug use or sexually transmitted diseases (Community Tool Box Team, 2002). Each community is unique. For example, a community-based sexually transmitted disease (STD) education program for teenagers in Los Angeles may differ considerably from a program planned for a small Appalachian community in West Virginia.

Just as patients should be taught in the context of what they perceive they need to know, any type of health education or health promotion program should be requested by the community. Hospitals may use community programs to promote goodwill, market hospital network services, or promote their image as invested in health promotion. When insurance companies use capitation to contract with providers, preventive programs may both attract customers and maximize profitability by decreasing the need for illness care. The community must recognize and express a need for services. Planning and implementing community-based patient education programs requires significant time and financial expenditure, and the community as a whole, directly or indirectly, will probably pay for all or part of the program.

There are several ways to assess community needs. One way to gather data pertaining to health education needs is to ask the health care providers who deliver community health care, such as the public health department. Next, formal and informal community leaders should be asked about their perceptions of health education needs. Patient advisory groups, focus groups, or surveys can be used. The congruence between the needs as identified by health care and other professionals and the needs as identified by lay community members should be determined. Community health education programs often fail when the program is perceived by health care professionals as needed, but the population does not perceive a need or desire for the program. To be successful, community-based education must involve community members in determining the priorities of the educational program. Chapter 6 presents a model and a tool for conducting a community needs assessment, and Table 13.1 summarizes methods for learning about the community.

TABLE 13.1 Methods for Community Needs Assessment

METHOD	DESCRIPTION
Literature review	Learn about community and social demographics as well as lifestyles, health beliefs, and health behaviors of the community. Types of literature include nursing and health care references, health intervention articles about the health problem, and behavioral and social science literature. Other sources include local telephone book, newspapers and magazines, census data and maps, and government reports.
Observations	Observations can occur at community gathering places, businesses, worksites, and clinics. Explain who you are and why you are there.
Informal conversations	Informal conversations can reveal what goes on in the community, and other issues that might be relevant to the delivery of educational programs. Talk with a variety of individuals that represent the population. Developing trust takes time. Listen carefully and take notes after you have left the interaction.
Written surveys	Surveys community members, community organization representatives, and local professionals. Ask regular folks to help identify what they see as the most important issues facing their community.
In-depth interviews	In-depth interviews may be done in person or by telephone. Interviews offer an accurate and thorough communication of ideas between you and the person from whom you're gathering information. You have control of the question order, and you can make sure that all the questions will be answered.
Focus groups	In focus groups, a trained moderator guides a group of community members through a series of questions designed to gather in-depth information.

Adapted from Community Tool Box Team. (2003). Assessing Community Needs and Resources. Retrieved August 20, 2003, from http://ctb.ukans.edu/tools/en/chapter_1003.htm

A comprehensive community assessment provides information about a community's strengths, health problems, and needs. After assessing the community's perceptions, educational priorities and community strengths and resources that can contribute to the educational process should be listed.

Planning and Implementation

Breckon, Harvey, and Lancaster (1998) have identified seven principles for planning (Table 13.2). Financing of the community-based education program needs to be considered early in the process. Is the community willing and able to pay for the educational service? Financing may be obtained through foundation grants, or federal or state governments. Because healthier patients use fewer health resources, managed care plans may support health promotion programs, if they can demonstrate cost savings.

CASE STUDY 13.1

PROGRAM PLANNING IN A RURAL COMMUNITY

Laura is a nurse who works in the health department of a rural county in Pennsylvania that needs community-based case management and patient education services to promote the growth and development of low-income children and families in the geographical area served by the department. The director of the health department has asked Laura to plan a program to meet this need. Laura uses the seven principles of planning for community-based educational programs from Table 13.2 to develop a comprehensive plan for the program.

TABLE 13.2 Principles of Planning for Community-Based Educational Programs

PRINCIPLE	DESCRIPTION
Plan the Process	The planning process itself takes careful thought and preparation. Consider community needs, strengths, and possible resistances. Establish timelines.
Plan With People	The involvement of community members is essential. Consider using a planning committee.
Plan With Data	The data obtained from a careful and comprehensive community needs assessment should provide a sound foundation for planning.
Plan for Permanence	Planning for community-based education takes time and resources. Plan for programs to occur on an ongoing basis to make the most of valuable planning time.
Plan for Priorities	Use your time to plan programs to meet the highest priority needs. Maintain a list of priorities that is reviewed and revised periodically. Continue to assess community needs and opportunities and incorporate this information into the planning process.
Plan for Measurable Outcomes in Acceptable Formats	Developing measurable objectives is a vital part of the planning process.
Plan for Evaluation	Develop the way in which you will evaluate the outcomes of your educational program as part of the planning process. Also, evaluate the successes and areas for improvement of your planning processes.

Source: Breckon, Harvey, & Lancaster, 1998.

Adapted from Breckon, D. J., Harvey, J. R., & Lancaster, R. B. (1998). *Community health education: Settings, role, and skills for the 21st century. (4th ed).* Gaithersburg, MD: Aspen.

PLAN THE PROCESS
Laura develops a written document to use in the planning process. She talks with colleagues to identify the specific needs of low-income children and families in the area. She lists the strengths of the community, the potential resistance to a new program of services, and the factors that may enhance the success of the program. Laura thinks about which members of the community and health care personnel should be involved, and what data are needed for planning. Finally, she lists the steps and activities of the planning process and develops a written timetable for each phase of the project.

PLAN WITH PEOPLE
By talking with her colleagues, Laura identifies two community agencies in the area that serve low-income families and children that need to be involved in planning the new program. In addition, two churches and one temple deliver support and advocacy services to low-income families and children, and there is a child-care center located in the county's largest town. An ambulatory care clinic run by the county hospital provides most primary care to the potential patients of the new program. Laura asks one representative of each of these organizations to serve on a planning committee for the new program.

PLAN WITH DATA
Laura meets with the health department's assistant administrator to obtain data and reports that pertain to the needs that the program is intended to address. She discovers that a comprehensive needs assessment was conducted more than 1 year ago. She updates this with recent vital statistics and asks her planning committee members to supplement her data with reports they

may have. She also researches the literature to gather information on similar programs, their interventions, and the evaluation of their services.

PLAN FOR PERMANENCE
Laura meets with the director of the health department to determine the department's long-range commitment to the program once it is developed. The director assures her that the department is prepared to fund the program for at least 3 years.

PLAN FOR PRIORITIES
Based on a careful review of all data and discussions held during multiple meetings of the planning group, priorities for program development are determined. The planning committee decides to focus on developing programs for families with children from the prenatal stage to 3 years of age. Within this overall priority, more specific priorities for program development are delineated, and the committee agrees to review and revise the list periodically as the program planning process proceeds.

PLAN FOR MEASURABLE OUTCOMES IN ACCEPTABLE FORMATS
Laura consults *Healthy People 2010* (U.S. Department of Health and Human Services, 2000) to ensure that the program addresses the objectives related to maternal, infant, and child health and those objectives related to access to quality health services. She uses the Healthy People objectives as a foundation for writing a set of program-specific objectives that cover both the processes of care and services that the program will provide and the expected patient-centered outcomes for the families and children served by the program. These objectives are reviewed, modified, and approved by the planning committee.

PLAN FOR EVALUATION
Laura builds an evaluation plan into her program proposal. She specifies what data will be collected, who will collect it, and how the data will be used to determine if the program objectives have been met.

After the completion of the seven steps of planning for the community-based educational program, Laura revises and adds to the document she developed in step one. She submits a comprehensive written program proposal to the health department director for her review and approval.

Models for Community-Based Health Education Programming

The use of a model for community-based health education programming provides direction to the process and helps organize the various phases of the project. Examples of four models are summarized in Table 13.3.

Types of Community Settings

Patient education can occur in many types of community settings (Breckon, Harvey, & Lancaster, 1998). Here are examples of several settings, and services they may offer.

Health Departments and Other Tax-Supported Agencies

Public health nurses organize and provide health education programs for health promotion, disease prevention, and disease management.

Traditional and Emerging Voluntary Health Agencies

Agencies such as the American Cancer Society, the American Diabetes Association, and the

TABLE 13.3 Health Education and Promotion Models

MODEL	DESCRIPTION	RESOURCE FOR FURTHER INFORMATION
PRECEDE-PROCEED Model for Health Promotion	This model is comprised of two phases: 1) A diagnostic or needs assessment phase called PRECEDE (Predisposing, Reinforcing, and Enabling Constructs in Educational/environmental Diagnosis and Evaluation), and 2) a developmental stage of health promotion planning that includes the implementation and evaluation processes (Policy, Regulatory, and Organizational Constructs in Educational and Environmental Development). The two phases work simultaneously and provide a multidimensional assessment process that guides the policy, implementation, and evaluation components of the model.	Green, L. W., & Kreuter, M. W. (1999). *Health promotion planning: An educational and environmental approach* (3rd ed.). Mountain View, CA: Mayfield Publishing Co.
PATCH (Planned Approach to Community Health)	The PATCH process was developed by the Centers for Disease Control and Prevention for use by communities as they plan, conduct and evaluate health promotion and disease prevention programs. A hallmark of the PATCH process is the active participation of many community groups and leaders. The five stages of the process are 1) mobilizing the community, 2) collecting and organizing data, 3) choosing health priorities, 4) developing a comprehensive intervention strategy, and 5) evaluating the process.	Centers for Disease Control and Prevention. National Center for Chronic Disease Prevention and Health Promotion. (1995). *PATCH Planned Approach to Community Health.* Atlanta: CDC.
Ten-Step Planning Model	The ten-step planning model provides a step-by-step approach to program planning, development and evaluation. The ten steps are 1) development of mission statement, 2) assessment and evaluation of organization, inventory of resources and review of regulations and policy, 3) writing of goals and objectives for needs assessment, 4) conduct of needs assessment, 5) determination of priorities, 6) writing of goals and objectives for project, 7) development of step-by-step activities and procedures, 8) development of timeline charts, 9) implementation of the project, and 10) evaluation and feedback.	Timmreck, T. C. (1995). *Planning program development, and evaluation: A Handbook for health promotion, aging, and health services.* Sudbury, MA. Jones & Bartlett.
Five-Stage Model of Organizing for Health Promotion	This model has as its foundation the developer's own community work, general principles of social and community change, elements of organizational development and strategic planning, and community empowerment theory. The five stages, each of which have several interrelated steps and activities, are 1) community analysis, 2) community intervention design and initiation, 3) implementation, 4) program maintenance and consolidation, and 5) dissemination and reassessment.	Bracht, N., Kingsbury, L., & Rissel, C. (1999). A five-stage community organization model for health promotion: Empowerment and partnership strategies. In Bracht, N., (Ed.) *Health promotion at the community level* (2nd ed., pp. 83–104). Thousand Oaks, CA: Sage.

National Stroke Association recruit, train, supervise, and reward volunteer workers.

Medical Care Settings

Medical care settings include primary care clinics, health care providers' offices, health maintenance organizations, urgent care, and same-day surgery centers.

Worksites and Employee Assistance Settings

Nurses working in business and industry sites provide education on occupational health and safety, employee wellness, disease prevention, and disease management. Employee assistance programs provide services (often educational) to help prevent or solve problems that might interfere with an employee's job performance.

School Settings

Programs that provide comprehensive health services in schools have increased access to health services for many children and adolescents. A major role of these programs is to educate students about healthy lifestyles, disease prevention, and the management of health problems (Lowe et al., 2001).

Faith Community Settings

Churches, temples, and other faith community settings are often effective sites for health-related educational programs.

Other Community-Based Organizations

In a community-based organization, a group of individuals have organized for a common purpose. The purpose is identified by the community and the potential solutions are based on the values, traditions, and culture of the community. Leadership and decision-making are controlled by the community

members. Any given community may have many community-based organizations with differing views on how to identify and approach a community problem. Examples of community-based organizations include adult learning centers, local health and human services councils, organizations for the homeless, and family service centers. Partnerships with community-based organizations can provide an important avenue for the delivery of health promotion and disease prevention educational programs.

Evaluating Community-Based Education Programs

Community-based educational services need to have a continuing connection with the community during all phases of the evaluation process. Box 13.1 presents a set of questions to evaluate community participation. An important consideration in evaluating

---

BOX 13.1 Questions to Evaluate Community Participation

1. Is there open and frequent communication between educational program staff and community group members?
2. Have community group members participated in the community needs assessment process?
3. Did the community group members participate in the setting of educational priorities?
4. Have the community group members agreed upon the measurable objectives for the educational program(s)?
5. Do community group members support the educational interventions?
6. Are evaluation results shared with participants and community group members?

community-based educational programs is the extent to which they can be sustained within the community after the initial planning and implementation efforts have been completed. The plan should address the potential for sustainability, and the evaluation should measure the program's progress toward self-sufficiency. Developing program sustainability is part of working with communities to influence the community's ability to identify, mobilize, and address social and health problems. This process is called creating community capacity.

A detailed presentation of these concepts is beyond the scope of this chapter. For more information on the dimensions of community capacity, refer to the suggested reading list following the references for this chapter.

Another measure for evaluating community-based educational programs is financial outcomes. A comprehensive review of the literature revealed many correlations between health promotion programs and reduced health care costs (Aldana, 2001).

CLINICAL RELEVANCE: TWO COMMUNITY-BASED HEALTH EDUCATION PROJECTS

The following are two community health projects that could be adapted to other communities. One is a program of educational services delivered by a school-based health center. The other is a peer advisor program for unpartnered elders recovering at home in the community after a myocardial infarction.

Mission High School Health Center

The Mission High School Health Center (MHSHC) is a school-based nursing center that provides health care services to 1,200 students, considered to be among the city's most at-risk youth, in a San Francisco high school. The school has a diverse ethnic distribution; its students speak more than 20 languages.

About one-third of the student population is Hispanic, one-third is Asian, approximately one-sixth is African American, and the rest are from other ethnic groups. More than half of the students have no health insurance.

The Health Center operates under the aegis of the San Francisco State University (SFSU) School of Nursing and in collaboration with other university departments, community and government agencies, the University of California at San Francisco, and the San Francisco Unified School District. The clinic is staffed by a nurse director, two nurse practitioners, a registered nurse, a licensed social worker, and a health intake coordinator. A physician provides medical consultation and 24-hour backup. Two SFSU School of Nursing faculty members serve as the project director and the consultant for educational services, quality management, and program evaluation.

The services of MHSHC are organized according to four care delivery objectives:

1. To increase access to health services for students
2. To provide primary health care services
3. To case manage at-risk students
4. To provide a comprehensive health promotion and education program

In this text, we will focus on the fourth objective. Specific components of the health promotion and education program include the development of a learning resource center, the provision of organized classes at the Center and in the classroom, and individual staff contacts with students during the delivery of medical and mental health services. The Teen Advisory Board, established to provide a formal liaison between MHSHC staff and high school students, is also an important venue for health promotion and education.

Learning Resource Center

The Learning Resource Center is a collection of print and video health education materials for use by both MHSHC staff and high school students. The development of the Learning Resource Center began with an analysis of existing patient health records to determine potential health promotion and health problem educational needs. In addition, a needs assessment of students was conducted. Commercial print and video materials were located and evaluated for developmental and cultural appropriateness. For topics for which commercially prepared materials were unavailable, MHSHC staff and students developed pamphlets, flipcharts, and other resources. Examples of the educational materials located in the Learning Resource Center are the Nutrition Education Resource and the Tobacco Education Resource Binders. Both binders contain a comprehensive collection of educational brochures, pamphlets, fact sheets, articles, posters, stickers and other items for both students and staff. Many materials are bilingual and culturally sensitive.

Classes in the Center and the Classroom

Various group educational and health promotion classes were organized and presented in the MHSHC community room. The use of group instruction and the incorporation of peers as educators is an effective strategy in the health education of adolescents. Examples of programs include:

- **Girls Group.** Facilitated by a high school teacher and a MHSHC nurse, the content covers many issues identified by the young women, such as sexuality, self-esteem, and body image. Field trips, discussions, and outside resources are methods used to address the interests identified by the girls at the beginning of the program.
- **Male Responsibility Group.** This group was formed to increase the awareness of roles and responsibilities with issues such as safe sex, relationships, parenting, conflict resolution, and anger management.
- **Latina Group.** This group was formed to help young women deal with issues of domestic violence. Several women in the community, who have experience in the juvenile justice system, conduct this pro-

gram in Spanish with 13 young women. The participants learn strategies to recognize domestic violence situations, interventions to use in potentially violent situations, and resources in the community that provide help. The young women participate in self-defense courses, an outdoor challenge program, and peer education training workshops.
- **Freshman Drug Education.** This weekly class covers drug education on marijuana, alcohol, tobacco, and inhalants. The activities were designed to increase decision-making skills, explore possible consequences of drug use, and practice ways of dealing with peer pressure.

MHSHC nurses are invited into various high school classes to provide health education sessions. Examples include classes on health careers, safer sex, tobacco education, nutrition education, adolescent physical and emotional development, and CPR training.

Education During the Delivery of Other Health Services

Each student visit to MHSHC, whether for a physical examination or for intervention with an acute medical problem, is viewed as a teaching opportunity. Often, it is the information given to the student at a time of identified need that contributes most to the patient's health education and growth. When a student comes to MHSHC for the first time, an assessment of educational needs is conducted through the psychosocial and medical history. In addition to an assessment of students' medical history, students are asked about their support system, alcohol and drug use, and sexual history. Learning needs are identified, and educational protocols are implemented as indicated. With each subsequent visit to MHSHC, learning needs are reassessed and addressed. The MHSHC Patient Encounter Form (Figure 13.1) is completed by the provider at the conclusion of every visit, and includes specific sections for the documentation of health risk factors and education.

MHSHC Patient Encounter Form

ID:

Name:

DOB:

School:

Date of Encounter:

Insurance Info

MediCal: No
Kaiser: No
Other Ins:

IZ Records ☐   OpenCase ☐

Self Consent:
Guard Consent:
Last Physical:
History:
Pysch/Soc:
Condom Ed:

Illness

☐ New   ☐ Established   ☐ Sensitive Services   ☐ CHDP

New Patient	Established	Consultations
☐ Minor (10 m)	☐ Nurse Visit (5 m)	☐ Focused
☐ Low Complex (20 m)	☐ Minor (10 m)	☐ Expanded
☐ Mod Complex (30 m)	☐ Low Complex. (15 m)	☐ Detailed
☐ Comp; Mod Comp. (45 m)	☐ Mod Complex. (25 m)	☐ Comprehensive
☐ Comp; High Comp. (60 m)	☐ Comp; High Comp. (60 m)	☐ Complex (Sexual Abuse)

Complaint:

Diagnosis

DX/ICD-9:

DX/ICD-9:

DX/ICD-9:

DX/ICD-9:

DX/DSM IV: GAF:

Psychosocial
☐ Assessment
☐ Crisis
☐ Group Therapy
☐ Individual Therapy
☐ Family Counseling
☐ Case Management
Time:

Other Contact
☐ C.B.O.
☐ Clinic
☐ Oth Family
☐ Parent
☐ Teacher
Other: _____

Appt. Type
☐ Scheduled   ☐ Called down for F/U   ☐ Crisis: Walk In
☐ Drop In   ☐ Crisis: Called Out   ☐ Phone

Referred By
☐ Everett   ☐ School Admin.   ☐ Social Worker
☐ MHSHC   ☐ School Security   ☐ Teacher
☐ Parent   ☐ Self   Other: _____

On-site Labs
☐ 186: HCG Urine
☐ 183: Hct
☐ 320: Strep A
☐ 185: UA Dipstick/Micr
☐ 188: Wet Prep
☐ Oth:

Outside Labs
☐ 180: CBC
☐ 177: Chlamydia
☐ 181: Diff
☐ 182: ESR
☐ 176: Gonorrhea Culture
☐ 333: Hep Panel

☐ 190: HIV	
☐ 175: Pap Smear	
☐ 174: Throat Culture	
☐ 179: Urine Culture	
☐ 178: VDRL	
☐ Oth:	

Immunizations/Inj.
173: Hep B Ser: _____
169: MMR Ser: _____
168 OPV Ser: _____
171: TD Ser: _____
Oth: _____ Ser: _____

Medications/Supplies

Qty	Unit		Qty	Unit		Qty	Unit	
		216: Ace Bandage			196: Doxycyline			220: Throat Lozenge
		204: Acetaminophen			197: Erythromycin			218: Tinactin
		207: Albuteral MDI			209: Hydrocort. Cream			213: Tylenol
		202: Amoxicillin			205: Ibuprofen			214: Vitamin C
		191: Ampicillin			198: Metronidazole			Oth:
		208: Analgesic Balm			217: Miconazole			Oth:
		215: Antiacid			349: Multivitamin			Oth:
		211: Antibiotic Oint.			201: Penicillin			
		193: Benzoyl Peroxide			206: Pseudoephedrine			
		194: Bicillin			348: Septra			
		195: Ceftriaxone			219: Tetracycline			

Contraceptives

Qty	
	314: Condoms
	325: Depo
	315: Diaphragm
	316: Foam
	317: Gel
	318: Oral
	319: Sponge
	Oth:

Screenings/Other Procedures
☐ 313: Audiometry
☐ 321: Blood Pressure
☐ 341: Burn Treatment
☐ 334: Condylomata
☐ 335: Debride. Skin Les.
☐ 336: Diaphragm Fitting
☐ 337: Dressing Change
☐ 342: Ear Wash
☐ 324: Height/Weight
☐ 344: I D
☐ 345: Injection Antibiotic
☐ 346: Injection Med

☐ 339: Nebulized Rx
☐ 323: Pelvic
☐ 311: PPD
☐ 338: Rmve Foreign B
☐ 340: Venipuncture >
☐ 312: Vision Screen
☐ Oth:
☐ Oth:

Risk Factors

☐ 276: Abuse Neglect   ☐ 278: Drugs   ☐ 288: Peer Social Relation   ☐ 298: Sexuality
☐ 274: Abuse Physical   ☐ 283: Family Relations   ☐ 289: Peer Violence   ☐ 300: Sleep
☐ 275: Abuse Sexual   ☐ 284: Family Violence   ☐ 292: Pregnancy   ☐ 304: Stress
☐ 309: Abuse Verbal   ☐ 285: Financial   ☐ 291: Pregnancy Risk   ☐ 297: Suicide
☐ 303: AIDS   ☐ 290: Gangs   ☐ 293: School Performance   ☐ 279: Tobacco
☐ 277: Alcohol   ☐ 302: HIV   ☐ 301: S.T.D.s   ☐ 328: Truancy
☐ 305: Anxiety   ☐ 286: Housing   ☐ 294: Self Care   ☐ 308: Vocational
☐ 280: Crisis Boyfriend   ☐ 330: Hygiene   ☐ 295: Self Esteem   ☐ 307: Oth: _____
☐ 281: Crisis Girlfriend   ☐ 306: Medical   ☐ 296: Self Harm   ☐ 307: Oth: _____
☐ 282: Depression   ☐ 287: Nutrition   ☐ 299: Sexual Harassment

Education

☐ 228: Alcohol   ☐ 231: Nutrition   ☐ 237: Oth:
☐ 227: Drugs   ☐ 221: Pregnancy Counsel   ☐ 237: Oth: _____
☐ 223: Family Planning   ☐ 332: S.T.D.s   ☐ 237: Oth: _____
☐ 232: Fitness   ☐ 224: Safer Sex
☐ 235: Harm Reduction   ☐ 234: Safety
☐ 229: Health Maint.   ☐ 230: Self Exam
☐ 331: Hygiene   ☐ 226: Tobacco
☐ 233: Medical Problem
☐ 225: HIV
☐ 236: Mental Health

Follow Up

Location: Date/Time: Reason: Resolved

Referral Categories

☐ Alcohol Tx   ☐ Drug Tx   ☐ FP   ☐ lab   ☐ Mental health (In)   ☐ PHN   ☐ Primary Care   ☐ S.T.D.   ☐ X-ray
☐ Dental   ☐ Emergency   ☐ Gyn   ☐ Medical Specialty   ☐ Mental health (Out)   ☐ Prenatal   ☐ Social Services   ☐ Vision   ☐ Oth:

REMINDER!! <<No insurance information has been entered for this patient>> REMINDER!! <<Patient's Self Consent Form>>
REMINDER!! <<Guardian Consent Form>>

Provider: ☐ NP ☐ RN ☐ MD ☐ MSW ☐ Health Ed ☐ PHD Other _____   ☐ Student

Please write legibly   Primary provider Code:

FIGURE 13.1 MHSHC Patient Encounter Form.

Teen Advisory Board

The Teen Advisory Board (TAB) was developed to provide a formal linkage between the high school youth and the staff of MHSHC. The Board allows the youth to have a voice in the development of new programs and services offered by MHSHC. In addition, the Board unites motivated youth who can be taught about MHSHC and its services; in this way, they can serve as a cadre of peer educators. Interested students are interviewed using the questions listed in Box 13.2, and eight youth are chosen to represent various ethnic groups and ages.

BOX 13.2 Teen Advisory Board Interview Questions

1. Tell me a little bit about yourself, your interests, and any future plans that you have at this time in your life.
2. Why are you interested in being on the Teen Advisory Board for the Mission High School Advisory Board?
3. Do you have any experience or knowledge in the following areas that you believe would be helpful to the Teen Advisory Board?
   a) leadership
   b) club or organization involvement
   c) health care
   d) student government
   e) group projects
4. Are you comfortable talking about reproduction and contraception with your male and female peers?
5. Are you comfortable talking (presenting) in front of a group?
6. Can you contribute at least 8 hours to the Teen Advisory Board throughout this semester?
7. What do you want to learn from the experience of participating on the Teen Advisory Board?

TAB members are active participants in conducting an educational needs assessment of their peers using a printed questionnaire developed during TAB meetings. Other TAB meetings are devoted to educational sessions on topics, such as reproductive anatomy, sexually transmitted diseases, relationships, and self-esteem. All of the sessions incorporate many hands-on activities and lively group discussions. At the conclusion of the academic year, TAB members are incorporated into the staff of the high school's Peer Resource Center. Each fall, the process begins anew. Evaluations by TAB members are positive and several pursued health careers upon graduation.

Community Peer Advisor Program for Elders

An innovative, cost-effective program has been developed in the Cardiac Rehabilitation Program of a large New England teaching hospital. The program matches older patients without partners who have had a recent myocardial infarction (MI) to a peer advisor who has also sustained an MI in the past (Rankin & Carroll, 1999). The program is targeted to elders without partners, because this population is at higher risk for morbidity and mortality than partnered elders. The intervention consists of 8 to 12 weekly phone calls by peer advisors to the unpartnered elders for the purpose of providing information, problem solving, and social support.

The use of peer advisors has proven to be an effective educational intervention for risk reduction and health promotion, and for use in ill populations. Elders who have had an MI may offer a unique type of self-help to other elders who experience the same event. Access to another elder who serves as a confidante, a friend, and a trusted source of information provides a form of assistance not readily available to community-dwelling unpartnered elders. Talking with another age- and gender-matched peer who has similar health circumstances may be a more potent intervention than simply receiving social support and information from a nurse who does not offer an opportunity for reciprocation. Additionally, elders who serve as peer advisors may also experience improved quality of life and higher levels of perceived social support as a result of the benefits gained from giving social support.

Selection and Training of Peer Advisors

Potential peer advisors are identified by the director of the Cardiac Rehabilitation program, who is also an advanced practice nurse (APN). The peer advisors are required to be either active participants or graduates of a cardiac rehabilitation program. Criteria for selection include men and women who are 65 years of age or older, are at least 12 months post-MI, can speak and read English, have a telephone, and are deemed by the program director to be willing to undergo training for the peer advisor role. Qualifications considered in the selection of peer advisors include successful completion of phase three or four of cardiac rehabilitation, the ability to be an empathic listener, use of adaptive psychosocial coping skills, and a willingness to participate in a training program.

The focus of Peer Advisor Training Program is to help peer advisors to develop empathic listening techniques, to learn how to role model successful recovery behaviors, and to develop techniques for building a helping relationship (Box 13.3). A review of coronary artery disease, its management, and methods of problem-solving situations involving potential health crises are included in these sessions. The two 2-hour sessions are conducted by two APNs. Teaching methods include presentation of information, discussion, extensive use of role-play, and use of a study manual.

Ongoing Peer Advisor Support

Two mechanisms were put in place to support the peer advisors. One mechanism is the Peer

---

BOX 13.3 Peer Advisor Training Program

The overall objectives of the Peer Advisor Training Program.

1. To reinforce previously learned content relative to cardiac disease and rehabilitation.
2. To provide an opportunity for peer advisors to share their own successful and difficult experiences in the rehabilitation process.
3. To provide an opportunity for peer advisors to recall strategies and persons who have helped them achieve successful outcomes in their rehabilitation.
4. To develop strategies that may be helpful as they guide fellow elders through the process of rehabilitation.
5. To discuss overall strategies that promote effective communication in a supportive relationship.
6. To learn strategies to help a peer sort out recovery issues.
7. To develop strategies to help a peer discern the seriousness of symptoms, and take accompanying actions when symptoms develop.

Advisor Support Group. This group has the following goals:

1. Listening to concerns and using strategies that had been successful for the peer advisors
2. Providing the advisors with additional techniques for handling difficulties that might arise (such as how to respond with empathy during the death of a patient's child)
3. Supplying updated information on the program
4. Providing an opportunity for the peer advisors to socialize with each other and with program staff

Support group activities have included holiday parties and luncheons. The second mechanism of support is ongoing, frequent contact between the APN and the peer advisors. The nurse has been called upon to give advice to peer advisors on various issues of the advising process, the advisors' own health, and various psychosocial issues related to their well-being.

Program Implementation

Peer advisors keep logs of their telephone calls to recovering elders; these telephone logs allow for retrieval of data regarding the various types of socially supportive and problem-solving interventions that they initiated. Logs reveal that at the beginning of the intervention and recovery period, telephone calls last longer, whereas toward the end of the intervention, phone calls are usually briefer.

Some advisors identify problematic symptoms in recovering elders and telephone the APN for advice. For example, one peer advisor called the APN because he was concerned about the recovering elder's nitrite usage. The APN solved the problem so that contacting the physician was unnecessary, thus saving the recovering elder time and money and alleviating that patient's anxiety. In another situation, a peer advisor relayed her concern to the APN about an elder's weakness and fatigue. The APN telephoned the daughter of the recovering elder, who checked on her mother immediately. In all cases, appropriate follow-up is provided to the recovering elder, either through the intervention of the APN or through the advisor's suggestion to the participant that the physician be contacted.

Program Accomplishments

Many of the peer advisors find that being an advisor reinforces the healthy lifestyle changes they themselves had to make, deepening their understanding of themselves and contributing to a feeling of returning some of the care and support that they remember as an important part of their recovery. In addition to improving and reinforcing their own knowledge and skills about the subject matter, the elder peer advisors master important developmental tasks and add depth and fulfillment to their own lives.

This program provides a unique, community-based model for providing support, encouragement, and monitoring of recovering unpartnered elders in a cost-effective fashion. This type of program provides a linkage between nurses and other health care providers in the acute care setting and community-based nurses (visiting nurses). The results of this program demonstrate that peer advisors can provide meaningful support and monitoring of other elders and provide a model for unpartnered elders experiencing other chronic illnesses.

SUMMARY

This chapter describes concepts relevant to developing educational programs to serve patients in community settings. Types of communities include health departments and other tax-supported agencies, traditional and emerging voluntary health agencies, medical care settings, worksites and employee assistance settings, school settings, faith community settings, and other community-based organizations.

The first step in developing community-based programs is to perform an assessment of the community's needs and strengths. The needs of communities can be determined in various ways, including interviews, patient advisory groups, focus groups, or surveys. After assessing the community's needs, develop a list of educational priorities that take into consideration the community's strengths and resources. Planning and implementing community-based education involves paying special attention to the input of community members and coordination with other programs that serve the community. Developing the way in which the outcomes of the program will be evaluated is an essential part of the planning process. The extent to which a community-based program can be sustained within the community after the initial planning and implementation phases is a major goal of program evaluation. Two examples of community-based programs, a health promotion and education program for adolescents in a school-based health center, and a peer advisor program for elders recovering at home from a myocardial infarction, were presented to demonstrate the application of the principles of community-based health education.

STRATEGIES FOR CRITICAL ANALYSIS AND APPLICATION

1. Identify a need for health education in your community, which might be met by a community program.
2. How would you gather information about the health need and verify a need for the program?
3. Describe how you might involve patients, family members, community leaders, and health care professionals to plan the program.
4. How would you evaluate the outcomes of your community-based program?
5. Develop a list of specific settings in your community in which patient education could occur.

To find the latest information

Key search terms
community program, community health, health promotion program

Websites
- Planning, Assessment, & Evaluation Resources (Association for Community Health Improvement): http://www.hospitalconnect.com/ communityhlth/resources/planning.html
- Community Toolbox: Bringing Solutions to Light (Community Tool Box Team): http://ctb.ku.edu/
- React (Division of Epidemiology): http://www.epi.umn.edu/react/main/ community_org/community_org.html
- Interfaith Health Program: http://www.ihpnet.org/

REFERENCES

Aldana, S. G. (2001). Financial impact of health promotion programs: A comprehensive review of the literature. *American Journal of Health Promotion, 15*(5), 296–320.

Breckon, D. J., Harvey, J. R., & Lancaster, R. B. (1998). *Community health education: Settings, role, and skills for the 21st century* (4th ed.). Gaithersburg, MD: Aspen.

Centers for Disease Control and Prevention. (2002, August 30, 2002). *Planned approach to community health (PATCH)*. Retrieved June 8, 2003, from http://www.cdc.gov/nccdphp/patch/

Community Tool Box Team. (2002). *Community context and planning*. Retrieved August 20, 2003, from http://ctb.ukans.edu/tools/en/ sub_section_main_1002.htm

Green, L. W., & Kreuter, M. W. (1999). *Health promotion planning: An educational and environmental approach* (3rd ed.). Mountain View, CA: Mayfield Publishing Company.

Lowe, J. M., Knapp, M. L., Meyer, M. A., Gall, G. B., Hampton, J. G., Dillman, J. A., et al. (2001). School-based health centers as a locus for community health improvement. *Quality Management in Health Care, 9*(4), 24–32.

Rankin, S. H., & Carroll, D. (1999). *Improving health outcomes for unpartnered MI patients*. R15NR4255, National Institute of Nursing Research.

Rissel, C., & Bracht, N. (1999). Assessing community needs, resources and readiness: Building on strengths. In N. Bracht (Ed.), *Health promotion at the community level* (2nd ed.). Thousand Oaks, CA: Sage.

U.S. Department of Health and Human Services. (2000). *Healthy People 2010: Understanding and improving health*. Retrieved, July 10, 2004, from http://www.health.gov/healthy-people; http://www.healthypeople.gov/

SUGGESTED READINGS FOR COMMUNITY CAPACITY

Bartle, P. (2003). *Community self-management, empowerment, & development*. Retrieved June 8, 2003, from http://www.scn.org/cmp/site.htm

Francisco, V. T., Fawcett, S. B., Schultz, J. A., Berkowitz, B., Wolff, T. J., & Nagy, G. (2001). Using Internet-based resources to build community capacity: The Community Tool Box [http://ctb.ku.edu]. *American Journal of Community Psychology, 29*(2), 293–300.

Labonte, R., Woodard, G. B., Chad, K., & Laverack, G. (2002). Community capacity building: A parallel track for health promotion programs. *Canadian Journal of Public Health. Revue Canadienne de Sante Publique, 93*(3), 181–182.

Mitchell, R. E., Florin, P., & Stevenson, J. F. (2002). Supporting community-based prevention and health promotion initiatives: Developing effective technical assistance systems. *Health Education & Behavior, 29*(5), 620–639.

Raczynski, J. M., Cornell, C. E., Stalker, V., Phillips, M., Dignan, M., Pulley, L., et al. (2001). Developing community capacity and improving health in African American communities. *American Journal of Medical Sciences, 322*(5), 269–275.

Veazie, M. A., Teufel-Shone, N. I., Silverman, G. S., Connolly, A. M., Warne, S., King, B. F., et al. (2001). Building community capacity in public health: The role of action-oriented partnerships. *Journal of Public Health Management & Practice, 7*(2), 21–32.

INDEX

Page numbers followed by a "t" indicate table, "b" indicates box, and "f" indicates figure.

A

Abuse, assessment and discharge planning and, 160–161
Acculturation, assessment of, 62–63
Acquired immunodeficiency syndrome (AIDS), education of patients with, 13
Acquisition, as learning phase, 89
Acute care setting, 9
  patient education needs in, 196b
Adaptation to stress, 80–81
Adherence, as compliance outcome, 11
Admission assessment, 108b
  documentation of, 303
Admission practices, analysis of, in needs assessment, 108b
Adolescents
  culture-specific education for, 64
  ecological niche for, 286
  Internet in education of, 286
  patient education for, 63–64
  school-based health education program for, 346–349, 348f, 349b
  teaching of *versus* teaching adults, 127–129
Adult learning (andragogy), 196–197
  application of, 197t
  creating climate for, 219, 222
  emotional needs affecting, 192–193, 220–221
  empowerment and, 75–76
  goal setting and, 196–197
  participative, 222
  physical comfort level affecting, 219–220
  problem-centered, 221–222
Adults
  older (*See* Older adults)
  patient education for, 124–125
Advanced beginner nurse, promoting skill acquisition of, in patient education, 120, 121t
Advanced practice

patient education in, 7–8
  in prenatal education program, 257–258
Advisory board, teen, 349, 349b
Advocacy
  motivation to learn and, 87–89
  promotion of change in, 90–92
Affect, in health promotion, 32–33
Affective learning, 87
  affective objectives in, 203, 204b
  instructional methods and media and, 224
  selection of activities for, 229b
Age
  in culture-specific assessment, 50, 50b
  implications for older adults, 84–85
  and normative age-related factors in life-span development frameworks, 84–85, 85f
Agency for Health Care Policy and Research (AHCPR), Clinical Practice Guidelines developed by, 39
American Academy of Nursing Management Panel, recommendations for culturally competent care, 60–63, 61b
American Nurses' Association
  health care delivery and, 11
  nurse's responsibility to teach, 9
Andragogy. *See* Adult learning (andragogy)
Anxiety, learning affected by, 220
Apperception theory of learning, 93t
Apprehending phase of learning, 89
Assessment, 158–187
  of acculturation, 62–63
  of admission practices, 108b
  application of
    diabetes case, 179–186
    premature twin case, 175–179
  of care process, 108b

case studies showing skill acquisition in, 175–186
collaboration with health care team in, 171
community
  for health promotion program, 133, 140, 141b–143b, 143–144
  of patient education resources, 109b
continuing edcation and, 170–171
cultural, 49–59, 50b, 164b, 167–168 (*See also* Cultural assessment framework)
data gathering for, 162–171
  planning and, 190
discharge planning and, 158–160
of existing patient education programs, 108b
formulating nursing diagnoses and, 171–172
guides/instruments for
  for community assessment, 141b–143b
  for patient/family teaching, 162–163, 164b–165b, 166
of hospital goals, 108b
of hospital philosophy, 108b
of hospital policies, 108b
of hospital staff, 108b
of in-hospital resources for patient education, 109b
instruments for, 162–163, 164b, 165b, 166
of Internet materials, 280–282, 282t
interview in, 168–169
learning during, 173
literature review and, 170–171
needs
  for community-based patient education, 340–341, 351t
  for community health program, 135, 136, 340–341, 341t
  prioritizing of, 172–173
observation in, 168

Assessment *(continued)*
  of outcomes, 291
  of patient care process, 108b,
      158–159
  of patient population character-
      istics, 108b
  patient records review in, 170
  priority setting and, 172–173
  problem areas in, identification
      of, 300, 301f
  process of, 161–172
      management of, 172–173, 173f
  of "red flag" patients, 159, 160b
  summarizing data gathered in
      (nursing diagnoses), 171
  time management and, 174–175
Assimilation
  assessment of, 62–63
  defined, 156
Asthma
  adult, goal setting for, 200–201
  pediatric, patient education for,
      14–15
At-risk patients, assessment of,
      160–161
Attention deficit disorder, teaching
      children and adults with,
      91b
Attitudes, change in, 151b–152b
Audio materials, as instructional
      media, 234
Auditory learners, teaching, 91b
Autonomy (self-determination), 7

B
Bargaining, as change-agentry
      skill, 328
Barriers
  to changes in behavior, 150
  to health promotion, 134
  to learning, 192b, 192–193
  in teaching, 117–119
Behavior. *See also* Motivation
  care-seeking, 34–35, 38
  changes in
      barriers to, 150
      self-evaluation of, 152f
  in health promotion, 32–33
  patient education influencing
      agenda of education and,
          75–76
      compliance orientation and,
          74–75
      empowerment and, 75–76
  Prochaska's theoretical model of
      change and, 90–92, 92t

  strategies for changing
      in workplace health promo-
          tion, 150, 151t–152t
Behavioral objectives (learning
      objectives). *See also*
      Objective(s)
  components of, 203–205
  in learning process, 202f
  for prenatal education classes,
      259b–260b
  statement of, 202
Behavioral outcomes, 33
Behavioral theory of learning, 94t
  case study application of, 96–97
Belief(s)
  about illness, 36
  assessment of, 58b, 164b,
      167–168
  culture-specific, 48, 56–57, 65
  religious, 52, 167
Bipolar illness, patient education
      in, 212–213
Boolean logic, in Internet search
      strings, 277, 278f, 279b
Boston College health promotion
      program, 148–153
Breast cancer, stress process in, 79,
      81b
Breast feeding, self-efficacy theory
      in, 77b
Bulletin boards, as instructional
      media, 232

C
Cancer
  screening for, 65
  stress and, 79, 81b
Cardiac rehabilitation
  case management and patient
      education for, 315, 316f,
      317f
  for older adults
      community peer advisor pro-
          gram for, 349–351, 350b
      patient education for, 14
Care maps
  in case management, 315, 316f,
      317f
  in teaching, 227–228
Care plan
  documentation of education and,
      304
  education needs in, 19
Care-seeking behavior theory,
      34–35, 38
Caring role of nurse

  and characteristics of excellent
      nurse teacher, 191b
  patient education as dimension
      of, 4–5
Case management, 21
  in acute care setting, 315, 316f,
      317f, 318–319
  benefits of, 315, 318
  care maps in, 315, 316f, 317f
  case studies of, 331–332
  case type in, 315
  defined, 314
  diagnosis-related groups in, 13
  in disease management pro-
      grams, 318
  documentation of, 318–319
  early discharge affecting, 319
  individualization in, 319
  leadership in, 21
  nurses as case managers in, 320,
      321, 322
  nursing responsibilities and, 320,
      321, 322t
  patient education in, 314–315,
      319
      patient input in, 319
  philosophical issues in, 318–323
  power/political issues in,
      323–326, 325b
  process of, 319–329
  products of, 315–319
  quality of care and, 314
  traditional *versus* progressive
      health professionals and,
      320–321
  variances in, 318, 318f
Challenge program, for workpace
      health, 148–150, 153
Change
  model of, 92t
  phases in, 149
  planned
      coercion in, 319
      collaboration in, 328
      confrontation in, 328
      consultation in, 327–328
      coordination in, 327
      miscellaneous strategies in,
          329
      negotiation and bargaining in,
          328
      reframing in, 329
      strategies for, 150, 151t–152t,
          153
  promotion of, in patient educa-
      tion, 90–92

stages of, 90–92
Change-agentry skills, 327–329
Charismatic power, 326
Chart. *See* Patient records
Charting. *See* Documentation
Chat rooms, 272
Childbirth classes
    community-based, 257–265
    objectives for, 258–259,
        259b–260b
Children
    Internet in education for, 286
    with learning disabilities,
        patient education for, 91b
    teaching, 125, 126t
Chronically ill persons
    case management of, 323
    community health and, 143
    goal setting and, 198–199
    patient education for, 13–15, 323
        needs in, 196b
Chronosystems, in ecological sys-
    tems theory, 83, 84
Clinical decision-making, 19
Clinical judgment, 19
Clinical practice guidelines, 218
Clinical preventive services guide,
    39–40
*Clinician's Handbook of
    Preventive Services,* 39–40
    case study, 41–43
Coercion, as change-agentry skill,
    329
Cognition, behavior-specific, 32–33
Cognitive appraisal approach, to
    stress/coping/social support
    theories, 78–79, 80f
Cognitive learning, 87, 94t–95t
    case study application of, 96–97
    instructional methods and media
        and, 224
    selection of activities for, 229b
Cognitive objectives, 203, 204b
Cognitive-perceptual factors
    in community health promotion,
        142b
Cognitive stages, approach to pedi-
    atric patient education, 125,
    126t
Collaboration
    in assessment, 171
    as change-agentry skill, 327
    of health care providers, 74–75
    interdisciplinary, in patient edu-
        cation, 17–18, 23t
    JCAHO standards for, 15–18

Communication
    as characteristic of expert nurse
        teacher, 191b
    culture and, 167
    in team work, 24
Community-based patient educa-
    tion
    assessment of community health
        education needs and,
        340–341, 351t
    case studies illustrating, 341–343
    evaluation of, 345b, 345–346
    home recovery and, promotion
        of, 246, 250
    models for, 343, 344t
    planning interventions for,
        341–343, 342t
    for prenatal care, 257–265
    programs for
        cardiac rehabilitation,
            349–351, 350b
        school, 346–349, 348f, 349b
    settings for, 343, 345
Community empowerment, 136
    case study of, 136–137
Community enhancement, in
    health education, 135
Community health promotion
    assessment of community for,
        133, 140, 141b–143b,
        143–144
    Blossom Park project, 136–137
    Consortium for the
        Immunization of Norfolk's
        Children, 137–139
    definitions and, 133–134
    education and, 133, 134
    Falmouth Safe Skin Project, 138
    implementation of, 145–146
    improving success of, 134–135
    intervention in, 145
    legal influences on, 136
    marketing affecting, 138–139
    nursing diagnoses for communi-
        ty and, 145, 146b
    outcomes of, 133, 134, 148
    political influences on, 136
    Por Cristo–Boston College
        School of Nursing
        (BCSON) health project,
        139–148
    teaching strategies in, 147
    workplace program for, 148–150,
        153
Community resources
    for instructional media, 236

for patient education, analysis in
    needs assessment, 109b
Competence
    as characteristic of excellent
        nurse teacher, 191b
    cultural, 58, 59b
    technological and Internet use,
        283
Competent nurse, skill acquisition
    in, for patient education,
    121, 121t
Compliance (patient), 9–11, 74–75
    as behavior choice, 74
    defined, 29
    early approaches to, 29–30
    factors in, 30
    fear and, 35–36
    partnership compared with, 9–11
    patient education affecting,
        9–11, 74
    as political/power issue, 323–324
Concurrence, 11
Conditioning, in learning, 94t
Confidence, as characteristic of
    excellent nurse teacher, 191b
Confrontation, as change-agentry
    skill, 328
Consortium for the Immunization of
    Norfolk's Children, 137–138
Consultation, as change-agentry
    skill, 327–328
Consumer responsibility, 11
Content
    determination of, 217
    of Internet resources, 280
    preparation for teaching, 20
Continuing education, 122–123.
        See also Staff development
    assessment and, 21, 22, 170–171
Contracts, learning, 88, 207–209,
    208f
Cooperation, 10–11, 74–75. *See also*
        Compliance
Coordination
    as change-agentry skill, 327
    staff, JCAHO standard for,
        113–114
Coping. *See also* Stress
    assessment of, 143b
    resources for, 78, 81b
Coronary heart disease. *See also*
        Cardiac rehabilitation
    case study of, 310
    in older women, 84
    normative history-graded
        influences and, 84–85

Cost benefit/cost effectiveness
  in community health program,
    135
  in patient education program,
    329–330
Cost containment
  case management and, 329–330
  patient education and, 111,
    329–330
Critical incidents, learning evaluated by, 300
Critical pathways
  for case management, 315, 316f,
    317f, 318
  documentation of, 304
Cultural assessment framework,
    49–59, 50b
  cultural competence in, 58, 58b
  culture-specific demographic
    factors in, 49–55
  customs in, 55
  demographic factors in, 49–53
  domains of influence in, 60
  epidemiologic and environmental influences in, 53–54
  group characteristics in, 49–50,
    54–56
  health beliefs and practices in,
    56–58, 58b, 167
  Kleinman model in, 59b, 59–60
  occupation and income in, 52
  time orientation in, 55
  views of universe in, 54–55
  Western health care organization
    and service variables in,
    58–59
Cultural competence
  in effective patient education,
    61–62
  in health care provision, 58, 58b
  stages of, 58f, 585
Culturally competent care
  general principles of, 60–63
  patient education in
    for families with adolescents,
      64
    for families with children,
      63–64, 64b
    for seniors, 66–67
    for women, 64–66
  principles of design and implementation in, 60–63
Cultural negotiation/brokering in
    culturally competent patient
    education, 61–62
Culture (cultural background)

  assessment of, 164b, 167–168
  intergenerational parenting and,
    67
  interpreters and, 67–69
  patient education affected by, 20
    explanatory models of illness
      and, 57
    patient education issues and,
      63–67, 64b
Customs, in culture-specific
    assessment, 55

D

Data, categorizing and sorting of,
    171
Data gathering, for assessment,
    162–171
  assessment guide to, 162–163,
    164b–165b, 166
  continuing education and,
    170–171
  healthcare team collaboration
    for, 171
  interviewing in, 168–169
  literature review in, 170–171
  observation in, 168
  patient records review in, 170
  planning and, 190
Day surgery unit, patient education in, 307–310
Death and dying, culture and, 67
Decision-making
  clinical, 19
  in family, assessment of, 168
  patient, 76
Demographics
  in cultural assessment, 49–53,
    50b
  in Health Belief Model of patient
    education, 31
Demonstration, for teaching, 230,
    233, 235
Development, Erikson's stages of,
    adult learning and, 197, 198t
Developmental frameworks, as
    bases for patient education,
    81–87
  ecological systems theory, 81–84
  life-span frameworks, 84–87
Diabetes, patient education in
    behavior change in
    case study of, 205–207
    documentation of, 306b, 307b
  case histories in, 305–307
    application of learning theory
      in, 96–97, 205–207

  assessment skill and nursing
    diagnoses in, 179–186,
    184f
  research in, 205–207
  in children
    Internet information resources
      for, 286–287
  evaluation of, 305–307
  normative age-graded factors
    affecting, in older persons,
    85
  research in, 334–335
  teaching and learning priorities
    and, 193
Diagnoses
  community, 145, 146b
  learning about, 191–192
  medical, 18–19, 158
  nursing, 18–19, 145, 146b,
    171–172
Diagnosis-related groups (DRGs),
    discharge planning affected
    by, 12–13
Dietitian, role of in patient education, 22t–23t, 102b
Disabled persons, community
    health and, 134
Discharge creep
  critical paths affected by, 319
  patient education affected by,
    319
Discharge planning, patient education for
  critical learning needs and, 193
  identification of "red flag"
    patients and, 159–160,
    160b
  increasing importance of, 159
  for older and chronically ill
    patients, 12–14
  vital information in, 160b
Discharge summary, documentation of patient education in,
    305
Disclosure, Internet, 280–281
Disease
  defined, 29
  explanatory model of, 57
  illness *versus*, 59
  patient perspective on, 59b
Disease management programs,
    318
Disease prevention, defined, 29
Displays, as instruction media,
    232, 236
Documentation

admission assessment, 303
care plan, 304
of case management, 318–319
by computer, 318–319
of cost of education, 111
discharge summary, 305
of domestic violence, 160–161
flow sheets, 304
JCAHO standard for, 114–115
patient contracts, 88, 208
problem list, 303–304
problem-oriented record, 304
progress notes, 304
SOAP note, 304, 305b
Domains of influence, culture-specific, 60
Domestic violence
assessment of, discharge planning and, 160–161
culture-specific education and,
66
Drawings, as instructional media,
233
DRGs. *See* Diagosis-related groups
(DRGs)

E

Ecological systems theory
adolescents in, 82
as basis for patient education,
81–84, 82f
chronosystems in, 83
exosystems in, 83
interactive systems in, 82–83
macrosystems in, 83
mesosystems in, 83
microsystems in, 82–83
Ecomap, 176f
Education. *See also* Continuing
education; Patient educa-
tion; Staff development
culture-specific, 51
empowerment in, 75–76
reforms in, 12
Elderly. *See* Older adults
Electronic mail, 271
Electronic media, instructional, 235
Emotional needs, learning climate
for, 192–193, 220–221
Employee assistance programs,
patient education in, 345
Empowerment
of adult learner, 75–76
community, 136–137
electronic media in, 231
individual/psychological, 75–76

Environment, in assessment, 69–70
Environmental influence, culture-
specific, 53–54
Environmental limitations, patient
education affected by, 53–54
Environmental racism, 53
Environment–person mismatch,
stress and, 80, 80f
Epidemiologic factors, culture-
specific, 53
Erikson's stages of development,
adult learning and, 125,
126t, 197, 198t
Ethnicity
cultural assessment framework
for, 49–59, 50b
patient education affected by
explanatory models of illness
and, 57
interpreters and, 67–69
migration status and, 53
Evaluation
checklist for, 297b
of community-based patient
education programs, 345b,
345–346
of community-based prenatal
education classes,
260–261, 261f–262f, 263b
critical incidents and, 300
direct observation in, 298–299
documentation of patient education and, 302–305, 305b
feedback in, 301–302, 302b
identifying needs and performance problems and,
300–301
of Internet information, 270,
279–282
interview and questionnaires in
with patients and families,
299–300
with staff, 300
learning outcomes in, determination of, 293–296, 294b
length of stay in, 300
levels of, 293–296
comparison of, 295–296
measurement methods in,
298–302
needs identification and,
300–301
outcome assessment in, 291, 292f
of patient education interventions, 291–292, 292f,
296–302

of patient education materials
checklist for, 297b
for videotape, 234–235
patient/family reports in, 299
patient record review in, 299
patient's participation during
interventions and,
293–294, 294b
patient's performance in
at home, 291, 295, 297–298
identifying problems in,
300–301
immediately after learning
experience, 294–295
overall self-care and health
management and, 294b,
295
scope of, 291–293
tests in, 299
Exosystems, in ecological systems
theory, 83
Expert nurse
promoting skill acquisition in,
for patient education,
121t, 122
Expert power, 325
Explanatory models of illness,
patient education approaches affected by, 56, 57

F

Faith community, health education
program in, 345
Falmouth Safe Skin Project, 138
Family
culture-specific education and,
63–64
in decision-making, 168
education of, 63–64
JCAHO standards for,
104–105, 105t, 106t
Internet resources for, 287
involvement in interventions,
293–294
Family physician, patient education expectations of, 102b
Family system, in assessment,
164b–165b, 166f, 166–167
Farm Workers' culture-specific
assessment, 52f, 52–54, 58–59
Fatigue, patient education affected
by, 210
Fear
as barrier to learning, 192, 192b
in compliance, learning affected
by, 35–36

Fear-arousing information, and Self-Regulation model of patient education, 35–36
Feedback
  constructive, guidelines for giving and obtaining, 302b
  in learning evaluation, 301–302
  as learning phase, 90
  negative, 302
Financial issues, in patient education, 112
Five-stage Model, for organization of community health education, 344t
Flipcharts, as instructional media, 232
Flow sheet, documentation of patient education and, 304
Forced relocation, as stressor, in patient education situations, 62–63
Force-field analysis, workplace health promotion program and, 149
Frye Readability formula, 237, 248b–249b

G
Games, as instructional media, 236
Gender, in culture-specific assessment, 51
Generalization, as learning phase, 89
Gerontologic patient. See Older adults
Gestalt learning, 94t
  case study application of, 96–97
Global health promotion, 139
Goals
  in chronic illness, 198–199
  of patient and family education, 13, 191
  patient–centered, 192–199
  setting
    adult learning and, 196–197
    with asthma patient, 200–201
    Health Belief Model applied to, 197–198, 199b
    patient and family involvement in, 191, 205
    prioritizing needs in, 194, 195b
    targeting outcomes for learning and, 190
  stating, 199
Gordon's functional health patterns, 133, 140, 141b–143b
Graphics, as instructional media, 232–233

Group discussion, as teaching method, 230
Group teaching, 225–226
  benefits of, 253–254
  individual teaching combined with, 226
  situations for, 253
Growth and development, Erikson's stages of, adult learning and, 197, 198t

H
Habits, in community health, 134
Handouts. See Instructional materials and media
Health agencies, voluntary, patient education and, 343, 345
Health Belief Model, of patient education, 30–31, 37, 76
  factors in, 30
  goal setting and, 197–198, 199b
  planning and interventions and, 225t, 254, 255t
  in research, 31
Health beliefs, culture-specific assessment of, 56–58
Health care
  consumer responsibility in, 11
  Internet incorporation in, 269–270
  reform of, patient education in, 11–15
  for special populations, patient education in addressing needs of, 63–67
Health care team
  assessment and, 171
  in patient education, 6
Health consumers
  Internet health and medical information searches by, 269, 283
  responsibility of, 11
Health departments, community-based patient education and, 343
Health education
  community-based models for, 343, 344t
  empowerment in, 75–76
  purpose of, 73
Health information databases, 275
Health maintenance
  defined, 29
  evaluation of, 298
Health professionals
  as information searchers, 283

  as Internet intermediary, 283–284
  paternalism of, 324
  patient education standards for, 101, 102b
  role in patient education, 22t–23t
    nursing staff, 320
    patient education expectations of, 102b
    physician specialist, 320
  as role models, 20–21
  traditional versus progressive, 320–321
Health promotion. See also Community health promotion
  in community, legal influence on, 136
  defined, 28–29
  global, 139
  workplace program for, 148–159
Health Promotion Model, 31–33
  components of, 32–33, 37
  research studies of, 33
Health promotion model(s), 30–38
  current, 37
  history of, 36–37, 37
  patient education and, 37–38
  Precede-Proceed Model, 33–34
  Self-Regulation Model, 35f, 35–36
  theory in, care-seeking, 34–35, 38
Health promotion projects, Por Cristo–Boston College School of Nursing (BCSON)
  acceptance of, 145
  burn prevention and treatment program, 147
  preparation for, 145
  water purification program, 148
Health promotion projects, The Challenge program, 148–153
Health screening, 40–41, 85f, 85–86, 129
Healthy People 2000, initiation of, 39
Healthy People 2010, objectives of, 39
Heart disease, 14
Holism, as philosophical issue, 322
Home health care (home visits)
  discharge and, 246, 250
  patient education for, 246, 250
Home health care nurse, 7
Homeless clients, patient education for, 210–211

Home visits, assessment skills in, 179

Hospital
  length of stay in
    critical paths affected by, 315
    discharge planning affected by, 13
  patient care maps in, 227–228
  patient care support staff of, needs assessment of, 108b
  patient education and resources in, 109b
    support of, JCAHO standard, 113
  perceptions of patient education programs, in needs assessment, 108b
  philosophy/goals/policies of, needs assessment of, 108b
  social workers, role of, in patient education, 22t–23t
  staff of
    interview and questionnaires for, in evaluation, 299–300
    motivating for patient education, 122–124
    needs assessment of, 108b
    perceptions of patient education programs in, needs assessment of, 122–124
    preparation for teaching, 224
    workshop for, on patient education, 115t, 116
Hospitalization, patient concerns during, 192b, 192–193
Hot and cold theory of disease, 57, 62
Human immunodeficiency virus infection, patient education and, 13, 331–332

I

Illness
  beliefs about, 36
  disease *versus,* 29
  explanatory models of
    patient education affected by, 56, 57
  patient education needs in, 196b
  patient's perspective of, 36, 57, 59b
Immigration, as stressor in situations involving patient education, 62–63
Implementation
  adult learning climate and, 222

application of learning and, 232
case studies illustrating, 221
determining content for, 217
emotional needs and, 220–221
instructional methods and media in
  learning and activities, 228–231, 235, 236
  media use in, 231–235, 232b
  for patients with low literacy skills, 250–251, 251b
  selection of, 219
  teaching/learning methods, 224–228
for organization-wide approach to patient education, 105–112
participative learning and, 222
physical comfort and, 219–220
priority setting and, 219
problem-centered learning and, 221–222
scope of teaching and learning and, 217–218
staff preparation for teaching and, 224
teacher-learner relationship and, 222–223
teaching style and, 223–224
Incentive programs, for patient education, 123
Incentives, staff motivation and, 123
Individual empowerment, 75–76
Individual learning theories, 94t–95t
Individual teaching, 224–225, 252–253
  group teaching combined with, 226
Information overload, 193
Information retrieval process
  application to Internet, 270–282
  definition in, 270
  evaluation and information in, 270
  searching in, 270, 275–279
  use of, to meet patient needs, 283–287
Information sharing, as philosophical issue, 321–322
Information sheets, as instructional media, 246, 250
Informed consent, 12
Inpatient setting. *See also* Hospitalization
  diagnosis-related groups and, 12–13

discharge planning in, 159–160, 160b
psychiatric patient education in, 211–212
Instructional materials and media, 228. *See also* Teaching
  audio materials, 234
  bulletin boards, 232
  closed circuit TV, 234–235
  community resources for, 236
  demonstrations, 235
  displays, 232, 236
  drawings, 232
  electronic, 235
  flip charts, 232
  games, 236
  graphics, 232–233
  guidelines for use of, 231–232, 232b
  low literacy skills and, 250–251, 251b
  models, 235–236
  one-page instruction sheet, 246, 250
  overhead transparencies and slides, 233
  photographs, 233
  posters, 232
  printed materials, 236–237
    readability of, 248b, 249b
  selection of, 219
  for self-directed learning, 228–229
  simulations, 236
  suitability assessment of, 238b–246b
  videotapes, 234–235
Instructional method(s). *See also* Teaching
  demonstration, 230
  group discussion, 230
  group teaching, 225–226
  individual and group formats combined, 226
  individual teaching, 224–225
  learning activities, 228
    selection of, 229b
  lecture, 229–230
  low literacy skills and, 250–251, 251b
  programmed instruction, 231
  return demonstration, 230–231
  role play, 230–231
  selection of, 219
  self-directed learning, 228–229
    electronic media for, 235
  tests, 231

Instructions
  for home care, 246
  writing and review of, 251–252,
    252t
Instruction sheet, one-page, 246, 250
Interdisciplinary teams, in patient
    education, 17–18
Internet, use of
  barriers to, 283–284
  by children and adolescents, 286
  factors in, 283
  by family, 287
  by health care providers, 283
  patient access and, 283
  in self-directed learning,
    284–286
Internet information
  defining, 269–275
    chat or chat rooms, 272
    communication tools, 271
    databases, proprietary health
      information, 275
    electronic mail, 271
    Internet Relay Chat, 272
    listserves, 271–272
    newsgroups, 272
    portal sites, 275
    search engines, 273, 279b
    search tools, 273f
    selection guide for, 275
    subject directories, 272, 274,
      274t
    Web video conferencing, 272
  evaluation of, 279–283
    for content, 280
    for credibility, 280
    criteria for, 280–281
    for design, 281
    for disclosure, 280–281
    at a glance, 281
    for interactivity, 281
    for links, 281
    materials for patient popula-
      tions, 281–282, 282t
    suitability assessment of mate-
      rials in, 281–282
  searching, 276. See also Internet
    search, steps in
  sites for patient education, 282t
    evaluation of, 280–282, 282t
Internet Relay Chat (chat and chat
    rooms), 272
Internet search, steps in, 276f
  Boolean logic in, 277, 278f, 279b
  define problem statement, 276
  execute, 278–279

identify search concepts,
    276–277
  modify, 279
  review help or tips screens, 278
  review results, 278
  search statement in
    construction of, 277
    revision of, 278
  select key words, 277
    identify related terms, 277
  select search tool, 277–278
Internet sites, for patient educa-
    tion, 67–69
Interpersonal learning theory, 95t
  case history example of, 96–97
  as patient education basis, 95t,
    96
Interpreters, for patient education,
    67–69
Interview
  for assessment data gathering,
    168–169
    note-taking in, 169–170
    open-ended questions for, 170
    patient input for needs and
      problem in, 169
    setting and timing for, 169
    trusting environment for, 169
  for evaluation, 299–300
Isla Verde. See Por Cristo–Boston
    College School of Nursing
    (BCSON) health project

J

Joint Commission on Accreditation
    of Healthcare Organizations
    (JCAHO) standards, 15–17,
    17b
  for collaboration, 15–18
  compliance challenges in studies
    and, 116, 116b
  for family education, 104–105,
    105t, 106t
  focus of, 113b
  outcomes and, 111
  for patient education, 101,
    104–105, 105t, 106t
  scoring guidelines for, 101,
    112–115, 113b
  staff development and, 101
    challenges for, 103–104, 104b
    need for innovation and, 101,
      103
    teaching program and,
      115–122
  team approach, 209

K

Key words, in Internet search, 277
Kleinman Model, of cultural
    assessment, 59b, 59–60

L

Language
  in culture-specific assessment,
    51
  translation and, 68
Language disabilities, teaching
    children and adolescents
    with, 91b
Learner–teacher relationship,
    222–223
Learning. See also Patient educa-
    tion; Teaching
  ability and, 220
  acquisition of, 89
  activities in, 228–237
  adult, 219
    empowerment and, 75
  affective, 87, 224
  anxiety affecting, 220
  application of, 222
    during assessment process,
      173–174
  barriers to, 134, 192b, 192–193
  cognitive, 87, 224
  in combination individual and
    group teaching, 226
  contracts in, 88, 207–209, 208f
  defined, 87
  empowerment and, 75–76,
    136–137
  evaluation of, 298–302
    four levels of, 293–296, 294b
    identifying needs and per-
      formance problems in,
      300–301, 301b
    patient interventions in,
      296–302
    tests in, 231
  feedback in, 90, 293
  generalization of, 89
  in group teaching, 225–227, 230
  in individual teaching, 224–225
  motivation in, 87–89, 92t
  objectives in, 203, 204b
  with one-on-one teaching,
    224–225
  participative, 222
  performance in, 90
  priority setting in, 219
  problem-centered, 221–222
  process in, 93t–95t

psychomotor, 87, 224
recall in, 89
scope of, 217–218
self-directed, 228–229
electronic media for, 235
sequence in, 87–90, 88f
style of, 223
tests in, 231
theories of, 92, 93t–95t, 96–97
Learning contracts, 88, 207–209, 208f
benefits of, 209
case study illustration of, 208f
components of, 208f, 208–209
design of, 207f
as motivator, 209
Learning disabilities, teaching children and adults with, 91b
Learning materials. *See* Instructional materials and media
Learning needs
critical preparation for discharge and, 193
physiological and survival needs and, 195b
prioritizing, 194, 195b
Learning objectives (behavioral objectives). *See also* Objective(s)
components of, 203–205
development of, 202–205
Internet and, 276, 276f
Learning outcomes. *See* Outcomes
Learning overload, 193
Lecture, as teaching method, 229–230
Legal influence, on health promotion, 136
Length of stay
diagnosis-related groups and, 13
learning evaluated by, 300, 319
Lifespan development frameworks (life course perspective)
as bases for patient education, 84–87
factors in, 84–85, 85f
implications for patient, 86
Listserves, 271–272
Literacy level, in culture-specific assessment, 51
Literacy skills, low, instructional methods and media and, 250–251, 251b
Literature review, in assessment, 170–171

Long-term memory disabilities, teaching children and adults with, 91b

M
Macrosystems, in ecological systems theory, 83
Mail lists, 271–272
Maintenance stage of learning, Health Promotion Model of patient education and, 32
Marketing, of community health programs, 138–139
Maslow's hierarchy of needs
priority setting and
in assessment, 172–173, 173f
in planning, 193
Massachussetts Tobacco Control Program, as marketing strategy, 138–139
Mastery learning, 95t
Media
in community health promotion, 135
guidelines for use, 231–232, 232b
Medical care settings, health promotion education in, 345
Medical diagnosis, patient education and, 18–19, 158
Medical model of illness, in patient education, 321, 322
Memory disabilities, teaching children and adults with, 91b
Mental discipline theory of learning, 93t
Mesosystems, in ecological systems theory, 83
Metasearch engines, 273, 275t
Migration
as forced relocation, 62–63
as stressor in situations involving patient education, 62–63
Models, as instructional media, 235–236
Motivation, 209
for behavioral change, 151b
as learning phase, 87–89
peers in, 349–351, 350b
in planning, 209
staff, 122–124
transtheoretical model of, 90–92, 92t
Motor disabilities, teaching children and adults with, 91b
Myocardial infarction

cardiac rehabilitation for older adults following, 14
in older women
normative history-graded factors in, 84–85, 85–86
stress process in, 80

N
NANDA (North American Nursing Diagnosis Association), nursing diagnoses approved by, 171
Natural unfoldment theory of learning, 93t
Needs assessment
for community-based patient education, 340–341, 341t
for community health program, 135, 136
for organization-wide patient education program, 107, 108b–109b
Needs (patient)
in acute and chronic illness, 194, 195b
anticipation of, 19
emotional teaching climate and, 192–193, 220–221
identification of
in outcome evaluation, 300–301, 301b
prioritizing
in assessment, 172–173
in planning, 194, 195b
Negative feedback, 302
Negotiation
as change-agentry skill, 328
with ethnocultural groups, 62
Newsgroups, 272
Noncompliance, 30, 74
as nursing diagnosis, 172
Nonnormative factors, in life-span development frameworks, 84, 85, 85f
Normative age-graded factors, in life-span development frameworks, 84, 85, 85f
implications for older adults, 87
Normative history-graded factors, myocardial infarction in older women and, 85–86
North American Nursing Diagnosis Association (NANDA), nursing diagnoses approved by, 171

Note-taking, in assessment interview, 169–170
Nurse midwives, patient education by, 8
Nurse practitioner
  patient education expectations of, 102b
  patient education in practice of, 7–8
  preventive services handbook for, 39–40
Nurses
  advance practice, 7–8, 257–258
  as case managers, 320, 321, 322
  development as educators, 120–122, 121t
  home health care, 257
  as midwife, 8
  promoting skill acquisition in, for patient education, 119–122, 121t
  responsibilities of, 9, 61
  role in patient education, 22t–23t, 102b
    as caring dimension, 4
    clinical judgment and, 19
    integration into nursing practice and, 18–19
    nurse midwife and, 8
    nurse practitioner and, 7–8
    nursing process and, 18–19
    overview of, 6–20
    skills needed for, 7
    teaching program for, 115t, 115–122
  as role models, 20–21
Nurse's notes. See Documentation
Nursing care plan. See Care plan
Nursing diagnoses, 171
  for community, 145, 146b
  learning needs and, 18–19
  NANDA approved, 171
  as summary of assessment findings, 171–172
Nursing homes, patient education in, 12
Nursing practice, role of patient education in, 6
Nursing practice education, patient education included in, 18–19
Nursing process, planning in, 18–19
Nursing skills, for change, 191
Nutrition-metabolic pattern, community health assessment, 141b

Objective(s). See also Behavioral objectives (learning objectives)
  affective, 203, 204f
  cognitive, 203, 204f
  components of, 203–205, 204b
  domains of, 204b
  evaluation of
    criteria for, 203–204
  learning contract and, 207–208, 207f, 208f
  in learning process, 202f
  performance in writing of, 203
  in planning, statements of, 202–205
  for prenatal education classes, 258–259, 259b–260b
  psychomotor, 203, 204b
  statement of, 199
Observation
  in assessment data gathering, 168
  for evaluation, 298–299
Occupation, in culture-specific assessment, 52–53
Older adults
  age-graded factors in lifespan development frameworks and, 84, 85, 85f
  cardiac rehabilitation program for, community-based, 349–351, 350b
  patient education for, 13–14, 24–25, 66–67
    cardiac rehabilitation program for, 349–351, 350b
  teaching, 124–125
One-on-one teaching, 224–225
  group teaching combined with, 226
One-page instruction sheet, 246, 250
Open-ended questions
  in assessment interview, 170
  in education for change, 329
Outcomes
  assessment of, 291
  behavioral, 33
  of community health prevention programs, 133, 134, 148
  determination of
    overall self-care and health management in, 295–296
    participation during interviews in, 293–294
    performance at home in, 295

performance immediately after learning experience, 294–295
  evaluation of, 291–296
  in evaluation of patient education program, 291, 292f
  for learning, 190
  in patient education program, 13
  in research and patient education, 330–332
Overload
  information, 193
  learning, 193

P
Pain, patient education affected by, 210
Parenting, intergenerational, 67
Participation
  in health promotion programs, 137–138
  in learning, 222
Participative learning, 222
Partnership
  in community health, 135
  versus compliance, 9–11
Paternalism, of traditional health professionals, 324
Patient and family education assessment guide, 163, 164b–165b
  components of, 163, 166f
  perspective of, 165–166
  theoretical basis of, 165–167
Patient care maps, in case management, 315, 316f, 317f
Patient care process, analysis of, in needs assessment, 108b
Patient case management. See Case management
Patient compliance. See Compliance (patient)
Patient decision-making, 76
Patient education. See also Education; Learning; Teaching; specific aspect
  adequacy of existing programs, 108b
  in advanced practice, 7–8
  agendas for, 75–76
  assessment for, 158–187
  barriers to, 117–119
  beginnings of, 5–6
  in case management model, 313–352
  challenge in, 20–21, 24
  for change, 90–92

for chronically ill persons, 13–15, 20, 196b, 323
community-based, 132–153
content in, 20
developmental frameworks as bases for, 81–87
as dimension of care, 4–5
discharge planning and teaching and, 12–13, 159–160, 193
empowerment in, 75–76
evaluation of, 109–111, 296–302, 329–330
for families with children and adolescents, 63–64
financial issues affecting, 112
goals and priorities for, 13, 107, 109, 116
health care reform and, 11–15
health promotion models in, 30–38
health screening and, 40–41
interdisciplinary collaboration in, 17–18
Internet in, 269–288 (*See also* Internet)
JCAHO standards for, 101, 104–105, 105t, 106t
materials for (*See* Instructional materials and media)
models of, 37–38, 76–87, 321
needs in, 196b
nurse's role in, 6, 8
in nursing practice education, 18–19
for older adults, 13–14, 66–67
organizational approach to, 108b–109b
partnership *versus* compliance and, 9–11
for pediatric patient, 125, 126t
    with asthma, 14–15
    culture and, 63–64
    with learning disabilities, 91b
philosophical issues in, 258, 321–323
political issues in, 112, 322–325
power development in, 326
as process, 72, 119–120, 120f, 158f, 158–159
resources for, 198b–199b
for self-regulation, 35f, 35–36
settings for, 343, 345
skill acquisition in, 119–122, 121t
for special populations, 63–67
staff development for, 100–131, 104b

continuing education in, 17–18, 21
staffing for, 17–18
for substance abuse, 15
team approach to, 6, 17–18, 209–210
theoretical basis of, 76–96
timing of, 319
for women, 64–66
Patient education steering committee, for implementation of organization-wide education program, 107
Patient record
    discharge instructions in, 115
    in evaluation, 299
    review of, in assessment, 170
Patient rights, 12
Pediatric patient education, 125, 126t
    for asthma, 14–15
    for children and adolescents with learning disabilities, 91b
Peer support
    for cardiac rehabilitation for older adults, 349–351, 350b
    and staff motivation for patient education, 123–124
Perceptions
    in culture-specific assessment of, 55
    of health, 141
Performance
    as behavioral objective, 203
    identification of problems with, in learning evaluation, 300–301, 301b
    as learning phase, 90
    patient education interventions evaluated by
        immediately after learning experience, 294–295
        overall self-care and health management and, 295
Personal mastery, in self-efficacy theory, 77b, 78, 79b
Person-environment mismatch, stress caused by, 80, 80f
Persuasion, verbal, in self-efficacy theory, 77b, 78, 79b
Pharmacist, role of, in patient education, 22t–23t, 102b
Philosophical issue(s)
    education for chronically ill persons, 313

holism, 322
information sharing, 321–322
patient–education models, 321
in prenatal case management, 258
self-care approach, 321
traditional *versus* progressive health professionals and, 320–321, 323
Photographs, as instructional media, 232
Physical comfort, learning climate and, 219–220
Physical limitations
    Internet use and, 284
    patient education affected by, 210
Physical therapist, role of, in patient education, 22t–23t, 102b
Physician
    refusal of patient education by, 324
    role of, in patient education, 22t–23t, 269
    specialist, attitude toward patient education, 320
Physiologic feedback, in self-efficacy theory, 77b, 78, 79b
Planned Approach to Community Health model, of community health education, 343, 344t
Planning
    assessment data used in, 190
    basic needs of patients and, 294, 295b
    case studies illustrating, 202–203, 212–213
    characteristics of adult learner and, 196–197, 197t
    clinical relevance of, 209–212
    community-based education and, case study, 341–343, 342t
    for community health program, community involvement in, 135
    critical learning needs and, 193–194, 195b
    discharge preparation and, 193–194
    empowerment of adult learning in, 136–137
    family involvement in, 205
    goal setting and, 194
    Health Belief Model applied in, 197–199, 199t

Planning *(continued)*
   outcomes for learning and, 190
   for patient and family education, 191
   statements in, 199
   learning contract and, 207f, 207–208, 208f
   learning priorities and, 194–195, 195b
   nursing skills used in, 191
   objectives and, 203
     rationale for using, 202
     statements of, 202–205
   outcomes targeted for learning and, 190
   and patient concerns during hospitalization, 192b, 192–193
   patient involvement and, 205
   teaching priorities and, 194–195, 195b
   for team coordination, 209–210
Political influence, on health promotion, 136
Political issue(s)
   compliance, 323–324
   patient education referrals, 324–325
   in staff education, for patient education, 112
   teaching responsibility, 324
POR. *See* Problem-oriented record (POR)
Por Cristo—Boston College School of Nursing (BCSON) health project, 139–147
   assessment in
     conducting, 140, 143–145
     guide for, 140, 141b–143b
     community diagnoses for, 145, 146b
   outcomes of, 148
   programs in, 137–139, 147–148
   teaching strategies in, 147
Positional power, 325
Positive feedback, 302
Posters, as instructional media, 232
Power
   charismatic (by personality), 326
   defined, 325
   determining sources of, 325b
   development of, 326
   expert, 325
   positional, 325
   social, 326

   types and sources of, 325b, 325–326
Power issue(s)
   compliance, 323–324
   patient education referrals, 324–325
   teaching responsibility, 324
   traditional *versus* progressive health professionals and, 320–321, 323
Precede-Proceed model, of health promotion patient education, 33–34, 37–38, 343, 344t
Prevention
   clinical
     guide to, 39–40
     handbook for, 39–40
     Clinician's Handbook of Preventive Services and, 39
     Guide to Clinical Preventive Services and, 39
   patient education for, 13
   primary, 29
Printed material, as instructional media, 236–237
   evaluation of, 237, 238b–246b, 247f
   readability of, 248b–249b
Priority setting
   in assessment, 172–173
   in implementation, 219
   for patient learning needs, 194, 195b, 196b
   for staff development, 107, 109
Problem areas
   assessment of, 300–301, 301b
   prioritizing, 172–173
Problem-centered learning, 221–222
Problem list, documentation of patient education and, 303–304
Problem-oriented record (POR), 304
Problem statement, in Internet search, 276
Prochaska's transtheoretical model of motivation and change, 90–92, 92t
Professional domain, and patient's understanding of illness, 60
Proficient nurse, promoting skill acquisition for patient education, 121t, 121–122
Programmed instruction, 231

Progress notes, documentation of patient education and, 304
Psychiatric setting
   case study, 212–213
   patient education in, 211–212
Psychological empowerment, 75–76
Psychomotor learning, 87, 203–204
   instructional methods and media, 224
   objectives in, 203–204, 204b
   selection of activities for, 229b

Q

Quality of care, case management and, 330, 330f, 331
Questionnaires, for evaluation, 299–300
Questions, open-ended
   in assessment interview, 170
   in education for change, 329

R

Racism, environmental, 53
Readability of instructional materials, 237, 248b–249b
Reading skills, minimal, instructional methods and media and, 250–251, 251b
Recall, as learning phase, 89
"Red flag" patients, assessment of, 159, 160b
Referral, as power/political issue, 324
Reframing, as change-agentry skill, 329
Refreezing, as behavioral change strategy, 149
Reinforcement, as change strategy, 329
Religious beliefs
   in assessment, 52
   culture-specific, 167
   health care and, 52
Reports, patient and family, for evaluation, 299
Research, patient education
   characteristics of, 329
   in diabetes education, 334–335
   on Health Belief Model, 31
   on health outcomes, 330–332
   human subjects clearance for, 336
   proposal development for, 333–336
   on Self-Regulation Model, 36
   summary of findings from, 336

Research proposal, 333
  background and significance of, 334
  design and methods in, 335–336
  human subjects clearance and, 336
  preliminary studies in, 334–335
  specific aims in, 333
  writing of, 336
Resistance, to health promotion, 134
Responsibility
  of consumer of care, 11, 269
  in learning, 89
  of management, 103b
  of nurse, 61
  for teaching, as political issue, 324
Retention, as learning phase, 89
Return demonstration, as teaching method, 230–231
Reward and incentive programs, for staff, 123
Role play, as teaching method, 230–231

S
School
  health education program in, 345
  patient education in, Mission High School Health Center, 346–349, 348f, 349b
Screening, health, 40–41, 85f, 85–86, 129
Searching the Internet
  search engines in, 273, 274t, 279b
  steps in, 276f, 276–279
Self-actualization, in Health Promotion Model, 31
Self-care
  evaluation of, patient's performance in, 298
  as philosophical issue, 321
Self-determination, community, 136
Self-directed learning, 228–229
  electronic media for, 231
  Internet in, 284–286
Self-efficacy, patient perception of, 142b
Self-efficacy theory
  clinical applications of, 77b, 79b
  as patient education basis, 77–78
  personal mastery in, 77, 77b

Self-evaluation, 150, 293
Self-help groups, 226–227, 324–325
  success of community health programs and, 135
Self-knowledge, in behavior change self-evaluation, 150
Self-management groups, 227
Self-Regulation Model, of health promotion, 35–36, 38
Seminars, in nursing education, 122–123
Senior adults. *See* Older adults
Sex (gender), in culture-specific assessment, 51
Sexuality-reproductive pattern, in community health assessment, 143b
Short-term memory disabilities, teaching children and adults with, 91b
Simulations, as instructional media, 236
Skill
  acquisition of, in patient education, 119–122, 121t
  Internet use and, 270
  nursing, for change, 191
  teaching and, 254
Sleep-rest, community health assessment of, 142b
Slides, as instructional media, 233
SOAP format, for problem-oriented records, 304, 305b
SOAPIER format, for problem-oriented records, 304, 305b
Social marketing, 138–139
Social power, 326
Social support
  patient resources for, effect on patient education, 78–80, 81b
  as stress mediator, 80
Social worker, hospital, role in patient education, 22t–23t
Socioeconomic status, in culture-specific assessment, 51
Sociologic approach, to stress/coping/social support theories, 78, 80, 80f
Specialists (physician), attitude toward patient education, 320
Staff development
  assessment and, 21, 24
  continuing education for, 21, 24
  JCAHO standards affecting, 101, 106t, 112–115, 113b

scoring guidelines and, 112
for patient education, 111–112, 224
  challenges for, 103–104, 104b
  evaluation of patient learning and, 109–111, 300
  financial issues affecting, 112
  goals and priorities of, 107, 109
  JCAHO standards affecting, 101–104, 112–115
  need for innovation and, 101, 103
  needs assessment and, 107, 108b
  organization-wide approach to, 105–107, 108t
  political issues affecting, 112
  staffing and, 111–112
  steering or advisory committee for, 107
  task forces for, 109
  teaching program for, 115–122
  workshops for, 115t, 115–117
Steering committee, for implementation of organization-wide patient education program, 105–107, 107
Stress, 78–80, 80f
  person-environment mismatch in, 80, 80f
  sociologic view of, 80
Substance abuse, health promotion and prevention and, 15
Subsystems, in assessment, 166
Support groups, 226–227
Suprasystems, in assessment, 166
Symbols, teaching low-literacy population and, 51
Systems theory, as basis for patient and family education assessment guide, 165–166

T
Tactile learner, teaching, 91b
Task forces, for staff education program, 109
Teacher-learner relationship, 222–224
Teaching. *See also* Instructional materials and media; Instructional methods; Learning activity—content matching in, 254
  barriers to, 192b, 192–193

Teaching *(continued)*
  case study, 255–257
  content preparation for, 19–20,
      217
  demonstration in, 230, 235–236
  evaluation of, 217, 296–297
  formats for, 224–227, 230, 252
  group, 225–227, 230
    benefits of, 253–254
    situations for, 253
  Health Belief Model and, 254,
      255t
  individual, 224–225, 252
  individual—group combined,
      226
  lecture method in, 229–230
  low literacy skills and, 250–251,
      251b
  one-on-one, 224–225
  process in, 93t–95t
  protocols for, 254
  responsibility for, as
      power/political issue,
      324
  role-play in, 230–231
  scope of, 217–218
  setting stage for, 218–224
  style of, 223–224
Teaching aids. *See* Instructional
    materials and media
Teaching programs
  JCAHO standards for documen-
      tation and visibility in,
      114–115
  for patient education, 115t,
      115–122
    barriers to teaching in,
        117–119
    compliance in, 116b
    haphazard efforts and, 118
    skill acquisition in, 119–122,
        120f, 121t
    teaching skills in, 117
    workshop in, 115t, 115–122
  protocols for, 254

scope of, 217–218
Team approach, to patient educa-
    tion, 6, 17–18
  coordination and, 209–210
  criteria for, 24
  promotion of, 21, 24
Teen Advisory Board, in school-
    based health education pro-
    gram, 349, 349b
Telephone calls, in patient educa-
    tion, 225
Ten-step Planning Model of com-
    munity health education,
    343, 344t
Terminally ill patient, culture and,
    67
Tests
  in learning evaluation, 299
  as learning experience, 231
Time management
  in assessment, 174–175
  prioritizing teaching and, 219
Time orientation, cultural, 55, 167
Time restriction, as barrier to
    teaching, 117
Timing, of patient education, 319
Translators, for patient education,
    68
Transparencies, overhead, as
    instructional media, 233
Transtheoretical model of behavior
    change, 90–92, 92t
Tuberculosis, 13

U
Unfreezing, as behavioral change
    strategy, 149
Universe, cultural view of, 54–55

V
Values, in culture-specific assess-
    ment, 55
Variances, in case management
    model, 318, 318f

Verbal persuasion, in self-efficacy
    theory, 77b, 78, 79b
Vicarious experiences, in self-effi-
    cacy theory, 77b, 78, 79b
Videotapes, as instructional media,
    234–235
Visual displays, as instructional
    media, 232–233
Visual learners, teaching, 91b
Visual perceptual disabilities,
    teaching children and adults
    with, 91b
Voluntary health agencies, 343, 345

W
Web sites for patient education,
    282t
Web slide show, 233
Western health care, organization
    and service variables in,
    58–59
Women, culture-specific education
    issues for, 64–65
  cancer screening, 65
  domestic violence, 65
  family planning, 65
  pregnancy/birth/postpartum
      period, 65
Workplace health, Challenge pro-
    gram, 148–153
  behavioral change strategies for,
      151t–152t
  enhancers of, 150, 153
  force-field analysis for, 149
  health promotion strategies in,
      150
  patient education and, 345
  personal barriers to, 150, 153
Workshop, for organizational
    approach to patient educa-
    tion, 115t, 115–122